Effective Staff Training in Social Care

Shifting values and practice dilemmas place unique demands on those providing services within social care settings. These distinctive demands should influence the management and delivery of training for the social care workforce. Yet existing theoretical frameworks are usually based on industrial approaches to training and ignore the specific issues that social care trainers are likely to encounter. *Effective Staff Training in Social Care* recognises the organisational, professional and emotional challenges of social care training. This book provides a theoretical framework for training and professional development, with particular emphasis on group learning in the social care context.

The opening chapters examine the organisational context of social care training, including issues related to inter agency training. Consideration is given to the tensions and dilemmas, for those engaged in training activity, of a contract culture, a climate of continual change, and a mixed economy of welfare. The second part of the book focuses on delivering training by exploring the application of theoretical perspectives of learning to the planning, design and delivery of training courses.

Effective Staff Training in Social Care will be essential reading for educators, trainers and managers engaged in the education and training of professionals in social care settings.

Jan Horwath is a lecturer in Social Work and Professional Studies at the University of Sheffield. **Tony Morrison** is an independent social care trainer and consultant.

Effective Staff Training in Social Care

From theory to practice

Jan Horwath and Tony Morrison

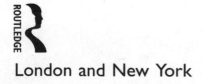

London and New York

To
Baz, Luke, Kate and Rachell
Jacquie, Christopher, James and Anna

First published 1999
by Routledge
11 New Fetter Lane, London EC4P 4EE

Simultaneously published in the USA and Canada
by Routledge
29 West 35th Street, New York, NY 10001

© 1999 Jan Horwath and Tony Morrison

Typeset in Galliard by J&L Composition Ltd,
Filey, North Yorkshire

Printed and bound in Great Britain by
Biddles Ltd, Guildford and King's Lynn

British Library Cataloguing in Publication Data
A catalogue record for this book is available from the British
Library

Library of Congress Cataloguing in Publication Data
Horwath, Jan.
Effective staff training in social care: from theory to practice/
Jan Horwath and Tony Morrison.
Includes bibliographical references and index.
1. Social workers – In-service training. 2. Team learning
approach in education. I. Morrison, Tony. II. Title.
HV40.5.H67 1999
361.3'071'5 – dc21 98–19535

ISBN 0–415–16030–8 (hbk)
ISBN 0–415–16031–6 (pbk)

Contents

Figures and tables

Figures

Tables

Foreword

I often reflect on the question 'What makes a healthy and successful organisation?'. There is a wealth of academic literature which explores the answer to this question. When one asks the question, 'What makes a healthy and successful social care organisation?', then the literature is much more rare. The literature on successful organisations will discuss the importance of organisations being clear of purpose and of the structures and processes to achieve that purpose. If one was to ask the question of staff who work in the social care agency, I would be very surprised if those staff did not state that the success of a social care organisation is dependent on the staff who work within the organisation. A number of academic texts identify the importance of organisational learning to the development of healthy and successful organisations. In organisations such as social services departments it is the staff who need to be part of organisational learning. I am convinced that the way in which individuals learn and indeed the way in which organisations learn is critical to an organisation becoming a successful one.

Learning is about growing and changing. We also know, from our school days, that most people learn in an environment where they feel secure. However, with the volume and scale of change in social care organisations over the past twenty years, many people feel anxious and threatened by the change. Therefore a successful organisation is an organisation that has learning at its core. That learning should be about change and growth.

How do we create an appropriate environment for this individual and organisational learning to occur? When I reflect on my own development as a worker and a manager, I recall the people I have worked with who have helped me to learn, grow and change. As a Director of Social Services I hold a responsibility for a large number of staff from a variety of backgrounds, disciplines, experiences and cultures. One of my responsibilities is to establish a culture within the organisation which values learning at both an individual level, a team level and at an organisational level. My task is to create what Peter Senge refers to as a 'learning organisation'. I would argue that every senior manager has a duty to 'make a difference' to their organisation by the creation of a culture which values learning.

However, the commitment of senior managers alone will be insufficient to deliver effective change within organisations. It is dependent on a range of individual managers and groups of managers who will work together. It is therefore crucial that all managers within organisations are able to answer the question 'How do individuals learn and how do organisations learn?'

To achieve this it is absolutely imperative that there is a close relationship between managers and trainers. Managers must understand that training and the individual competencies which are promoted through training are more than just technical processes and issues.

Training must be part of a change strategy in helping staff to learn and to transfer their learning in the delivery of services to some of the most vulnerable people in our society. However, training must be supported by a range of other activities. Social work has well-developed systems of supervision. Increasingly, appraisal systems are being introduced in social care organisations as are other performance management techniques. These performance management tools are essential if organisational learning is to occur.

One of the responsibilities of senior managers is to manage 'upwards' and 'outwards'. Senior managers need to be looking to the future and anticipating changes which are likely to occur in order that organisations and individuals can be prepared for the changes which are anticipated. Most managers recognise this strategic dimension to their role. Organisations which value learning and see the growth of individuals within the organisation will also see the training function as part of the wider strategic team anticipating and preparing for change. Senior managers must have a passion for the future. Similarly, this passion must be shared by trainers. Both senior managers and training managers must have a clear view as to how learning can be used appropriately to enable an organisation to change, develop and grow.

Jan Horwath and Tony Morrison have produced a book which explores these questions and issues. In so doing, they have produced a text which brings together a body of theory on social care training which is unique. Previous texts on this issue have been based on industrial models. For the first time a text is available to those who work in social care and health agencies which draws on a wide range of developmental literature, knowledge and theory which is specifically related to social care. The authors explore important practice issues for all those involved in delivering training in social care agencies, especially about the application of theory and knowledge in practice. With major change taking place in the way that social care training is organised within the UK, through the creation of a national training organisation and the creation of a General Social Services Council, this is a timely publication. The book has implications not just for all those involved in training but for people on the Diploma in Social Work courses, practice teachers, for staff who are considering pre-qualification training as well as those considering post-qualification training. There are important messages for senior managers of social care agencies as well as for the civil servants within the Department of Health who are responsible for the management of the training support grant.

I believe that change will only take place in organisations where individuals in those organisations are aware of the practical steps to achieve change. Similarly, with the development of learning organisations I believe they will only occur where senior managers create a climate of the culture which values learning, but where managers and trainers are aware of the practical steps that are required to create learning opportunities for a range of staff working in a variety of settings. Horwath and Morrison have made an immense contribution in providing managers and trainers with the practical steps which are required to help individuals and organisations learn. They have taken on a range of challenges which confront all of us who work in social care organisations. They acknowledge that training is not a quick fix for the ills of an organisation.

However, the single and most significant contribution of this book is the framework it provides with which senior managers and trainers can make an impact in delivering social care services to the most vulnerable people in our society, through linking the theory on how adults and individuals learn to the practice of training and learning in our own organisations. It should be required reading for all those in social care organisations responsible for the training and development of staff.

David Behan
Director of Social Services
London Borough of Greenwich

Acknowledgements

This book would not have been written without the support and encouragement of the many social care trainers and their managers with whom we work on a regular basis. In particular we wish to thank the participants in the Advanced Child Protection Training, The Trainers' Course which we facilitated for the National Children's Bureau Child Abuse Training Unit in 1995. These trainers identified the need for this publication and motivated us to write it. We would also like to thank Rod Thompson from Sefton Health Authority and Stephanie Irwin, independent consultant, for their advice and suggestions regarding content. We wish to acknowledge the contribution of the Promoting Inter-Agency Training (PIAT) development group, Anne Davies, Ann Godfrey, Tilly Jones, Jean Lockley, Sue North and Sara Glennie, who were happy to share their ideas on training evaluation which are included in Chapter 11. Finally we would like to thank Joanne Crossland for her secretarial help in completing this book.

Introduction

'I thought training would be much less stressful than being a practitioner but that is not the case. I find the problems I encounter in training just mirror the problems I encountered as a practitioner.'

'A training job must be the only job in social care where you receive such little training and preparation but are evaluated as soon as you take on the role.'

'Training feels a bit like painting the Forth bridge; you no sooner feel you are on the way to completing the task then something in the organisation changes and you have to start again.'

'If anything goes wrong in the organisation, the immediate response seems to be sort it out with some training. There seems to be a lack of appreciation that training is not the solution to all ills.'

These comments, made by trainers at a recent training convention, highlight the burden that is currently placed on trainers in social care settings. Yet the complexities of the training task are frequently unrecognised by colleagues and managers within social care organisations. There exists a belief that training is a cushy number. All you have to do is stand up, speak for a short time, set a few exercises, send the course participants off and go home. Maybe you need to read a few books and ensure you are aware of current developments in the field, but what a luxury! As a trainer you do not have to deal with complex cases or the aggression and negative responses of service users, life must be easy. Anyone who has been involved in social care training, as the comments above suggest, knows that training is anything but a cushy number.

It is not only the job of the trainer that is seen in a naïve and simplistic way, but training itself can be seen as the solution to all ills. Many trainers and their managers will have had the experience of being asked to plan and deliver training with the expectation that the training will provide a quick and effective solution to a whole range of diverse problems. For example, if there are concerns regarding the quality of care provided in a residential unit for older people, a common response is to send those working in the unit on a training course. While this may be part of the solution, training alone can be of little benefit if other factors such as staffing levels, resources within the unit, and supervision and management of the staff are not also addressed. A major task for many trainers is convincing others within the organisation that training cannot be delivered in a vacuum.

The focus of social care training also adds to the complexity of the task for a number of reasons. Trainers are engaged in the activity of developing the knowledge, values and skills of a workforce working with service users who each have different and often unique problems. The focus of the training also means recognition of the morally contested and critical role of values and judgements in directing practice. This requires trainers to provide learning opportunities that empower the learner to adapt their learning to meet a whole range of diverse situations. In addition, learners need to consider the use of authority and power in situations where there is potential for discrimination. Trainers also have to consider the impact that working in social care can have on the workforce. It is a stressful area of practice that affects workers at an individual level. Learning can only take place if these feelings are recognised and managed. The focus of social care training consequently demands a completely different approach from that of a trainer who prepares the workforce to produce a clearly identified end product such as car components.

The different approach is perhaps most obvious in the area of inter-agency training. In this arena trainers are not only managing the complexities of social care training but are also delivering the training to professionals from a range of different disciplines. This provides an additional challenge, as these professionals have different values and attitudes, roles and responsibilities and levels of status. They will approach the learning situation with a range of differing expectations regarding the way in which the training should be delivered and the knowledge and skills of the trainer.

Social care training is being delivered in a climate of continual organisational change. As described in one of the quotations above, the trainer is often left in a situation feeling that before they have met one training need that need has changed and they are having to respond differently to a newly identified need. A cause of frustration for trainers is the disparity between the time it takes to ascertain and respond to identified training needs and the speed at which these needs are likely to change. Continual change is also likely to provoke a level of insecurity amongst the workforce and this may influence their capacity to engage in learning. These changes will affect the role of the trainer. For example, changes within the probation service have had a major impact on the brief of the probation trainer. Their new role is influenced by a changing agenda focusing on public protection and the management of risk, the introduction of national standards and the removal of the Diploma in Social Work as a required qualification for probation officers.

Over the last ten years social care training itself has become a far more structured activity. Since 1988, for example, the government has sub-stantially increased investment in social services training through the Training Support Programme (TSP). As more money has been invested in training there have been greater expectations placed on trainers and their managers. Our experience of social care training in the mid 1980s was one of *ad hoc* courses often provided as a reactive response to an incident or a request by practitioners or managers, with little attention paid to recruitment, selection and the impact of learning on practice. The picture has changed in a number of ways. Although the influx of TSP moneys provides opportunities for training sections to expand alongside this training, managers are expected to demonstrate their ability to use the moneys effectively through the production of annual training plans which are monitored by the Social Services Inspectorate. This has required training managers to analyse, quantitatively and qualitatively, training that has occurred and to plan strategically to meet future training needs. The introduction of the purchaser–provider split within social care agencies has also affected the approach towards training. In many agencies training units have had to take a more structured approach to the purchasing and provision of training to meet the needs of the operational services. This has often resulted in complex arrangements for the commissioning and delivery of the train-ing. For example, within the health services the structures for training are not as much part of the infrastructure as in social services. The purchaser–provider split has resulted in small units or teams commission-ing training for their staff groups, often with little guidance.

Training has also become linked to performance management. This has resulted in more attention being paid to the outcomes of training and impact of learning on the quality of work with service users. There is an increasing emphasis on learning outcomes, competencies and universally recognised qualifications. This means that trainers are under pressure to demonstrate their effectiveness, i.e., to show that training works. The focus has shifted from training as part of a process of learning to training being defined as a product.

It is in this climate that the social care trainer operates. Yet the trainer is in a similar situation to the cobbler whose family are the most ill shod in the neighbourhood. Those who are in the business of training and staff development are often those who have received the least training to prepare them for the task. It is notable, for example, that the SSI report on training (SSI 1997) considers training for all service areas but does not consider training for the actual trainers. Advertisements for trainers and training officers in social services and health trusts still stress the need for practitioner experience, rather than training experience, and the salaries offered are commensurate with that of an experienced practitioner or front-line manager. This results in trainers being recruited who have a wealth of practice wisdom but often very little, if any, training experience. Some may have acted as practice teachers to students or undertaken short presentations within training courses but few will have received any training as trainers. In addition, trainers are frequently expected to negotiate with senior managers within the organisation, and yet the level at which they are recruited means that they are unlikely to have any experience of operating at this level within the organisation.

Once in post trainers may be expected to obtain the Training and Development Lead Body (TDLB) National Vocational Qualification training qualifications, and increasingly experienced social work trainers are being encouraged, and in some cases expected, to obtain the Central Council for Education and Training of Social Workers Advanced Award. However, our experience of acting as training consultants, internal assessors for candidates working towards the TDLB qualification, undertaking the Advanced Award ourselves and running training the trainers courses highlight the lack of any clear conceptual framework for social care training. Our experience also indicates that there are no clear frameworks for the induction, supervision or development of trainers. Trainers are often expected to get on with the task with no clear performance standards.

In these situations those engaged in training activity frequently turn to books. Books on training seem to fall into a number of categories. There are training manuals which usually consist of a series of proposed programmes on a specific topic and a series of exercises with notes as to how these can be utilised. While there is a place for these manuals they often presume that the trainer has some understanding of the training task. Their focus is content and methods of delivery. There are a number of workbooks which are designed almost as 'cookbooks' – for example, when planning a training course you should do the following. These books provide a framework highlighting what is required of the trainer in particular situations but they do not provide a theoretical analysis. There are books which do address the training task. Some of them consider the broader context of training such as undertaking a training needs analysis, others consider issues related to the actual face-to-face delivery of training. The problem with these books is that their focus is largely on industrial or business settings and they do not consider some of the specific issues related to training in social care settings. In addition, there are many books that are written on the subject of adult learning. Most of these have been written by educationists, and few consider the application of adult learning to training, outside of schools and further education establishments.

This book arose out of our frustrations at attempting to find a text that specifically met the needs of those engaged in social care training, enabling us to understand the organisational (macro) and training room (micro) issues involved in the design and delivery of social care training. We also recognised the need for a text that identified relevant theory and its practical application for all those engaged in social care training. We consequently decided to write a book which considered the powerful interaction between theory and practice and macro and micro issues. In writing the book we had the following aims in mind:

- to apply explicitly the research and application of knowledge of adult learning gained from further and professional education to social care training – our hope being to provide an underpinning framework for those engaged in training activity in social care settings;
- to identify the features that make social care training unique at an organisational, professional and individual level and to consider the issues for organisations, trainers and learners;
- to consider the impact of legislation, national and local guidance, and organisational expectations and culture on the role of trainers, training units and learners;
- to acknowledge the changing context of social care and to consider the challenges and dilemmas this raises for trainers, learners and their managers.

We hope this book will be of relevance to a range of people involved in the commissioning, planning, delivery and support of training. We have tried to consider the dilemmas for trainers working in a range of social care settings, including health, social work and probation. We have also attempted to consider issues from a range of perspectives, the full-time or occasional trainer, the training manager, senior managers within organisations with responsibilities for training and internal and external trainers. As we are both actively engaged in inter-agency training we have also attempted to consider the particular issues for those involved in this challenging area of training. The book is also a valuable resource for those engaged in the education of social care professionals and their trainers.

We were confronted with some hard choices regarding the focus of this book. Rather than attempting to cover too wide a range of staff development methods and therefore not give sufficient attention to theory we decided to set our perimeters on in-service training courses. We made this decision as these courses centre on group learning, which remains the form of learning which attracts most funding, occupies the largest share of trainers' and learners' time and is subject to most evaluation.

Throughout the book we have attempted to apply theory to context and consider the implications for social care training. The book begins by exploring the broad framework in which social care training is delivered. Consideration is given to the changing context and value base of social care work. The structural changes for the delivery of social care training and the psychological impact on training of changing context are identified. The consequences in terms of changing demands for training, and the impact on the human resource framework, are discussed. In Chapter 2 we focus on the ways in which adults learn and apply this to social care training. Particular attention is placed on the concept of professional competence and the nature of professional development. These two chapters provide the framework on which the rest of the book is based.

The following three chapters begin to apply this conceptual framework to the macro issues of social care training. In Chapter 3 the focus is on the commissioning of training. Consideration is given to the wide range of training commissioner and provider arrangements that exist in social care settings. The implications for undertaking a training needs analysis are identified and key principles for commissioning training are provided. In the following chapter we consider one of the more complex areas of social care training: inter-agency training. We consider what is meant by inter-agency training, explore the challenges and barriers and provide a framework for effective inter-agency training. Chapter 5 centres on creating a climate for learning. Consideration is given to organisational conditions required for adult learning, blocks to learning are identified and the notion of a 'learning organisation' and a 'learning team' are explored. The roles of the individual learner as a reflective professional, the trainer and the manager in terms of creating and maintaining a learning environment are discussed.

Having considered the contextual framework in which social care training is delivered we then move on to focus on the micro issues; that is, the actual planning and delivery of training. The focus of this section of the book centres on learning through training courses rather than other forms of learning such as on-site learning. We consequently begin by considering the implications of group dynamics on the learning group. This includes an exploration of the impact of anxiety, status, power and discrimination on group process and learning. Models for managing conflict within group settings are provided, as is a framework for assessing learning group dynamics. The ways in which adults learn in group settings will not only be determined by the group dynamics but also by the way in which the trainer facilitates group learning. In Chapter 7 we consider the impact of the training style on group learning and explore the roles and responsibilities of the trainer as facilitator of learning. As a significant number of social care training courses are co-facilitated, attention is given to the benefits and pitfalls of co-facilitation as well as ways of managing the co-facilitation partnership. We also explore the dilemmas for external trainers and visiting speakers in terms of meeting the needs of the learning group. In Chapter 8 we have applied the learning from the previous chapters to the planning of training. The importance of programme design is explored and a framework for course design based on adult learning theory is provided. Utilising this framework, the next chapter considers the methods for facilitating learning, identifying the principal training methods and how they produce different types of learning. Potential pitfalls and process issues are also considered.

The final two chapters move beyond the training room. In Chapter 10 we discuss the importance of learning transfer and consider models and research about the transfer of learning. Strategies for maximising the transfer of learning from training to job performance are offered. The final chapter focuses on an area that is increasingly demanding the attention of trainers and their managers – that is, ways of evaluating the effectiveness of training. The purpose of a training evaluation is discussed and a model for evaluation is provided. Consideration is given to factors that influence the effectiveness of evaluation and attention is given to the specific issues related to evaluating inter-agency training.

As can be seen from a description of the contents, the book has been constructed in such a way that each chapter builds on the learning from previous chapters. We hope that this will provide a framework for the reader, enabling them to analyse and reflect on their own practice. We also hope that the strategies offered in many of the chapters will enable the reader to develop their practice based on their own analysis and reflections. Our key message is that properly planned training, clear models and theoretical principles delivered in a skilful and empathetic manner can make an impact which endures despite the difficult circumstances in which we are operating.

Chapter 1

Context, challenges and agendas for training in social care

> By the time you know where you ought to go, its too late to go there.
>
> Charles Handy

This chapter explores:

- the changing context and value base of social care work;
- structural changes to the delivery of social care training;
- changing demands for training;
- the psychological impact on training of the changing context;
- a human resource framework for effective training.

It is estimated there are nearly a million staff involved in the delivery of personal social services in England (LGMB/CCETSW 1997). Together with their counterparts across the rest of the UK, they are responsible for the provision and quality of personal social services. They face the challenge of providing better quality and more services in the context of rising expectations, continuous change and mostly static resources. In this rapidly changing climate the workforce's needs for effective training in order to be able to function resourcefully are greater than ever.

Increasingly the key to quality and standards in social care will be the way that human resources are managed and trained. The partnership between management and training is therefore critical, if staff development and training are to be properly embedded within a robust system of performance management. For it is this fundamental linkage that ensures that training contributes to the achievement of organisational and service user goals, by integrating training within an explicit framework of service standards, competences, values and quality assurance. Without a strong partnership between management and training, individuals may develop, but the workforce as a whole cannot. Moreover, training may buckle under the weight of excessive expectations, for it alone cannot ensure the competent workforce that the organisation requires. Only through managers, staff and trainers sharing the responsibility can the whole workforce become competent, both to carry out their current roles and to learn and adapt continuously.

In this opening chapter the role of training in the changing organisational and professional climate of social care is explored. The nature of recent reforms in the social care field is reviewed, with their implications for the value base, structures, demands and agendas for training. The chapter concludes by presenting a human resource framework designed to maximise the effectiveness of the role of training within social care organisations, which underpins the structure of the rest of the book.

ORGANISATIONAL REFORMS AND CHANGING EXPECTATIONS OF PERSONAL SOCIAL SERVICES

Much space has been devoted elsewhere to the nature and effects of the raft of recent reforms in social care, health, education and the criminal justice system (Parton 1996), so this review will be brief, for it is the implications for training that concern us more. The past decade has seen a radical recasting of the role of the state in relation to individuals, which has affected every aspect of public sector service. The welfare state, the so-called 'nanny state', has been under constant attack for curtailing personal freedom, draining the public purse, and being inefficient and ineffective. Howe summarises much of the underlying philosophical rationale:

> The apparent failures of the welfare state to guarantee safety, personal growth and improved behaviour coupled with their alleged undermining of initiative, independence and creativity have seen a swing back in the 1980s to . . . human freedom . . . personal responsibility and choice, prepared only to recognise the individual. In its extreme form, radical liberalism sees no need for external

constraints or welfare experts who attempt to set boundaries around . . . self determination.

(Howe 1996: 85)

The principal regulator is therefore seen as the market place which, through competition, it is hoped, will drive out inefficiency and drive up standards. At the time of writing, however, it remains to be seen just how far the new Labour government will reverse any of these Thatcherite trends.

The result right across the public sector has been the establishment of a mixed economy of welfare based on the contract culture. Thus, purchasers and providers are separated; market ethos and competition have been introduced; care has been commodified; a proliferation of voluntary and private sector providers has arisen; decentralisation has drastically reduced the role of the centre, especially in education and health; and there is an increasing emphasis on standards, quality assurance and auditing.

At the heart of this have been two driving forces, one economic and the other ideological. The economic motivator has been driven by the three Es of efficiency, economy and effectiveness – the search for value for money. The ideological motivators have been consumerism and personal/family responsibility. The consumer has been empowered by increasing choice, involvement in decision making, making expectations about standards transparent, and monitoring and publicising outcomes. There has been a move to change the boundaries of social care welfare provision between formal and informal care (Clarke 1996: 46). Personal and family responsibility for care has been emphasised though social security, housing and criminal justice reforms, which have sought to divest the state of responsibilities that have proved too expensive or intractable to manage. However, as we shall explore later, the ideological tensions beneath these changes have been transmitted into the day-to-day management and practice realities of social care work, raising major issues about values and the nature of the professional task.

Benefits of reforms

The balance of power

Despite these philosophical tensions, and the turbulent experience of staff and agencies undergoing these reforms, the potential and emerging benefits are extremely important for service users. Whatever the real difficulties of translating the language of consumerism into the context of social care, the underlying philosophy that agencies exist to serve their users, and not vice versa, cannot be over-stated. Concerns in the 1980s about paternalistic practice, in which users were not consulted, decisions were made behind their backs, and their needs defined by powerful professionals, were increasingly understood as being part of wider structural forces that were oppressive and discriminatory. The result was further disempowerment and marginalisation among user groups, experiencing a high degree of vulnerability, dependency and isolation, whose political voice and ability to influence powerful agencies and professionals was already very limited. Hatch put the case powerfully when she stated:

> There is a gap between the professionals who make policies and deliver care services and those who use and depend on those services. The gap seems to be based on power: who has it; how they get it; what they do with it. Professionals of all disciplines have the power to define the lives, abilities, and needs of clients. This power has been acquired by professionals through their academic and practical training. The distribution of power is systemic: it is embedded in the system of community and primary care, and as such is widely accepted both by the professionals and those who need their help.
>
> (Hatch 1994: 158)

There was therefore a pressing need to redress this imbalance on social justice and moral grounds – e.g. that it was wrong in principle, as well as on professional grounds, in that good outcomes for users could not be achieved if users were not fully involved and making informed choices about their needs and services. Thus one of the fundamental aims of the reforms has been the rebalancing of power between professionals and users, in favour of the latter, either towards equality of power or at least in reducing the disparities. Thereby the concept of partnership was born, an ideal that has come to permeate every aspect of public sector service.

Partnership

The essence of partnership is about sharing power, user participation, and placing the user in the forefront of agency thinking. It is about users and their needs shaping the nature of the services they require. It is about the user's definitions of their own experiences, needs, strengths and resources being central to agency responses, and agencies striving to see the world from the user's perspective.

To do this demands a much more self-critical agency culture that seeks to recognise the multitude of ways in which service delivery systems and workers impose, knowingly or not, their own frames of reference upon the user. Agency cultures must therefore be embedded in an anti-oppressive framework that has the courage to expose practice and policy to user scrutiny, and to an analysis that understands the individual's experience in terms of socially structured power differences (Shardlow and Doel 1996: 16–23) that result in individuals having unequal life chances. To achieve this, organisational changes and user involvement are required at every level: in the assessment, planning, delivery and evaluation of services. Key elements in this restructuring of power relations are transparency of process, and the involvement of users, even when, in mental health or child protection, there are competing user rights and responsibilities, and where the scope for negotiation may be more limited.

Other reforms have sought to underpin the partnership ethos by creating a clearer and more coherent service delivery framework:

- improved strategic planning based on detailed assessment of need;
- greater clarity of professional roles;
- clearer eligibility for services and fairer distribution of resources;
- increased emphasis on, and structures for, inter-agency collaboration;
- increased professional accountability, reduction of inappropriate autonomy;
- increased focus on outcomes, effectiveness and inspection;
- increased avenues for user views and concerns to be expressed via complaints and consultative mechanisms;
- more accurate and strategic targeting of resources;
- localisation of services;
- improved standards and greater consistency.

Finally, of course, 'partnership' and anti-oppressive principles have wide implications for training, both in terms of how users can be involved in an area that has traditionally been seen as a 'professional' zone, e.g. the organisation of training, as well as in the content and conduct of training. In the same way as services have become far more involving of users, there is a need for the same to happen in training at both the strategic (macro) and delivery (micro) levels. Changes have already begun, particularly in services to adults where both users and carers have been involved in training – for instance in mental health. In children's services progress has been slower, but recent examples include the involvement of young people from the 'looked after' system, in child care training, sharing their experiences and telling workers what helped or what was needed.

Conflicts in values

While there are many things to be welcomed in these reforms, conflicts over values in social care services have been and will always be present. None the less, the recent reforms have both exposed and deepened the debates. The freedom that individual professionals used to have to practise with relative autonomy has largely been eroded as both resources and managerial scrutiny have become tighter. Therefore values have become far more contested as agencies and staff have to make hard, practical choices between competing needs and views of priorities. Understanding these key debates is essential for the trainer, as values are the cornerstone of social care practice. Indeed the significance, complexity and conflicts of values in social care work are among the features that distinguish social care training from industrial and commercial models of training, and stand out even by comparison with training in health and educational sectors.

Banks describes four traditional value positions in social care, although even these are not straightforward, either in their meaning or implications for practice:

- *Respect for and promotion of individual's rights to self-determination.* This principle contains both notions of empowerment and participation in the sense of promoting people's involvement in decision making and building on their own strengths and abilities.
- *Promotion of welfare or well-being.* This is the duty to work in the user's interests, and not to cause harm. Often, however, workers are faced with conflicting needs of different users; for instance, between carers and their elderly relatives. There are also the needs to ensure that the promotion of one person's well-being is not at the expense of that of another, and to safeguard the rights and safety of the vulnerable.
- *Promotion of equality and the removal of disadvantage.* This has

three components, which together constitute the basis for anti-oppressive practice:

1   equality of treatment and access to services without prejudice or favour;
2   equality of opportunity through removing disadvantage in competing with others in order to meet socially desired ends;
3   equality of result so that disadvantage is removed altogether, such that all people with similar needs receive the same high-quality care. As Banks states, equality of treatment is easier to achieve than the other two, which require both more resources and deeper structural changes.

● *Promoting distributive justice in the allocation of resources.* This concerns allocating publicly funded resources according to clear criteria concerning rights, deserts and needs.

(Banks 1995: 42; my emphasis)

Even without the effects of the recent reforms it can be seen that these four principles contain conflictual elements. How far should the self-determination of one user be assisted at the expense of another person? How far can services only be focused on individuals when the removal of disadvantage requires addressing social and structural forces? How should 'needs', as opposed to 'wants', be defined and who should define these anyway?

However, Banks describes four new agendas which have emerged from recent reforms, that have exacerbated these value tensions:

1   The new managerialism (Banks 1995: 133–4).
2   The new authoritarianism (1995: 133–4).
3   The new consumerism (1995: 104–6).
4   The new professionalism (1995: 104–6).

The new managerialism

Social care has become increasingly regulated by managerial processes, to the detriment of professionals' discretion over individual cases. In support of this is cited the degree to which work patterns are prescribed through the purchasing process, and practice is circumscribed by increasingly detailed procedures and the formulation of occupational competences, and is subject to vigorous audit. The result, according to Hopkins, is one in which 'professional judgement and discretion are refined as a technical process' (Hopkins 1996: 31). Practice becomes defensive and bureaucratic, as the agency becomes preoccupied by the management of risk.

The new authoritarianism

The social control function of welfare has been strengthened, particularly in the management of risk and danger, as a result of heightened public concern. Although this has long been an accepted feature in child protection work, more recently this agenda has been widened to the management of certain mental health patients, while public protection has taken centre stage in the work of the Probation Service. For probation officers this has threatened their traditional rehabilitative and befriending ethos (Lancaster 1995) as compliance with national standards has come to dictate probation practice.

The new consumerism

Already mentioned above, this sees the worker's role, not in terms of making a relationship with the user, nor as a professional who exercises judgement. Rather, the role of the worker becomes more akin to that of an official, or broker, distributing resources according to certain prescribed criteria. Inherent in this are elements of anti-professionalism, challenging the perceived power and exclusivism of the professional. Howe comments on the demise of the therapeutic aspects of relationships between users and workers, being replaced by a focus only on the immediate performance of the client (Howe 1996: 89). Psychological and sociological contexts are de-emphasised in favour of a short-term and immediate focus on eligibility, task and role definition, contract compliance and turnover. Rationing and the testing of competing claims for service against explicit eligibility criteria have become formalised as a central social care task, not just in community care, but increasingly in children's services.

The new professionalism

Although related to the new consumerism, this agenda sees the professional as seeking to increase user involvement and participation in decision making, protecting the user's rights, while preserving a professional role for the worker. As Bamford states: 'The new professionalism does not deny the existence of professional knowledge and skill, but seeks to bridge the gap between worker and client, and widen the range of choices open to the client' (Bamford 1990: 57).

In summary, the new welfarism, with its emphasis on consumerism, and its focus on distributive justice combined with efficiency, has exposed real conflicts about the nature of the task. The moral basis of social care is not only becoming more contested, but at the same time it is becoming more exposed as decision making is made more open, and users have far greater scope to challenge professional judgements, and make complaints. Multiple interests and stakeholders are involved, each with differing priorities. Key questions arise:

- Who is the 'client' – purchaser, user, employer or community?
- What is valued – outputs or outcomes, throughput or involvement?
- Where to focus – immediate crisis or the longer term, surface or depth? (Howe 1996)
- What to assess – risks or needs?
- What to measure – equity or individual responsiveness?

Anti-oppressive practice

Social care work brings together powerful professionals and vulnerable individuals and communities, in circumstances where poor-quality services – or worse, exploitation – may be difficult and sometimes almost impossible to challenge until it is too late. This is why anti-oppressive practice should be at the heart of the training agenda if the aspirations of partnership are to be achieved, and power relations between professionals, users and carers are to be reformulated on a more equal basis. However, the changing political context for social care, with its increased emphasis on individual responsibility, and a de-emphasis on structural solutions to issues such as poverty and inequality, has served to dilute and dissipate some aspects of anti-oppressive philosophy and practice. Preston-Shoot describes conflicting expectations for workers in terms of three very different agendas:

1 Reformist/therapeutic – helping individuals cope with the conditions in which they live their lives and assisting them to access services.
2 Radical/social justice – challenging and changing the structures which create those conditions.
3 Social control/bureaucratic – influencing and sometimes controlling

individuals to conform to legal or other socially sanctioned standards.

(Preston-Shoot 1995: 12)

Increasingly staff are working in more bureaucratically led agencies in which the pressures on resources create thresholds for service which can become so high that, by the point at which services are provided, the crisis of the moment is likely to result in interventions which control and contain, rather than liberate, or change the conditions which produce such crises.

Yelloly and Henkel state: 'professional education and training are operating amidst radical external change: a reappraisal of professionalism itself. The powers of the professions to impose their needs, priorities, skills and good practice is being questioned' (1995: 10). For trainers, all of the above raises profound issues, for which easy answers do not exist. Indeed they may never have existed, but what is different now is that the relative autonomy of professionals to plough their own furrow has gone, so that these questions have become the subject of much more public debate. Such questions include:

- What is the nature of the professional task?
- What are the relevant values, knowledge and skills?
- What is good practice?
- What are the standards, and who defines them?

Although the answers to these questions will not easily reveal themselves, and will always vary depending on who is answering them, one clear implication for training is that in this climate workers will need to be able to explain more clearly than ever before the reasons and the rationale for their actions and decisions. For there will be an increasing number of occasions on which workers will face conflicting demands and competing entitlements. However specific performance competences or eligibility criteria for services are drawn, the need for professional judgement cannot be eliminated, either in the assessment of need or the prediction of risk. Nor can the need for high-quality interpersonal helping skills be bypassed, for the vast majority of services are still delivered primarily through the medium of a relationship between worker and service user. The fact that the terms of such relationships are becoming more prescribed, and their length shortened, only increases the importance of such inter-personal skills. All of us seek to see the GP who we experience as relating to us, even though her or his list will almost certainly be busier, for we know within minutes whether we are in the hands of a reflective and sensitive professional or a bureaucrat.

Having considered the changing expectations upon the delivery of social care services, the shifting value base, and ambiguities about the nature of the professional task, the focus moves now to the specific consequences for, and context of, training in the light of these changes.

TRAINING IN SOCIAL CARE: CONTEXTS AND CHALLENGES

Issues for training arising from welfare reforms

Social services departments and probation services have since 1971 built up an impressive staff development track record, focusing primarily on in-house training. Social services have also benefited hugely in recent years from training support programme funding from central government. In contrast, most NHS Trusts appear to rely more on external programmes and have far fewer dedicated in-house trainers. Outside of social services departments, arrangements in the voluntary sector agencies tend to vary depending on agency size, while in the rapidly expanding private sector it is as yet unclear what training provision exists. However, the recent reforms are bringing sweeping changes and new demands across the whole landscape of training.

Structures for training

Social services departments now have four different roles in relation to training, in terms of commissioning, purchasing, providing or inspecting training. Bell has identified three different models for the staff development departments:

1   *Corporate model.* This crosses the whole organisation and is driven from a local authority central training unit. This has the advantages of ensuring consistency across the authority, can be used by the Chief Executive to drive change throughout an authority, and offers possible economies of scale. However, there is a danger that needs, and the uniqueness of social services and its users, may become secondary to those of the authority, or lost altogether.

2   *Independent model.* This is when training units are 'responsible only for the provision of services on a contract or commissioned basis, operating on a separate trading account'. Here the purchasing and commissioning of training are separated from its provision. Its advantages, however, depend on the quality of the commissioning process, and the commitment of senior management, to ensure that staff development does not become separated from organisational development. Its dangers are that the broader staff development function may be diluted, as it is much easier to calculate the unit costs of training courses and to generate income by running them.

3   *Organisational model.* Here training and staff development are integrated within the human resource development function and thus into the development of the organisation as a whole. This does not preclude purchasing training from external providers. Senior managers recognise the strategic importance of training and are active in implementing effective human resource development strategies which create the conditions in which training can really make a difference. More detailed discussion of the pros and cons of the different models can be found in Chapter 3, but it will be clear that the structural arrangements and location of the staff development and training function are crucial to its role. It is the organisational model which Bell considers as being most advantageous in the personal social services.

(Bell 1993)

Changing boundaries

The pace and complexity of organisational change has resulted in a myriad of new boundaries, roles, accountabilities and responsibilities between and within agencies. The boundaries between nurses and care workers in residential care are becoming increasingly blurred, with the prospect that there will be increasing demands for hybrid health-and-care workers. In some areas unwaged workers, such as volunteers equivalent to family aides, provide services for which other workers are paid. Moreover, there are increasing numbers of salaried foster carers who have become independent contractors and self-employed. Employment agencies act as the broker in the relationship between foster carers and employers. There are also unresolved issues around the roles and required qualifications of education and social services in day services for the under-5s (LGMB and CCETSW 1997). All these situations raise questions about the competences and training needed, if uniform standards are to be set and maintained, so that the needs and rights of vulnerable users will be protected. Other boundaries may shift too, particularly between health and social care, if, for instance, GP fund holders are allowed total purchasing.

Changes in workforce profile

The workforce has not only expanded, particularly as a result of community care, but also its profile, and therefore its training needs, have changed considerably, especially through the dramatic expansion of the private sector. The following figures come from Human Resources for Personal Social Services (LGMB and CCETSW 1997). In 1995 it is estimated that out of a total social care workforce of 931,000 in England, 315,000 staff were employed in social services departments, 152,000 in the voluntary sector and 464,000 in the private sector. Two-thirds of staff work in adult care. The growth in the private sector, focusing largely on residential adult care, has seen care workers in independent care homes increase by 23,000 between 1993 and 1995. The other major expansion area has been in day services for the under-5s, both in terms of child minders and in day nurseries. In both areas continued expansion is predicted. It is also estimated that 90 per cent of the workforce is white; 85 per cent are women (although only 22 per cent of Directors of Social Services are female); 58 per cent are part-time; 50,000 staff possess social work qualifications, of whom 44,000 work in social services departments. In 1996 it was estimated that under 5 per cent of the personal social services workforce had an NVQ certificate.

From these crude figures some of the challenges for training can be seen: the need to increase qualifications and established competences, especially in the private sector; the need to ensure that training offers equal access to part-time, mainly female staff; and that the needs of black staff are not marginalised. All of this underscores the importance of ensuring that training provision reflects the needs of the whole workforce and not just those working in high-profile services, such as child protection.

Competition

Increasing competition between training providers, for qualifying and post-qualifying training and NVQ training, as well as training not leading to qualifications, means that commissioners will need to become more explicit regarding standards and contract-awarding processes. It also means that some training providers will not survive. In addition, given the proliferation of providers, especially from the private sector, there is an urgent need for commissioners and purchasers to specify, as part of the contract for services, what training and qualifications service provider staff should have, and to set workforce targets to achieve such levels.

Flatter management structures

Decentralisation and the drive to reduce management costs has led to flatter management structures, with significantly increased spans of control. The consequent reduction in supervisory time and increase in managerial and administrative tasks, have serious implications for the ability of managers to exercise their vital developmental role with staff. This has implications at all stages of the training cycle if managers cannot contribute fully to training needs analysis, selection of staff for training, and the transfer of learning after training. The SSI Inspection report on training highlighted variable management understanding and commitment to their staff development role: 'Achieving Bell's aims requires the commitment of senior managers. In many departments, this requires a significant shift in the culture of the organisation' (SSI 1996a).

Strategic role of training

Given these shifting demands, the need for a strategic approach to training, integrated within a wider human resource planning framework, is becoming increasingly important. However, SSI inspections of training, while commending much good training practice, have highlighted serious concerns that the strategic and human resource function of training is as yet under-developed. Thus inspections found:

• poor linkage between training, agency policy and service delivery so that there was little specific evidence as to how training facilitated agency policies or services. For example, training staff experienced difficulties in 'breaking into' policy forums, and linkage between training and senior management was therefore over-reliant on individual networking and informal relationships;

• problems in identification of, and consultation about, training needs, so that too often training was based on an 'impression' of what was needed; thus workforce needs were 'largely unknown' except where formal appraisal or staff development schemes were in operation. In general, therefore, there was an absence of proper management information data to underpin the training strategies;

- an absence of systems to monitor access to and take-up of training. This meant in particular that it was hard to ensure equal access to training for disadvantaged staff groups such as home care, residential, ethnic minority and part-time staff, the majority of whom are women;

- problems in providing staff cover to release staff to attend training, leading to drop-outs and disruptions with the greatest effects on longer training courses. This is a particular problem in the residential sector;

- poor systems to evaluate training outcomes.

(SSI 1994, 1996a)

Standards

There is clearly much work to be done, not just on the strategic function and performance of training, but more widely in strengthening the whole approach to workforce planning and performance management. In a context of multiple providers, competition, a largely unqualified workforce, with rising public and professional expectations, the need to establish and ensure professional standards should be high on the management agenda. Concern about risk and public protection has given further impetus to this. Without clear standards about expected levels of competence, the link between training and improved practice cannot be easily improved.

Social services departments, utilising their commissioning role, have through the contracting process a mandate to set standards, but there are few areas of practice in which there are nationally agreed standards – the Probation Service being a significant exception. Although NVQs have sought to build a bridge between occupational standards and performance requirements, they are criticised on the grounds of being too wide, and too time-consuming to obtain (LGMB and CCETSW 1997). There are also unresolved questions about the relationships between NVQ levels 3 and 4 and the DipSW, as to the levels of work for which these qualifications are considered essential. None the less, occupational standards are the way forward in helping employers define uniform expectations from roles. These will be essential if skill mixing and more flexible working practices are to be promoted. However, it may well be that these standards will need to be developed more locally between purchasers and providers to reflect local situations, deciding what competences are required for what roles.

The competent workforce

In 1994–95 a total of £163 million was spent on training by social services departments, but only £28 million of the moneys spent led to qualifications (LGMB and CCETSW 1997). As a condition of the Training Support Grant, authorities are now required to set targets for the numbers qualified in NVQs, the DipSW, CCETSW Post-Qualifying Awards and Management Development Qualifications.

However, there are major debates about which arrangements for the certification of competence will be most appropriate, given the low qualification base in the personal social services. The low take-up of NVQ combined with criticisms of its high cost, inflexibility (for example, candidates must register for a whole NVQ), and concerns about variable standards of assessment, mean that it is unlikely that NVQs can fulfil this need. This is particularly relevant to the Probation Service where, since 1996, the Home Office has removed the requirement that probation officers should possess a social work qualification. A variety of pathways for certifying competence are likely to be needed covering full-time, part-time, open learning and employment-based routes on:

● national approved programmes of qualifying within higher education;
● NVQ/SCVQ systems for competence approval, with fewer mandatory units;
● local agreements to assess and recognise competence against occupational standards on a unit base;
● employment qualifications having local currency that might later gain national recognition, likely to carry a CATS (credit accumulation and transfer) rating (LGMB and CCETSW 1997).

Nevertheless, qualifications of any sort cannot ensure competence unless there is a vigorous system of performance management by the employer. However, the costs of sponsoring staff through qualifications in terms of fees, mentoring, supervision and appraisal, through any of these routes, is high. Therefore employers will only increase their investment in this process if they can see a clear return on it in terms of rising standards and improved services. In order to demonstrate that qualifications, and investment in training generally, do make this difference, there must be a strong link between training and performance management to ensure that training gains are translated into higher standards of job performance.

Future joint inspections by the Audit Commission and SSI will link the appraisal of services with a scrutiny of how the workforce is managed, including levels of assessed competence. This focus on the quality of performance management could well provide the impetus that has so far been lacking, to weld training and management much more closely together, and thus link training inputs to performance levels and service outcomes.

PSYCHOLOGICAL IMPACT OF CHANGES ON TRAINING

In addition to the structural and professional impacts of change already described, there is a third dimension: the psychological impact. While these changes do present opportunities and motivation for learning, it must first be acknowledged that the primary impact of such rapid change is insecurity and anxiety. If this is not acknowledged, then the anxiety cannot be harnessed in the learning process and will, instead, become debilitating and prevent learning. The role of anxiety in the learning process is thus of great significance for trainers, for it affects not only individual learners but, of equal importance, anxiety also affects organisational behaviour.

Another dimension is the way that external anxiety about organisational change can resonate with other, more personal sources of anxiety. The internal and the external do not exist in isolation of each other, but are inter-related. The organisational world inhabits the internal world of individuals, and this internal world is often projected onto the organisational world. Thus organisational insecurities, fears and fantasies can resonate with individuals' own historical and current fears and uncertainties. For instance, a group of managers undergoing considerable uncertainty during a re-structuring were asked what metaphors described their experiences. Almost all referred to a sense of bereavement, abandonment, separation, powerlessness and loss of control, which for several members resonated with earlier personal experiences of grief and loss. Only one person was able to perceive their experience as having any positive possibilities. Yelloly and Henkel (1995: 1) suggest that training will not be fully effective unless it facilitates reflection of the ways in which our internal and external worlds are inextricably linked, and how this impacts on our practice.

Menzies' research on the 'Social Defence Systems' based on a study of nursing in a hospital provides a compelling description of the organisational and human effects of working in an organisational environment in which anxiety is neither acknowledged nor managed. She writes:

> The success and viability of a social institution are intimately connected with the techniques it uses to contain anxiety. The needs of the members of the organisation to use it in their struggle against anxiety leads to the development of socially structured defence mechanisms, which appear as elements in the structure, culture and mode of functioning of the organisation. A social defence system develops over time as a result of collusive interaction and agreement between members of the organisation in order to avoid the experience of anxiety, guilt, doubt and uncertainty which are felt to be too deep and dangerous for confrontation.
>
> (Menzies 1970)

At an organisational level failures to contain anxiety appropriately can permeate every aspect of the agency's work as well as affecting its relations with the outside world and other agencies. This is demonstrated in the dysfunctional learning cycle described by Vince and Martin (1993) (see Figure 1.1).

In this environment anxiety is seen as unprofessional, a sign of weak-

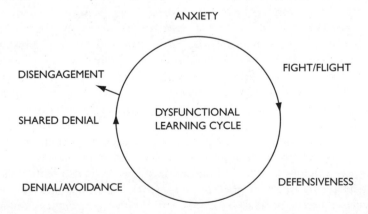

Figure 1.1 The dysfunctional learning environment
Source: Vince and Martin (1993)

ness or not coping. As a result uncertainty is suppressed through fight-and-flight mechanisms. There is an expectation that everything can be solved. The focus is on task or procedure, and there is an absence of forums where questions, feelings, difference and doubts can be safely expressed. Individuals struggling to make sense of their experience, or worried about their level of knowledge and skills in a changing world, feel isolated and wary of opening up. The consequence is defensiveness at every level, and a resistance to share and reflect. In this context the scarcity of peer group support, particularly for black staff or women, is significant. The environment also undermines confidence to experiment with new ideas and practice, and refuge is sought in old habits, loyalties and attitudes, for they are familiar. Emotional defensiveness then deepens into denial, whereby anxiety and changes are warded off through the rejection of dissonant information and attitudes, offering a temporary but false sense of security. Power relations are exploited in order to preserve the *status quo*, individuals are scapegoated, and attitudes become polarised in a struggle for dominance and control. Oppressive processes go unchallenged. If this process worsens, it becomes socially structured into the agency's social and cultural systems, making it even harder for individuals to challenge (shared denial). Unchecked, such processes may lead eventually to total disengagement, as parts of the organisation strive to keep things the same – perhaps proclaiming, for instance, about partnership that 'we are doing all this already – this is nothing new'.

It goes without saying how easily these processes can permeate the learning environment, both as a projection of painful organisational realities and as a defence against the challenge posed by change and the demand to review attitudes and acquire new skills. As can be seen, in this dysfunctional learning environment, engaging and reflecting on experience, the principal way in which adults learn, is deliberately rejected in order to ward off anxiety and fear of change. This may affect training in a range of ways at both an organisational level as well as at the level of the individual learner. Common examples at an organisational level include the following:

- training may be misused by the organisation to solve other problems such diversity in practice standards, poor performance, high turnover, low morale or the lack of services for a particular user group;
- training may be expected to shoulder the whole burden of helping the staff assimilate organisational changes, with the predictable result that it is the messenger who is shot;

- training may be used as a quick-fix presentational solution following public exposure, often in fields such as child protection after things have 'gone wrong'. (In one authority every social worker was instructed to tick a sheet sent round to ensure that all of them had read the Cleveland Report.) Meanwhile difficult questions about supervision, policy or resources can go unanswered;
- training may be used as a covert reward system, or dumping ground, when workers are struggling, burnt-out, or difficult to manage;
- training may become marginalised if it is perceived as too challenging to the *status quo*.

In all these scenarios the common denominators are: managers offloading responsibilities from the 'too difficult to do' tray onto training; reactive rather than strategic uses of training; placing excessive expectations onto training and then having an easy scapegoat when the problem remains unsolved. These organisational distortions of the training function can then in turn become reflected in the attitudes and behaviours of learners at an individual level. These may include:

- ambivalence or hostility to training;
- dumping negative feelings generated elsewhere in the organisation in training;
- an increase in dependency behaviours including negative projections about authority directed onto trainers;
- difficulty in 'joining' training and putting down psychological or organisational baggage;
- lack of personal safety/containment;
- unwillingness to raise issues of difference and inequality;
- heightened sensitivity and reluctance to any exposure or risk;
- a felt sense of de-skilling;
- reduced optimism about being able to apply learning back in the work place;
- more frequent withdrawal from courses, especially where a commitment over time is required;
- unwillingness to accept an appropriate level of personal responsibility for learning.

In addition to the effects on the training function in general, as well on individual learners, these processes inevitably take a toll on trainers, as their own responses to this environment are generated. Trainers may become absorbed in the same process, and feel abused, misused and unvalued. The extra amount of time, flexibility and emotional energy that groups bringing such baggage require may feel increasingly demanding to trainers, who may become more impatient with participants, more adversarial with the agency, or who may begin to disengage from the agency, pursuing their own pet 'courses' with little or no regard for organisational training priorities.

Training can thus become triangulated through a process in which the organisation and participants are felt alternatively to be persecutors and victims, with trainers cast in the role of inadequate rescuers, destined to disappoint, and who themselves then become the object of persecution. In response, just at the very point where training has such a vital role in helping the organisation negotiate major changes, training itself may become caught up in the organisation's dysfunctional responses to anxiety and uncertainty.

While such bleak scenarios may not take place in quite such an all-encompassing manner, the important point is that training is an easy target for the displacement of agency anxiety, if the role and function of training is either unclear or not owned by management.

OPPORTUNITIES AND MOTIVATORS FOR LEARNING

Such changes, destabilising as they have been, have also acted as a powerful opportunity for learning. Brookfield states that often the most significant learning we undergo results from some 'stimulus that causes us to engage in an anxiety producing and uncomfortable reassessment of aspects of our personal, occupational and recreational lives' (Brookfield 1986). At points of radical and imposed change, we must either learn, or suffer alienation and anomie.

In a climate of rapid and imposed change, organisations and individuals may be forced to relinquish previous certainties, assumptions and practices, in accepting the inevitability of continuous change. For some this may provide exciting new and creative opportunities.

Such changes create organisational structures that are embryonic and immature, and therefore potentially more available to influence and development. The new unitary authorities are a good example of this process. This may create the opportunity at the outset for training to become embedded at the strategic level of the organisation. At an individual level too, all of the above can act as a powerful motivator for learning and development, as staff seek opportunities for reflection about changes, affirmation of existing skills and the acquisition of new ones.

Training has a key role to play in the management of change. Staff experiencing organisational upheaval need opportunities to reappraise their value base, and frameworks to order their experience, as well as new skills and knowledge to carry out new roles. Properly commissioned training has a central role to play in helping staff through periods of upheaval and intense anxiety. It can provide the psychological containment to enable staff to engage in, and make sense of change, allow the expression of anxiety and begin to recover the confidence to translate existing skills and knowledge into a fresh context, as well as to become ready to learn new skills.

In summary, this is a learning environment in which threat and opportunity are finely balanced. The question then is how the learning opportunities in the current context can be maximised by training so that training really does make a difference. In the final section of this chapter, we examine ten key factors upon which the effectiveness of training depends.

HUMAN RESOURCE FRAMEWORK FOR EFFECTIVE TRAINING

Throughout this chapter, the significance of the link between management and training has been stressed as fundamental to the effectiveness of training. This is therefore at the centre of the model that is now presented, in which training is located within a strong human resource management framework.

It was Oscar Wilde who once stated that 'A map of the world without utopia is useless'. While the following framework is presented as an ideal type, it should not be forgotten that positive learning outcomes are regularly obtained in sub-optimal contexts. The difference is that in the less benign environments, these gains will be over-reliant on the efforts of individual trainers and learners, more likely to be short term, less easily generalised across staff groups, and therefore of less benefit to service users. The less supportive the learning context, the more individual rather than organisational are the learning outcomes. Valuable though these gains are at an individual level, they can never achieve competency at the workforce level. To achieve this, all the ingredients must be in play and working within a comprehen-

(10) Evaluation of learning outcomes
(9) Reinforcement and transfer of learning
(8) Skilled management of learning
(7) Strategic commissioning process for training
(6) Comprehensive training needs analysis
(5) Workforce planning
(4) Continuous performance management
(3) Clarity of training mandate, purpose and role
(2) Clear value base
(1) Positive organisational culture towards learning

Figure 1.2 A human resource framework for effective training

sive human resource framework that is owned by managers, trainers and practitioners.

As the model shown in Figure 1.2 underpins the structure for the book as a whole, the discussion here will largely be an introductory one, as the different elements in the model are described and expanded in the subsequent chapters. However, while all of the areas discussed within this framework are relevant to inter-agency training, Chapter 4 focuses specifically on this, and provides a framework which addresses the additional demands and complexities of inter-agency training. Therefore this discussion is focused on the framework required within a single social care organisation.

Positive organisational culture

If training is to be fully effective, the culture of the organisation and its attitude towards learning are critical factors in mediating both individual and organisational learning processes. This involves an organisational commitment to continual renewal and learning, rather than simply survival. Learning must be engrained and modelled within organisational goals, values, structures, cultures and working relationships. It is a culture in which complexity, uncertainty and ambiguity are confronted and not denied. Difference is seen as a strength not a threat. Vince and Martin (1993) describe such an environment in the functional learning cycle (see Figure 1.3).

In this culture, anxiety and uncertainty are seen as normative, allowing for the expression of feelings, doubts and uncertainties, where 'mistakes' are opportunities for learning, not punishment. Difference is utilised by exploring and valuing individuals' experiences and realities, appreciating how such realities are socially constructed, and reflective of

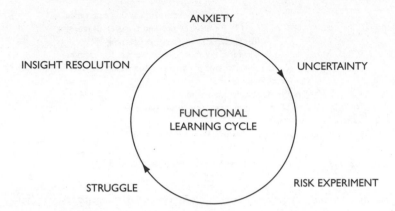

Figure 1.3 Macro model of the functional learning cycle
Source: Vince and Martin (1993)

broader socio-economic relations and inequalities. Contact is made between

> differing emotional realities, different systems of meaning and different types of bias. Consequently women and men, black and white, disabled and able bodied, gay and straight have to address differential experiences of power and powerlessness as aspects of the organisational practice and learning.
>
> (Vince and Martin 1993)

This culture also involves service users, not just at an operational level, but more widely in planning and reviewing processes, as well as in training. Risks are taken and innovations are attempted. The unresolvable nature of many issues is openly acknowledged and struggled with, from which unexpected or creative resolution may come. As a result, staff are empowered to tackle further demands. To put it more crudely, this is an agency culture in which 'thinking and feeling' and not just 'doing' are legitimised, and used in the organisation's whole approach to problem solving.

In the current political climate of reducing resources and of unpredictable demands, establishing and sustaining such a culture is a tall order in complex organisations. Concepts such as the 'learning organisation', while attractive in principle are in practice hard to achieve. Nevertheless the concept of the positive learning environment is a helpful and motivational one, even if its practical expression is much easier in smaller work units or specific learning situations. The very idea helps to maintain a vision of what can be, and to challenge bureaucratic and defensive organisational cultures. In Chapter 5 these ideas are explored in terms of creating a positive learning context.

Values

The opening section of this chapter explored some of the tensions regarding values which recent reforms have brought to the surface. Multiple stakeholders, conflicting views as to the nature of the task, competing priorities, all placing pressure on a limited pool of resources, have each contributed to shifting ideologies of welfare. Procedures and standards cannot prescribe what should happen in every situation, so the exercise of judgement will remain a central feature of social care work. Indeed it is this very aspect, the centrality of values, that distinguishes social care training from its industrial and commercial counterparts. Social care training cannot teach staff what they should do in every situation, or guarantee that the same responses will work in apparently identical situations. The vulnerability, dependency and powerlessness of many users of social care services mean that their capacity to challenge those judgements, or to recognise poor practice, may be very limited, however much agency policies seek to ensure that this is not the case. Social care staff, whether social workers, care managers or nurses, will remain in a powerful role. Therefore a strong value base in place for the management of performance, based on the twin pillars of partnership and anti-discriminatory principles must exist.

This value base must underpin training at all levels. There must be a clear anti-oppressive policy framework for the delivery of training that covers all aspects of the training cycle. This must ensure that in the analysis of training needs, the need of black staff, staff with disabilities or part-time staff are fully understood. It must ensure that learning events are organised so that such groups have equal access to training. It must ensure that the allocation of training resources does not favour parti-cular groups: for instance, full-time qualified field staff groups. It must ensure that the content of training is anti-oppressive and integrated into all aspects of learning programmes. It must promote anti-oppressive behaviour in learning events, first by ensuring that trainers model this, and second by agreeing and reinforcing these expectations with all staff who engage in training. Finally, it must enable minority groups to express their views through evaluation of the whole process.

Clarity of training mandate, purpose and role

Hinricks defines training as: 'Any organisationally initiated process which is intended to foster learning among organisational members, in a direction contributing to organisational effectiveness' (Hinricks 1976). Thus the training function is primarily to assist the achievement of organisational, rather than individual, staff development needs, and must therefore be part of the strategic planning and management of the agency. It also makes clear that training is not about 'courses' but about learning, which may be generated through a whole range of means, many of which will not imply the presence of a 'formal trainer'.

Leslie Bell spells out the purposes of staff development and training in social care as follows:

1   *To meet service users' and carers' needs.* To ensure all staff are equipped with the appropriate attitudes, skills, knowledge and competence necessary to provide a high standard of service.

2   *To contribute towards achieving organisational goals.* To ensure congruence between organisational development and staff development, to ensure that the right people are in the right place.

3   *To meet the professional development needs of individuals.* To maximise the abilities of staff, in particular those who may be disadvantaged, in order to increase motivation, reduce unnecessary staff waste and develop transferable skills.

(Bell 1993)

Linking these two definitions, we can define the role of training in or between social care agencies as: 'an organisationally initiated process intended to foster learning and competence throughout the workforce, in order to: meet the needs of service users; contribute towards organisational goals, and meet the professional development needs of individual staff.'

To fulfil these objectives Leslie Bell recommends an organisational model, as described earlier, in which the training and staff development function is integrated within the human resource function so that training can be strategically linked to workforce planning and performance management. However, in the organisational model the training role could potentially combine commissioning, purchasing and providing, so that it would be important for clear contracting and quality assurance arrangements to exist. A major advantage of this model is that it provides training with a clear authority because it is linked to the management of performance. But to make this work, it is crucial that a senior manager carries the human resources (HR) portfolio.

This in turn stresses the importance of an HR plan and policy for training (Garavan 1991), in order that the function and role of training are clear, and that they work to specific targets. Fletcher identifies five core roles for training:

● Identifying training and development needs.
● Designing training and development strategies and plans.
● Providing learning opportunities and support.
● Evaluating the effectiveness of training and development.
● Supporting advances in training and development practice.

(Fletcher 1991)

Continuous performance management

Training and qualifications alone cannot ensure a competent workforce. Moreover, as discussed earlier, there is considerable debate about the types of qualifications that are appropriate, and how to get a better match between national qualifications and the specific needs of employers. Finally there are unresolved questions even with certified competences as to the extent to which they certify capability as opposed to performance, a theme that is pursued further in the next chapter. The implications are therefore that the competent workforce cannot be achieved simply through raising the numbers of qualified staff alone. The management of human resources cannot be separated from the management of the organisation as a whole. Therefore training must be integrated within a vigorous framework of continuous performance management which requires:

● clear values;
● defined goals;
● definitions of accountabilities, responsibilities and areas of discretion;
● standards of performance;
● supervision and appraisal systems;
● skills and systems to handle individual issues of capability and conduct;
● quality assurance processes.

(LGMB and CCETSW 1997)

Workforce planning

Closely linked to performance management is workforce planning. Organisations will need to ensure that they have strategies for the recruitment, retention and career development of all staff, and appropriate pay and conditions within which equal opportunities can be promoted and monitored (LGMB and CCETSW 1997). As Bell states, there is a need to ensure that 'the right people are recruited, that the organisation has the requisite range of skills in the right locations, and that regular staff appraisal and training opportunities are provided to keep the organisation in peak condition' (Bell 1993). This requires a coherent approach to personal development, linked to the performance management systems just described. Additionally, the ability to monitor the management of the workforce needs a strong management database in order that information such as: turnover and vacancies, labour costs, absences, confirmed competences, complaints, conduct and capability proceedings, and exit interviews can be brought together and analysed.

Comprehensive training needs analysis

The SSI Inspection (1996a) of training commented that too often training was based on an impression of what was needed. In large organisations the completion of a full training needs analysis is a massive and lengthy task, often overtaken and delayed by fresh demands or crises that weaken the eventual outcome of the exercise and make the results hard to implement. The involvement of users in assessing the training needs of staff is also important. Their comments on the key skills and attitudes experienced as helpful are invaluable. There is therefore a need to use a range of measures and information gathered on a continuous basis both directly from the staff by questionnaires and sample interviewing, and indirectly from other management data of the sort just mentioned above. These methods, together with the commissioning of training, are discussed in depth in Chapter 3.

Strategic planning and commissioning of training

This cannot be fully effective if the previous steps are not in place. If training is to contribute to organisational, and not just individuals' development goals, then its strategic planning must be related to performance levels and service delivery aims, in terms of workforce targets and specific standards. These issues are also discussed in Chapter 3. At the level of training delivery, our own experience as trainers is that often it is the trainer who is asked to devise learning outcomes, and that the link with desired competences, specific performance standards or service outcomes is generally weak, unless training is part of an assessed piece of learning and competences exist. Moreover, it is not uncommon for commissioners and priorities to have changed between the point at which a piece of training is commissioned and when it is delivered. The result is that there can be lack of management interest in the organisational, policy or performance issues arising from the training, poor reinforcement opportunities and little or no evaluation.

Skilled delivery of training

The processes involved in professional learning are complex, and these are explored in Chapter 2. Individuals have different learning strategies and styles, and bring very different experiences, expectations, feelings and anxieties to the learning process. Therefore the awareness and ability of the trainer to attend to the power issues and to value difference in their relations with learners is critical. Moreover, training processes are frequently mediated by organisational and socio-cultural forces external to the immediate learning environment, which must be taken account of, if learning is to be anti-oppressive, relevant and meaningful. For the trainer this requires an understanding of how professionals learn, how to use this in the design of programmes of learning, and confidence with a wide range of ways to facilitate learning, including learning in groups. Co-worker competence and skills are also important, as poor co-trainer modelling can be a potent block to group learning. All these areas are variously discussed in Chapter 6 to 9.

Reinforcement and transfer of learning

The successful transfer of learning from a 'training' context to the work context, or from one work context to another, is probably the most difficult and important challenge for training. The relationship between training inputs and learning outcomes depends on multiple factors, many of which are beyond the trainer's control. Therefore it is vital that from the very outset, in the commissioning of, design and recruitment for training, rehearsal, reinforcement and transfer opportunities are ensured. It is simply not enough to tack this on as a final exercise for learners in the last session of a training event, not least because, without the practical support of their immediate manager and their work colleagues, many of the reinforcement and transfer strategies cannot be created. Chapter 10 tackles these questions.

Evaluation

Learner satisfaction, as expressed by the completion of a 'happy sheet' immediately after the end of a training course, is obviously inadequate in rating learning gains. However, evaluation is a time-consuming business which hard pressed trainers are given too little practical encouragement to undertake, despite the considerable amount of money invested in training and staff development. On the whole, all that is measured is outputs – for example, how many training courses there were, and who attended. Although determining what outcomes to measure, and how to identify the precise effects of training inputs on practice is no easy matter, models exist for evaluation, and these are described in Chapter 11. However, the most robust approaches combine self-report with observational feedback from managers, trainers, peers and service users.

SUMMARY

- The context and nature of social care work has radically altered in recent years, particularly as a result of the purchaser–provider separation and the introduction of market principles.
- Increased competition for resources has resulted in a reduction of professional autonomy and an increase in managerialism and accountability.
- The development of partnership and the promotion of anti-oppressive practices, through involvement of service users at all levels, is a key challenge. However, the emphasis on individual responsibility and a de-emphasis on socio-economic solutions threaten to dilute the anti-oppressive agenda.
- There are changes in structures for the delivery of training arising from the purchaser–provider separation, but social services departments have a key role to play through their commissioning arm in setting standards for training, especially given the expanding size of the private sector.
- There is a need to ensure that more training results in accreditation and qualification, and that part-time staff, staff from minority

groups and unqualified staff are not marginalised in terms of training provision.

- It was emphasised that the exercise of judgement, based on clear values, and high-quality inter-personal skills remain at the heart of good practice. It has also become more important than ever, in this turbulent context, to equip workers to be able to articulate clearly the reasons and rationale for their judgements.
- The impact and management of anxiety were seen to be powerful factors affecting the culture and commitment to learning.
- A central message is that if training is to be effective in achieving a competent workforce it must be embedded within a strategic human resource framework and underpinned by a strong performance management system.

Chapter 2

How people learn

This chapter explores:

- how people learn;
- the concept of professional competence;
- the nature of professional development;
- implications for training in social care.

INTRODUCTION: WHY THEORY IS IMPORTANT

In the opening chapter consideration has been given to the context in which social care is operating, in terms of structures, rationale, values and task, and the subsequent implications for training. It is now time to consider in more detail both general theories about how people learn and, more specifically, the nature of professional development. The importance of doing this is fourfold.

First, training is an expensive and precious resource, whose effectiveness will be badly blunted if trainers lack knowledge about the nature and complexities of learning and professional development. Indeed the need to strengthen the theoretical base available for trainers was a principal reason for writing this text. It is little use picking up a handbook of training exercises or applying clever 'techniques' without an underlying understanding of learning processes. Without an understanding of how adults learn, trainers have little to guide them in designing a coherent event. Being an expert in a field of practice and having much relevant information to share do not guarantee that effective learning will occur.

Second, learning theories remind us that the role of the trainer carries considerable power in relation to learners who may be feeling anxious, unsupported and vulnerable within their agencies. There is a potential for this power to be misused in the service of the trainer's own needs or ego, which can leave learners de-skilled, disempowered and reluctant to engage in future training, if trainers do not fully appreciate the range of ways in which this power can be exercised. Sometimes this can be in ways which are barely perceptible but none the less have great effect, to the extent of being considered actively harmful, and certainly oppressive. One participant recalled a training course which was compulsory to attend early on in his first post as a qualified worker. In front of thirty other colleagues he undertook a role play, which was then subject to a general critique by the whole group. He was so distressed by this that he fled the room in tears, and reported that ten years on he still could not look those who had been on that course in the eye – never mind participate in role play.

Anti-oppressive practice and the values of partnership-based practice have to be modelled and reflected in all that the trainer does, both in the curriculum and course content, and in relations with learners and co-trainers. Shardlow and Doel describe the ways in which socially structured difference can permeate learner–teacher relations through the exercise of power:

> Power is an inescapable part of the dynamic of relationships between all teachers and all students. Both teacher and student will have individual biography and affiliation to various social groups: male/female; black/white; disabled/able-bodied; gay/straight.
>
> (Shardlow and Doel 1996: 16–23)

Thus the relationship between trainer and learner will be mediated through the personal experience of each, and through the organisational values and culture in which each works. It is vital therefore that trainers have a real appreciation of the nature and sources of power relations in the learning situation. Trainers must model and conduct their relationship in ways which acknowledge openly the power dimensions and difference on both sides, in which the power of the trainer and difference is managed and utilised so as to empower learners.

Third, trainers need a strong theoretical base, not just to design an effective learning event, but to manage it. However carefully an event is designed, a myriad of other factors and processes can arise during learning events which cannot be planned for, and which require an immediate response from the trainer. This may result in a need to adapt the programme, address areas that had not been anticipated, or to manage powerful group processes, such as distress, immobilisation or conflict. For instance, a participant may disclose a traumatic personal experience in front of a large group. Knowledge of learning theory, and indeed group process (Chapter 6) is essential if the trainer is to transform such 'crises' into opportunities for learning. Without a sound grasp of theory there is the danger of the trainer responding defensively, or losing control of the situation.

Finally, learning theory is essential in the evaluation of training, as discussed in depth in Chapter 11. In order to evaluate training intelligently and comprehensively, the complexity of learning processes has to be appreciated. For instance, learning outcomes occur not just at a behavioural level, but at an intellectual and feelings level as well. Learning outcomes are strongly influenced by how supportive the context of practice is in utilising new skills and knowledge. Learning outcomes also occur over time. Thus an evaluation that measures changes in job behaviour alone immediately after a learning event may fail to detect other areas of learning – for instance, in attitude or feelings. The evaluation process may not recognise that the absence of behaviour change is to do with a lack of opportunity given to try out new skills in the worksite, rather than the failure of teaching or learning. Understanding the nature of the transfer processes between learning and practice, which is the subject of Chapter 10, is another vital part of the trainer's theoretical armoury.

LEARNING THEORIES

Having established the importance of a strong theoretical base for trainers, in this section four main approaches to learning theory are described. These are:

1   Behavioural
2   Cognitive
3   Humanistic/self-development
4   Socio-cultural.

The first two will be discussed relatively briefly, so that more time can be spent examining the two experiential learning approaches stemming from humanistic and socio-cultural origins from which notions of adult learning have been derived. However, it is important to recognise at the outset that the complexity and variety in how people learn is such that a single theory is unlikely to be satisfactory. Second, what follows are theories about how people learn, rather than about teaching. The vast majority of human learning does not involve teachers or trainers, for it is part of the process of continuous human adaptation to the world around us. Theories about designing training courses and methods of delivery are covered in Chapters 8 and 9, although some comments about the implications for training of different approaches to learning are introduced here.

Behavioural approaches

Behavioural approaches can be divided into two main groups: trial and error approaches, and conditioning approaches. Essentially, both see the human being in terms of a very complex machine, which can be programmed to respond in particular ways through types of conditioning. The trial and error approach states that if the learner discovers some act or explanation as valid, it will be repeated until the consequences no longer produce the desired or expected result (Jarvis 1995: 60). Pavlov's (1927) classical conditioning asserted that the learner comes to associate the reward with a stimulus that occurs just before it. In contrast, Skinner's idea of operant conditioning stated that learning is shaped by the reward that follows the behaviour. Good behaviour is thus rewarded (Skinner 1951).

The shortcomings of behavioural approaches to learning are that no account is taken of internal affective, cognitive or unconscious processes, such as feelings, beliefs and values, or historical influences from one's past. It is therefore a poor guide for learning and self-reflection. It may also result in patterns of learnt behaviour that are neither functional in the long term, nor helpful to maturity and development, as, for instance, in the case of a person who may learn always to adapt to the expectations of others. Moreover, the focus on behaviour reduces the learner's critical capacities. It also emphasises a very individualistic explanation of behaviour and experience, de-emphasising the socio-cultural context, and wider socio-economic factors that shape behaviour.

From a teaching perspective, a purely behaviourist approach results in a highly teacher-centred process based on the teacher as expert and conditioner. Thus the teacher defines what is 'good' and necessary for the learner to learn, the teacher defines the method and prescribes the outcomes. Power is very much centred in the hands of the teacher. Little attention is given to the role of the learner in defining needs or outcomes, and there is little opportunity for partnership between teachers and learners. Power relations, and value differences between learner and teacher, are ignored.

All of this is not to deny the very important role of positive reinforcement in both learning and teaching. Moreover, there is a very healthy emphasis in competence-based teaching on the behavioural application of knowledge, values and skills to job. It is changes in job behaviour that are the real test of effective training as far as service users are concerned. However, as a sole approach, behavioural-based teaching is not sufficient beyond those routinised tasks, such as lifting a patient or remembering information, that can be learnt by rote. For the vast majority of social care work, where prescribed solutions are not appropriate, responses depend on values, attitudes and judgements about the specific contexts and conditions.

Cognitive approaches

The origin of these approaches drew on the work of Piaget, who described five stages in cognitive development during childhood:

Stage 1 (0–2 years): Sensori-motor, when infants learn to differentiate between themselves and objects in the external world.

Stage 2 (approx. 2–4 years): Pre-operational thought, when children classify objects by single salient features.

Stage 3 (approx. 4–7 years): Intuitive, when children think in classificatory terms without necessarily being conscious of them.

Stage 4 (approx. 7–11 years): Concrete operations when logical thinking starts.

Stage 5 (approx. 11 years on): Formal operational thinking which is based on abstract conceptual thought.

(Piaget 1929)

Piaget examined the internal mental processes that shape behaviour, intellectual growth and the capacity to adapt. He identified two principal adaptive mechanisms: assimilation and accommodation. Assimilation occurs when we interpret experiences and incorporate their meaning within our existing mental frameworks. Thus no fundamental changes in attitude or beliefs are required. Accommodation occurs when experience is strongly dissonant with existing mental frameworks, causing re-evaluation, and change in our beliefs and ways of interpreting the world.

Gagne (in Jarvis 1995: 88) focused on the role of memory in developing a hierarchy of learning and built on Piaget's cognitive development framework. According to Gagne's hierarchy (shown below), cognitive skills must be acquired at each level before the next level can be properly mastered. Failure to do so may result in regression back to the previous level. Blocks in cognitive developmental in childhood may restrict learning in adulthood. Trainers will have encountered adult learners whose ability to generalise or conceptualise is very limited. Conversely, stressful experiences in adulthood – for instance, fear or anxiety – causing regression back to childlike approaches to learning, will also block learning. The result may be that the learner feeling threatened ceases to be able to analyse, and becomes instead dependent and rule-seeking – for instance, asking, 'Just tell me what to do'. Gagne proposed seven cognitive levels, which can be seen to relate to the different stages of child development described earlier:

1   *Signal learning* – classical conditioning as described above.
2   *Stimulus–response learning* – response shaped by reward, operant conditioning.
3   *Motor or verbal chaining* – basic skills or rote learning.
4   *Multiple discrimination* – intellectual ability to distinguish between similar types of phenomena so as to select what is appropriate.
5   *Concept learning* – thinking in the abstract.
6   *Rule learning* – ability to respond to signals by a range of responses.
7   *Problem solving* – drawing upon previously learnt rules to solve new problems.

(Gagne)

Here it can be seen that, in contrast to the behaviourists, the freedom to choose different responses based on memory, and the selective recall of information and experiences stored previously, are affirmed. The role of memory is also important for learning in terms of modelling. Thus Bandura (1977) saw that one way to learn complex patterns of behaviour is to copy others. The short-term memory is only able to store a limited amount of information, so that what is retained must be held in a long-term memory but coded in such a way as to be retrievable. This involves the acquisition and use of abstract concepts in order to aid recall, and to generalise from the particular to the universal. This is crucial in social care training, for it is the exercise of judgement based on the transfer of principles from one situation to another that is at the heart of social care work, because rarely are two situations identical. It is this that differentiates social care training from industrial-based training, in which routinised responses must be learnt to tackle identical situations, and in which the nature of the work is morally less contested and where there are fewer practice dilemmas.

In contrast to behaviourist approaches, cognitive approaches to learning focus on internal mental processes, and recognise that human beings have freedom to make choices and to select and analyse information to help them do so. However, cognitive approaches still pay little attention to wider socio-cultural influences on learning, or to the positive role played by emotions in shaping learning capacity and style. The emphasis is on the human being as an information processor.

Experiential learning

Experiential learning is based on the idea that learning is the continuous process of human adaptation to our physical and social environment. Knowledge evolves through the continuing relationship between individuals and the world around them. Therefore learning occurs through the accumulation and reflection on experience, which is an interaction between the internal world of the individual and what is going on externally. Jarvis states that all learning begins with experience, whether conscious or not, and defines learning as the 'process of transforming experience into knowledge, skills, attitudes, values and feeling' (1995: 59). Thus knowledge is not construed as objective 'out there' truth, apart from the individual, but as continually developing and always provisional while individuals continue the adaptive process throughout their lives. Thus an important distinction with behavioural and cognitive approaches lies in the fact that experiential learning theorists such as Kolb (1988) see learning much more as a process than as an outcome or product. Nevertheless, this does not mean that experiential learning rejects these earlier frameworks, but rather that it seeks to integrate them into a more holistic theory.

Characteristics of experiential learning

Kolb (1988) identifies a number of characteristics of experiential learning.

First, learning is a continuous process grounded in experience, more akin to a grafting and growth than the accumulation of knowledge. Every experience is influenced by and takes up what has gone before, and therefore modifies what comes after. Thus past and future are present in all learning. One implication of this for training is that to some degree all learning is re-learning. Learners are not empty receptacles into which teachers pour knowledge, but rather they bring, however unexplored, a deep reservoir of life experience. Therefore it is important that the facilitation of learning starts by exploring the learner's experience, existing beliefs, theories and actions. Not only does this validate their previous experience, it also brings such experience and beliefs, which may be held at an unconscious level, into conscious awareness, and thus available for examination. For instance, workers may have experience-based or culturally based beliefs that shape their practice, about which they have little or no conscious awareness.

Second, learning is an interplay between experience and expectation. Jarvis states that learning occurs when there is dissonance between our previous experience, and current demands and expectations (1995: 65). This dissonance produces a situation in which previous ways of thinking and responding appear inadequate, stimulating reappraisal of existing attitudes and ways of dealing with the world. It is this discomfort that causes us to reassess, creates the opportunity to learn from experience and to integrate new knowledge or values. However, as we shall see later, the presence of such opportunities does not mean that we necessarily learn from experience. We may choose instead to reject the experience.

Third, learning requires the resolution of conflicting ways of dealing with the world. Four principal conflicts have been described by Eraut (1994):

1   Accommodation versus assimilation.
2   Concrete experience versus abstract conceptualisation.
3   Observation versus action.
4   Impulse versus reason.

At the risk of over-simplifying the last three of these terms, another way of expressing these conflicts is to describe them as differences between approaches based on feeling (impulse-driven); thinking (reason, observation and abstract conceptualisation); and doing (concrete experience and action). Kolb (1988) suggests that the way in which the tensions between these different modes are resolved determines the style and approach to learning. Thus very different learning approaches and outcomes would occur depending on which of the following methods of resolving these tensions were used:

- imitation – simply copying another;
- substitution – giving up one's own thinking and behaviour in favour of another set of beliefs or behaviours;
- suppression – ignoring one's own beliefs or behaviour;
- integration – learning involves a continuous dialectic or healthy tension between the different adaptive modes.

For instance, if a particular social care competence is seen only in terms of a behavioural outcome, this could result simply in the imitation of the desired behaviour, and the suppression of the individuals' beliefs and other skills. In contrast, integration would involve grafting new skills onto the learner's existing skills, accepting both as valid and helpful to their work.

Different modes should be chosen according to what is most helpful in any situation. Thus active involvement in one situation as a way of adapting and learning may be changed to observation in another. In contrast, someone whose only way of responding is to 'jump right in' has no other choices about how to respond. In other words, the more flexible and greater the range of learning modes available, the more choices and capacity individuals have in learning situations.

It follows from the above that developing new knowledge, beliefs or skills will be most effective where the learner can engage in four types of learning. These are:

1 Concrete experiencing approaches, to involve oneself fully and openly in experiences.
2 Reflective observation approaches, to investigate the nature of one's experiences.
3 Abstract conceptualisation approaches, to analyse and create conceptual meaning and theoretical understanding from experience.
4 Active experimentation approaches, to make decisions, plan and try things out, which creates new experiences from which further reflection arises, and so on.

Fourth, individuals develop different learning styles and strategies in response to their life experiences. Dependent on an individual's adaptations to developmental, family, educational, and socio-cultural influences and intellectual ability, the individual will adopt different learning styles and strengths. Honey and Mumford (1982) have described four learning styles, which they describe as follows:

1 *Activists.* Activists involve themselves fully in the here-and-now experience, tend to be enthusiastic, gregarious and open minded – 'I'll try anything once.' They learn by doing. They act first and consider afterwards, but are likely to get bored once the activity stops. They are less interested in looking at what they have learnt via reflecting, than going on to the next experience.

2 *Reflectors.* Reflectors prefer to stand back and observe, collect data and consider all angles, past and present, before acting. This can result in cautiousness and delay. They are more likely to take a back seat in training, listening to others before contributing. Our experience also suggests that reflectors pay close attention to the emotional content of the situation.

3 *Theorists.* Theorists adapt, analyse and integrate observations into complex but logical theories, thinking things through in a systematic way. They like things to be 'right', and focus on underlying principles and models, asking whether 'its logical, or how does this fit with that?' As a result they can be detached, more objective and cautious about anything subjective, emotional or generated from lateral and creative thinking.

4 *Pragmatists.* Pragmatists are keen to try things out to see if they work in practice, wanting to experiment with new ideas. They can act quickly and confidently, but can be impatient with theorising and reflecting. Learning is about solving problems, therefore 'if it works It's good'.

Whereas Honey and Mumford seem to describe these styles as quite discrete and somewhat fixed, our experience is that there can be considerable range within individuals as to the style that is adopted, depending on the situation. Brotherton (1991) suggests that intelligence and ability are not fixed and general but variable and particular. In other words, different contexts will reveal different aspects of a person's abilities. Thus, how a person performs and their ability to learn is highly influenced by the context and the security of the learning environment. Learning styles can also be deliberately modified or improved so that, for instance, an 'activist' can practise reflector skills by spending time observing rather than doing. Seeking a healthy balance in learning styles is important if we are to maximise the capacity to learn.

In the context of a learning group, there is likely to be considerable variation in learning styles. Thus, where one person is stronger at reflective learning, another's strength lies in the ability to analyse and conceptualise, while yet another learns by doing. This has important implications for trainers who will need to design learning programmes bearing in mind the need to offer a range of learning methods which can complement the likely mix of learning styles in any group.

Fifth, past and present experiences and roles mediate our approaches to learning. Because of each person's unique past, one cannot know how an individual will respond to learning, and to what extent different learning experiences will be perceived as threat or opportunity. Adults have multiple roles, extensive and powerful life experiences, and undergo continuous processes of life transitions that lead to reinterpretation of prior experience and knowledge. Therefore adult learning is:

- lifelong;
- personal;
- a function of human development;
- related to our experience;
- partially intuitive;
- often triggered from the unexpected, or at times of crisis.

(Brookfield 1986)

Sixth, experiential learning is a cyclical process occurring through experience, reflection, conceptualisation and active experimentation. Kolb (1988) has described this in his Experiential Learning Cycle (Figure 2.1).

According to Kolb (1988) and Jarvis (1995), learning is triggered by experience, either in terms of a problem to be solved, a situation that is

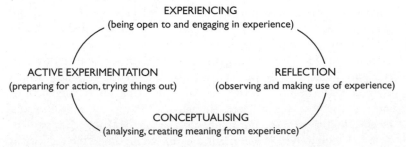

Figure 2.1 Kolb's Experiential Learning Cycle

unfamiliar, or a need that must be satisfied. These might be intellectual, emotional or physical demands or needs. However, it is not sufficient to have an experience to learn, for the experience may be suppressed, denied or rejected as irrelevant or of no significance. For instance, learners may be physically present at a training event, but psychologically absent. In order to learn from it, there must first be an engagement in the experience.

However, engaging in experience is not enough either. Without reflecting on the experience it may be lost or misunderstood. For instance, group members may be engaged in a powerful role play but if it is not debriefed and reflected on no learning, or negative learning may result. Reflection explores observations, feelings and thoughts arising from the experience. Failure to make careful observations of what actually happened during the experience may render the conclusions drawn from it partial and incomplete.

Reflection needs to lead to conceptualisation and analysis, so that meaning can be attached to the experience and generalisations can be generated. If this is not done, and the cycle stops at reflection, the lessons from one experience cannot be transferred to other situations, or erroneous conclusions may be drawn. Moreover, without conceptualisation, the conclusions drawn have not been exposed to the experience of the outside world – for instance, research, or other socio-cultural perspectives which might offer other ways of looking at the same experience. Thus the reflections of a white male manager on a role play with a black female staff member about her lack of confidence and how difficult she was to help might be reassessed when exposed to research on the general marginalisation experienced by black staff.

Finally, it is from generalisations that we become better able to tackle new situations, or to try innovative solutions to current situations. This is how theory is translated into practice. If this is not done, and we move straight from reflection into action, it is possible to get it 'right' but without knowing why. This will prevent us being able to replicate or adapt the learning to other situations (Further Education Unit 1988). If behaviour is to change, new concepts alone will not be sufficient, otherwise the learning will be purely intellectual or academic. The learning must be tested out in new situations through active experimentation.

Lastly, there are a wide variety of ways in which we respond to experiences, so that the capacity to learn from experience depends on how we respond. Therefore simply having an experience is no guarantee that learning will result. Jarvis (1995: 71) describes nine ways of responding to experience which he divides into three types: non-learning, non-reflective and reflective learning responses. Trainers will certainly be familiar with, and have been puzzled by seeing some of the responses described below despite their best endeavours to create experiences from which staff may learn.

Non-learning responses

Presumption

This is a typical response to a new learning situation which is seen as familiar. 'I take the structure of the world as constant, thus I can repeat my successful acts, on the basis that what worked for me before, will work now. I've done all this before, I have no need to learn.'

Non-consideration

Newness or difference is rejected out of hand. 'I don't need to bother with this, this doesn't apply to me, I am too busy or too fearful to respond to a learning situation.' There is a failure to engage in the experience.

Rejection

The experience is engaged with, but its implications are rejected or denied, whatever the evidence. 'Nothing will change how I think, whatever experiences I have.'

Non-reflective learning

Pre-conscious

This involves incidental/accidental learning that one is not aware of, occurring at the edge of consciousness. The significance of this form of learning is often over-looked, where there is an exclusive focus on tangible outcomes. This type of learning shapes attitudes, perceptions and behaviours without one being aware of it. It can thus have a power-ful effect on values, and self-beliefs. It can also result in the development of unconscious competences and changes in performance.

Skills

Mostly this describes the acquisition of manual or physical skills where reflection, thought or judgement is not required because it is repetitive and becomes automatic. This learning often takes place via imitation or role modelling, and is based on a behaviourist approach.

Memorisation

This involves learning by rote, such as multiplication tables, which are then stored in the memory so that it can be reproduced, for instance, in an exam. This leads to the so-called 'banking' concept of education, in which learning becomes a product rather than a process. A good example is where staff are being taught new legislation, where the task is to be able to recall information in practice situations – for instance, training for Approved Social Workers under the Mental Health Act.

Reflective learning

Although in general this type of learning is more likely to lead to change, this does not always follow.

Contemplation

This is learning pure thought or meditation, with no necessary link to action. It might, for instance, be associated with higher mathematics, philosophy or spirituality.

Experimental learning

This is a scientific approach to learning in which hypothesis and theory are tested in laboratory or experimental conditions.

Reflective skills

This is concerned with learning through problem solving, and involves both reflection-in-action and reflection-on-action. It is thus of central relevance to professional development, where staff have to be equipped to exercise judgement, often under pressure and at speed, because prescribed solutions are rarely found to be generally appropriate. Moreover, those judgements involve the translation of values, knowledge and skills in specific and continually changing contexts. Therefore the ability to think and act reflectively in the face of complex human and value dilemmas is crucial.

Awareness of the varied ways in which individuals respond to experience is very important for trainers, and provokes important questions about the factors which influence such responses to experience. Why might a normally thoughtful worker suddenly reject a learning experience out of hand as irrelevant? The reason might stem from previous learning experiences, socio-cultural or current organisational factors, all of which need to be anticipated in the design and delivery of training programmes if learners are to be enabled to make constructive use of their experience. In Chapter 5 these factors are discussed in detail.

Self-development versus socio-cultural approaches

Having provided an overview of the concept of experiential learning, we can now identify two main schools of thought within this concept: first, the self-development approach; and second, the socio-cultural approach. While both share a humanistic base, the self-development approach builds on the work of Rogers, who emphasises experiential learning as the process through which self-actualisation and maturity occurs (Rogers 1969: 279–97). Thus the goal is a fully functioning person. Knowles's work on andragogy – 'the art and science of helping adults learn' (Knowles 1978: 53–7) – also places the individual and their growth at the heart of the learning process. Thus Knowles sees adults as naturally motivated to learn and self-directed in their approach. This self-development ethos has underpinned much of the approach to the facilitation of adult learning.

The self-development theorists' emphasis on the self in the learning process neglects any consideration of the impact of socio-cultural forces on learning in terms of self-esteem, identity, motivation, opportunity and access. For instance, Brookfield (1986) points out that Knowles's assumption that adults are innately self-directed ignores totalitarian regimes in which this is not a reality and where learning is not by choice but is imposed. Similarly, poverty and other inequalities directly affect an individual's access to, expectations of, and capacity to learn.

Friere (1973), writing in the context of mass oppression in Brazil, constructed a more political and emancipatory role for learning. Thus education cannot be a neutral process, and teachers are, consciously or otherwise, powerful transmitters of culture. Therefore education either facilitates freedom, or it is 'education for domestication', to accommodate an oppressive regime's culture and control. This is therefore a social, not a self-actualisation theory of learning, focusing on the role of learning either in securing compliance with a dominant culture or enabling individuals and groups to reflect critically on an understanding of themselves within their socio-cultural context. It is here that liberationist educational and anti-oppressive values in social care come together, with an implicit social action orientation both for groups and individuals.

In social care training and practice both the self-development and the socio-cultural models of experiential learning are relevant. Staff require knowledge, and skills at both self-management and social action levels. Similarly, services for users will encompass meeting both inter-personal and environmental needs. Social care services are continually working with both the individual and their social context.

The nature of professional competence

So far we have looked in broad terms at how people learn. The second half of this chapter considers the nature of professional competence, and how it is developed. The link with the foregoing discussion on experiential learning is the proposition that the most appropriate model for social care training is one that emphasises experiential learning as the means by which professional competence is acquired and developed. As Winter suggests, a 'theory of professional competence must incorporate principles about the nature of professional work and the educational models best suited to promote it' (Winter 1991).

Therefore choices about approaches to training need to be informed not only by values and learning theories, but also by an understanding of the nature of the professional competence required in social care work. However, as Chapter 1 demonstrated, recent changes have raised major questions about the future direction of social care work and its value base, which in turn leads to considerable debate about the nature of professional competence.

Defining competence

The training revolution that has swept across all sectors of vocational education and training, both in the public and private sectors, has been driven by the concept of competence. This was generated from concern about the inadequacy and inconsistency of vocational training, the lack of attention in professional training to practical skills and domination of academic standards, and the low qualification base of most workforce groups. The result was the establishment of the National Council for Vocational Qualifications and the Scottish Council for Vocational Qualifications. The 1988 White Paper 'Employment for the 1990s' stated: 'Our training system must be founded on standards and recognised qualifications based on competence. These standards must be identified by employers.'

The main advantages sought from this approach were in providing the means of comparing levels across a range of occupations; an opening of access to professions; and a focus on outcomes which more closely matched the needs of the workplace and its users; and finally, a more transparent and therefore more just way of assessing.

In subsequent guidance, competence was described as 'the ability to perform the activities within an occupation or function to the standards expected in employment. Competence is a wide concept which embodies the ability to transfer skills and knowledge to new situations within an occupational area' (DOE 1991: Guidance Note 8). This definition follows the Job Competence Model, which has four components:

1   the specific technical aspects or tasks of the work role – activities with clear tangible outcomes;
2   contingency management – dealing with things that go wrong, or the unexpected;
3   task management – the over-arching management of all the tasks – for instance, through prioritising;
4   managing the job/role environment – including both the physical environment and the interactive environment: colleagues, customers, etc.

(Mansfield 1991: 14)

While this wider concept of competence is welcomed in beginning to address the complexities involved in social care work, where judgement, unpredictability and complexity are central features, it does not solve all the problems. Some vigorous critiques such as those by Ashworth and Saxton (1990), have been mounted, whilst others (Yelloly and Henkel 1995; Eraut 1994) have been more balanced in their commentary. These critiques have focused on a number of problematic themes:

● Do competences describe ideal or minimum standards?
● Are competences personal attributes or externally learnt behaviours, knowledge and skills?
● Do they describe capability or performance?
● Are competences inferred from performance or observation of process?
● Do they adequately describe the complex interaction between cognitive, affective and behavioural knowledge, values and skills that produces good practice?
● Can complex skills be atomised into their constituent parts when the overall skill is greater than the sum of the parts, and when it involves degrees of intuition and creativity?
● How wide can competence be predicted; e.g. to what extent is performance dependent on context?
● Are competences too individualistic in areas such as social care, in which successful action is likely to depend on team or inter-agency action?
● Can competence be either an action, outcome, piece of knowledge or an understanding?
● If competence is an outcome, does it matter how the outcome was achieved?
● To what extent do outcomes reflect individual performance when many outcomes in social care are mediated by multiple factors?

Joss expresses many of these concerns, in relation to social work education at least, when he writes:

> It denies the holistic nature of the work; shows what people must do but not how or why; completely fails to provide an explanation of the importance of the exercise of discretion and thus devalues the fact that equally competent performances can arise from quite different actions; it denies the importance of process and cannot handle abstract concepts such as reflective insight which are not easily amenable to observation; and similarly is a very poor training tool since it cannot shed light on the learning process, only on the acquisition of competences.
>
> (Joss 1991)

Despite these concerns, the competency focus has many emerging and potential benefits. The specification of competences and standards enables all involved to have a common understanding of what is expected, and how performance will be assessed. It makes the process of performance management potentially far more objective and transparent and less subject to personal bias and preferences. The link between standards and competences facilitates the accreditation of prior learning, enabling a range of earlier learning outside of qualification courses to be recognised and validated. For instance, many unqualified care workers, who make up a very large percentage of the social care workforce, have for the first time had their work experience and knowledge validated and accredited. Competency-based training ensures that training is continually linked to performance in the work place through its firm emphasis on the need to be able to demonstrate the application of knowledge, values and skills in the work place. Competences also provide a framework for training needs analysis, curriculum design and assessment of learning against measurable outcomes.

Although many questions remain about the degree to which a competence approach can reflect the true nature of the social care task, our understanding of competency is becoming more sophisticated. This is particularly necessary to ensure that the application of values and nature of decision making can be encompassed within the way in which competences are framed. Attitudes, emotional responses and critical thinking are thus as important as skills and actions. In other words, competences must recognise that the process by which outcomes in social care work are reached can be as important for the service user as the outcome itself. The way that competence is framed depends, in turn, on how the concept of professionalism is understood.

PROFESSIONAL COMPETENCE IN SOCIAL CARE: THE REFLECTIVE PRACTITIONER

Jones and Joss describe four professional types:

1 The *practical professional* or crafts person who is atheoretical acts on common-sense practical knowledge based on work, uses intuition and is organisation centred.
2 The *technical expert* who is sole possessor of technical/academic knowledge believes that there are right and wrong solutions. The expert's authority exists through expecting deference and dependence on their expertise. The expert denies the relevance of process, or the user's knowledge.

3 The *managerial expert* has a systematic or academic knowledge base based on management techniques; focuses on resource management, efficiency and effectiveness.

4 The *reflective practitioner* acts in the role of a facilitator who recognises there is no right answer or objective truth. The theory base includes relationships between external/social processes and internal/perceptual processes. Knowledge becomes manifest in working with users, and new rules are created out of practice to make sense out of uncertainty. The reflective practitioner is user centred, seeking partnerships based on the development of shared meanings, and a recognition of the uniqueness of each problem and its context.

(Jones and Joss 1995: 24)

It is possible to recognise all four types within social care practice – for instance, the 'management/systems' approach which is bureaucratically centred, or the technical expert or 'therapist'. In a study by Fisher (1995) it was found that social workers operating in the child protection field tended to act more in the role of the practical professional. However, it is our contention that the reflective practice model is the most appropriate in the current context, if professional values and skills are to be upheld and workers enabled to make increasingly complex decisions, and to work with wider ranges of responsibilities.

The concept of the reflective practitioner is eloquently described in the following analogy about social work practice from Yelloly and Henkel:

There are laws of harmony which the musician must follow; the act of musical creation or interpretation is grounded in and underpinned by accepted regularities which allows it to be heard and understood by the listener. But its precise form is in no way determined by these laws, and at some times they clearly do not apply, and a new musical language may be introduced. It is likely that the effective worker, like the accomplished musician, combines an informed understanding of principles and theories with an intuitive gift which enables her to tune in to the experience of troubled people. Knowledge, values, personal capacity and the practice of the craft are the essential elements of professional education.

(Yelloly and Henkel 1995: 7)

Thus professional competence for the reflective practitioner requires the ability to relate values, theory and knowledge to each new situation, together with a form of craft, highly tuned intuition and creativity. Without this, as Howe has pointed out, practice could be confined to performing surface responses according to pre-coded procedures, in which users must fit the batteries of checklists and guidelines, or to relegating service users to a passive or observer role while 'experts' fix their problems (Howe 1996: 92).

All of this implies the need for a definition of competence that incorporates the complexity both of the task and the problem-solving processes required of the professional. Wood and Powers, following the idea of reflective practice, describe a developmental model of competence:

> Competence must be distinguished from competences (specific capabilities). Competence rests on an integrated deep structure (understanding) and on the general ability to co-ordinate appropriate internal cognitive, affective and other resources necessary for successful adaption. In this way specific competences are integrated at a higher level, and accommodate to different contexts.
>
> (Wood and Powers, in Eraut 1994: 181)

Put more simply, this definition suggests that competence must integrate 'doing' with 'thinking' and 'feeling', and it is for this reason that experiential learning is so fundamental to the development of reflective social care professionals.

THE NATURE OF PROFESSIONAL DEVELOPMENT

In this final section, we consider what is known about the nature of professional development and its implications for training in social care.

Achieving a professional qualification is only the beginning point in becoming a learning professional. The pace of change means that staff must be able not only to do their current job well, but must also acquire skills and knowledge that will enable continuous learning and role adaptation.

Unfortunately, understanding about how staff develop after initial training, in terms of what knowledge and practice is affirmed, built up or discarded, is still very limited (Eraut 1994: 40). In other words, there is a lack of comprehensive and empirically based theory of how professional development occurs to guide training practice. However, we are not completely in the dark, as work, particularly by Schon (1987) and Eraut (1994), have provided considerable insight into the nature of professional development.

These writers have identified that professionals learn foremost through the processes of problem setting and solving, through which theories of practice develop. Therefore theory is built up based on experience, and is established in response to the context of its use, rather than being applied directly from academic or training contexts. Eraut states that 'knowledge cannot be defined independently of its use' (1994). This has considerable implications. If knowledge and learning occur in the context of their use, this means that the process of transferring and translating theory, values, knowledge and skills from training to the job is a highly complex one. The knowledge and skills acquired on a training course will not therefore be replicated in an exact way when they are utilised in the work place, as the work place is a different context of use. To understand this further, we need to explore Eraut's ideas about the nature of knowledge.

The nature of knowledge

Eraut distinguishes between three dimensions of knowledge, each of which affects the nature and application of knowledge:

1 Sources of knowledge.
2 Context of knowledge use.
3 Modes of knowledge use.

For the trainer these distinctions are important to understand when it comes to the selection of relevant knowledge to be taught, facilitating learners' reflection on their work, helping the transfer of training into practice, and assessing the potential effects of the work context on the transfer of learning into performance. As Figure 2.2 demonstrates, the nature of professional knowledge is more complex and wide ranging than the knowledge described in academic books or theories. It combines both academic and practical knowledge, as well as being dependent on the context (academic, institutional or practical) in which it is being applied and the manner in which the knowledge is used (imitation, application, interpretation or association). Each of the three dimensions are explored in detail in Figure 2.2.

The central message of Eraut's work is that learning is not a process of applying public knowledge taught in one setting, namely, academic or

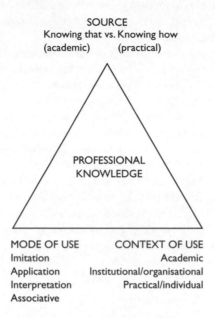

SOURCE
Knowing that vs. Knowing how
(academic)   (practical)

PROFESSIONAL
KNOWLEDGE

MODE OF USE	CONTEXT OF USE
Imitation	Academic
Application	Institutional/organisational
Interpretation	Practical/individual
Associative	

Figure 2.2 Framework for professional knowledge
Source: Eraut (1994); academic or practical knowledge

training, to another, practice. Rather, learning occurs in the process of transforming public knowledge – that is, that which can be codified and formally taught, into personal use, namely, that which an individual uses in their practice (Eraut 1994: 17–19). Thus learning takes place in its application.

For trainers this means that it is not possible wholly to predict what learners will learn, or do, in response to what is taught, for participants will transform that public knowledge in making personal use of it in their work. This means that the transfer of knowledge from the context of training to the context of work is rarely immediate or exact. Second, it means that learners will not use all the explicit public external knowledge they possess. Third, academics and trainers need be to alert to the danger that, by focusing exclusively on formal knowledge which can be academically codified and examined, the tacit (that which we know but cannot tell), intuitive, internal and practical knowledge accumulated by professionals over time may be ignored, invalidated, or left unexpressed and unchallenged. Under these conditions professionals may develop very divergent personal theories-in-use without any conscious appreciation of doing so, or of the consequences. For instance, a home care worker may hold beliefs about how younger family members ought to be able to care for elderly relatives, based on her own experiences which direct her responses to all other situations without her realising it. We now go on to examine Eraut's three dimensions of knowledge in more detail.

Sources of knowledge: academic vs. practical

In terms of source of knowledge distinctions can be made between *academic*, technical, propositional, formal knowledge and *practical*, personal and intuitive knowledge. Ryle calls these two types 'knowing that' and 'knowing how' (Ryle 1949). Eraut states: 'Important aspects of professional knowledge and expertise cannot be represented in propositional form and embedded in publicly accessible knowledge bases, such as books and research' (1994: 15). Practical knowledge includes case impressions, memories, or patterns built up over time, which become the prime source of a worker's expertise. This type of practical knowledge is crucial in making rapid and complex judgements in relation to problems for which there are no clear solutions, where theory is only partially helpful and where there is some uncertainty about outcomes – a common experience in social care work. It can be seen from these distinctions, between academic and practical knowledge, why staff find it so difficult simply to read professional texts, or hear new theory and apply this formal type of knowledge straight into practice, and conversely why it is so difficult to describe in book form the nature of professional practice.

These difficulties in translating theory into practice are worsened by the pace of change, so that the contexts in which formal and theoretical knowledge are being applied are constantly shifting, as well as becoming more pressurised. For instance, in training on supervision, it is not uncommon to find that in the time between training modules, one or more participants have had their span of control enlarged, thus reducing the time available for reflection, internalisation and application of their new knowledge.

In contrast to academic knowledge, Eraut describes practical knowledge as 'experience-derived-know-how' (1994: 42), or process skills (1994: 107). These are the skills which are essential in knowing how to conduct various processes that contribute to professional action, without which workers cannot be effective. Unfortunately, too often it is naïvely assumed that professionals either possess or will develop these skills without assistance. A further consequence is that if these skills are lacking, the transfer of learning into performance will be severely hampered. As this theme is explored in more detail in Chapter 10, process skills will only be discussed briefly here. Eraut lists five main process skills:

- *Acquiring information*: interviewing and observation skills, and interpretation of information.
- *Skilled behaviours*: a complex sequence of actions that becomes so internalised that it is performed almost automatically, so that workers can cope with high volume demand and rapid decision making.
- *Deliberative processes*: planning, problem solving, analysing and decision making, which require a combination of theoretical, situational and practical knowledge and judgement, and where reliance on procedures is inadequate.
- *Giving information*: the ability both to give information clearly and in ways that can be heard and understood by service users, and to provide the information that is likely to be most relevant to the service user. This relates to the ability to listen, pick up what is of concern to the user, and build on the user's definitions of her situation.
- *Metaprocesses*: self knowledge and self management to direct one's own behaviour to engage effectively in the processes described above. It requires the reflective capacity to critically self evaluate what one is doing, thinking and feeling – to stand outside oneself, and be prepared to examine assumptions and actions.

(Eraut 1994)

The assumption that these core skills exist and do not require teaching is a dangerous one. For instance, it is presumed that social workers have the skills to communicate with children, whereas in fact the introduction of the Memorandum of Good Practice demonstrated that this was not always the case. In fact, despite the critical need for high-quality interviewing skills right across social care work, the majority of workers have received little or no interviewing training. Indeed, there is little attempt even to define what is meant by interviewing, communication and listening skills. Once again it is assumed that workers possess these key process skills. Moreover, the opportunities to focus on deliberative and metaprocess skills are under increasing threat as practice becomes more prescribed by procedure and audit. However, the faster, more pressurised and more anxiety-ridden the context of practise, the harder it is to practise reflectively, and thus the more important 'skilled behaviours' become.

Context of knowledge use

The second dimension of knowledge concerns the context in which knowledge is used. Three contexts in which knowledge may be applied are described by Eraut, each with different implications for the type of knowledge used and its transferability to the other contexts. These three contexts are:

1   *Academic.* Knowledge is characterised by specialised language, a high value is placed on theories rooted in established academic fields of study, and there is the need to locate knowledge by reference to existing academic literature. Knowledge acquisition is seen as an on-going process and the importance of remaining open-minded is emphasised. Knowledge is dominated by written work, and it is through this that learning is expected to occur. However, the detailed application of academic knowledge to practice is left to the learner.

2   *Institutional.* This refers to the organisational context of knowledge use, and specifically therefore to the use of knowledge in policy making and the management of the organisation. Here the primary motivation for knowledge is to increase accountability, cope with external demands, and help the workforce adapt to change, rather than directly to improve practice. In this context therefore successful knowledge use depends much less on academic or practice skills, than on the social and political skills to manage organisational processes and politics in order to achieve sufficient consensus to make changes. Thus knowledge use has to be integrated with institutional life.

3   *Practice context.* Here knowledge is focused on its hands-on applicability to actual practice situations. Often this occurs where judgements have to be made under pressure and there are multiple and sometimes conflicting demands on the worker, who is moreover often practising alone. Written guidance on practice can offer only limited help, as the knowledge application process is an adaptive and problem-solving one, which must take into account individual style, and interpretation. For the successful application of practice knowledge, much depends on the degree of work-place support to

assist the process, not just at the practitioner level, but also to review agency policies and systems which are often crucial factors in whether new knowledge and skills can be utilised.

(Eraut 1994: 30–9)

Taken together, the different sources of knowledge (academic and practical), combined with the different contexts of use, underline Eraut's central theme that a significant proportion of learning associated with any change in practice takes place in the context of its use (Eraut 1994: 33). Trainers too, under pressure to deliver more, need to pay careful attention to the context of their own knowledge base and use, and the changing contexts of the staff with whom they work. Too often too much is demanded, expected of, or promised by the training process, and too little is understood about the complexities of professional knowledge and how it is developed. This takes us to Eraut's third dimension, which is how knowledge is used.

Modes of knowledge use

This third dimension describes the way in which we use knowledge and how theory is applied in practice. Broudy (1980), quoted in Eraut, suggested that there are four principal modes:

- *Replication*: mindless imitating, reproducing or copying of theory or practice.
- *Application*: following a simple set of principles without considering the context of application.
- *Interpretation*: selecting and varying the translation of theory into practice according to the situation.
- *Association*: this occurs when knowledge is made real via metaphors, or images which stimulate an emotional and experiential link with theory.

(Broudy, in Eraut 1994: 27)

From the perspective of social care work, where judgement must always take context into account, it is essential that the transfer of learning to practice is not simply a matter of replication or rule following but involves the interpretation and association levels. For this to happen effectively however, standards and supervisory systems need to be in place to ensure that knowledge and values are applied appropriately and consistently. In other words, the trainer alone cannot ensure that the knowledge and skills acquired during training will be appropriately interpreted and applied.

The exploration of Eraut's work has sought to explain why the journey between training inputs and outcomes is such a long and complex one. It should not therefore be a surprise that outcomes may range between being desired or undesired, planned or unplanned, transient or lasting. In Chapter 10 we will be exploring what other factors mediate the successful transfer of knowledge, values and theory from the training context into skilled behaviours in the work place. However, one important aspect for the trainer is related to understanding the process of how skills are acquired.

Skill acquisition

From the above it should now be clear why the provision of knowledge, values and theory through training does not guarantee how or whether it will be translated into skilled practice. Specific attention must be given to the development of skills. Haring *et al.* describe a four-stage skill development model, which will be illustrated with reference to the example of developing chairing skills:

1   *Acquisition.* This involves the first appearance of a desired behaviour, and the reasonably accurate performance of it under protected or simulated conditions such as on a training course. At this stage it may be more imitation or replication than integration. The worker will not have considered its application in different contexts. Thus the worker can chair a simulated meeting during a training course on chairing skills, following a structure presented by the trainer, in the presence of the trainer, and in which the worker can stop and re-start if she becomes stuck.
2   *Proficiency.* The skill can be used in meaningful ways, rather than in parrot fashion. Connections are made with the rest of the worker's practice, knowledge and values, and the worker is able to perform the skill of chairing under certain conditions. This might include chairing a small meeting of workers within the agency, all of whom are known to the chair, and in which nothing unexpected occurs. This might be akin to Broudy's second stage of application.
3   *Generalisation.* The skills can be applied in more complex situations, or when the conditions are more testing. For instance, the worker becomes able to chair more difficult meetings when there might be conflict, the participants come from a range of agencies

Table 2.1 Skill acquisition and learning methods

Level	Emphasis	Learning methods
Acquisition	Accuracy Rehearsal	Demonstration Modelling Role play Pairing/observing Video and feedback
Proficiency	Speed	Practice Reinforcement Video and feedback
Generalisation	New situations	Planning and rehearsal Consultation and feedback Differentiation
Adaptation	Complexity Range Modification	Problem solving Planning Consultation and feedback

and the process is less predictable. Some immediate interpretation of events and selection of responses must be made.

4   *Adaptation.* By this stage the worker is able to modify and adapt her chairing skills to an increasingly wide range of different contexts, where analysis, problem solving and on-the-spot strategies are required. For instance, the worker can chair a meeting involving service users, carers and staff over proposed cuts in residential provision for respite care.

(Haring *et al.* 1978)

Each stage of the skill acquisition process requires different kinds of learning methods, which are summarised in Table 2.1.

SUMMARY

● This chapter has provided an overview of learning theory, with particular emphasis on learning through experience.

- An underpinning theme has been the link between a humanistic educational value base and the anti-oppressive value base of social care work. The humanistic values underpinning experiential learning have been seen to integrate personal growth and social action approaches.

- Experiential learning approaches have been suggested as being particularly appropriate for the professional development of reflective professionals, who are able to respond to the individual meaning of each user's situation, concerns and needs.

- Professional competence has been defined as the ability to adapt continuously to changing contexts, and to integrate affective, cognitive and behavioural dimensions.

- Knowledge and learning occur in the process of its use. Therefore the nature and meaning of knowledge gained in the training context changes when transferred to practice within complex social care agencies.

- Professional development is most effective when focused on problem-based learning.

- A four-stage skill development was presented. If learners are not given the opportunities to complete these stages, the early tentative acquisition of a new skill during training may not progress to proficiency or wider generalisation, and may thus be lost.

Chapter 3

Commissioning training

This chapter explores:

- a training needs analysis: what it is and why do it?
- factors that impact on training needs analysis;
- techniques for undertaking a training needs analysis;
- commissioning training: the key principles.

A colleague was reminiscing about the 'old days', when as a trainer in a social services department he had more or less determined what training would be provided to the workforce. This was often decided on the basis of a worker contacting him saying they wanted training in a certain area. As the colleague said, if he felt like delivering a course on the subject the training was set up. There was no direction from managers, the approach was one in which the trainer took responsibility for all matters related to training. This *ad hoc*, reactive approach to meeting training needs has in the last ten years largely been replaced by a far more strategic process for commissioning training. In this chapter we examine how and why a more proactive approach is required in the current culture of social care organisations.

Perhaps the factor that has most influenced a change in attitudes towards the commissioning of training has been the introduction of the contract culture in the public services. This has resulted in an emphasis on effectiveness, with the aim of providing flexible, efficient, needs-led services. The contract culture has been present in community care since the implementation of the recommendations of the Griffiths Report (Griffiths 1988). Many of the principles have subsequently been applied to children's services. However, they have only recently affected the delivery of such support services as training and human resource management.

Training has traditionally operated within a mixed economy, some training being commissioned and purchased externally, while the rest has been provided in-house. However, as the contract culture has become established within health and social care settings, the increased use of competitive tendering has entered the training world. This has resulted in a shift of emphasis within certain training and development sections, from a mixed provider and commissioner function to sections that are predominantly responsible for either the commissioning or provision of training. There has been no standardised response to training within a contract culture. Crouch *et al.* (1995) describe in terms of a continuum the variety of arrangements that have been made for the commissioning and provision of training in the social care sector. At one end the emphasis is on training departments as providers of training, while at the other, as commissioners of training.

provide ———————————————→ commission					
in-house training unit providing all training	in-house training unit providing and commissioning training	in-house commissioning unit for training	training commissioners attached to operational units	operational managers commissioning all training	individual commissioning their own training
1	2	3	4	5	6

Figure 3.1 The commissioning and provision of training

The role of the trainer in terms of commissioning training will be determined by their position along this continuum. This is considered in more detail later in the chapter. Our concern here is to set the context for the commissioning of training.

The second factor that sets the context is that in a climate of organisational change it is crucial that training is targeted at meeting the changing needs of the workforce. The way in which the training is commissioned is a key factor in the targeting process. McMahon and Carter (1990) liken the commissioning process to a market gardener preparing the ground for planting. If the ground is not properly prepared then the quality of the harvest may be affected. They divide the commissioning process into three stages:

1   *Planning the crops.* This describes the identification of training needs through a training needs analysis. In the same way as certain

crops will not grow in particular ground, not all organisational needs can be addressed through training. The role of the commissioner is to determine which needs can best be met by training.

2   *Knowing the ground.* A gardener becomes familiar with her plot of land knowing the quality of the soil and what areas get sun. She is able to consider the implications for planting crops. In the same way the training commissioner needs to identify the organisational, professional and individual factors that will influence the training requirements, specifications and contracting arrangements.

3   *Providing the necessary nutrients.* A gardener decides what will assist the plants to grow. Likewise, the commissioner needs to identify the type of training that is likely to meet the training needs and to consider what additional support learners will require to ensure learning is put into practice.

These three stages should all form part of the commissioning process. If this groundwork is not done effectively, then the planting of the crop, which can be seen as the delivery of the actual training, is likely to fall on stony ground. The result is a poor harvest in which the training is likely to have little impact on meeting organisational goals. In this chapter each of these stages will be considered in detail.

The focus of the chapter centres on commissioning training in single agencies. However, the discussion is also very relevant to those involved in the commissioning of inter-agency training. If inter-agency training needs are to be properly assessed, each individual agency must have a framework for identifying and commissioning inter-agency training. It is only through an analysis of initial single agency training needs that the needs of the workforce, in terms of inter-agency training, can be identified. Further discussion of some of the particular issues in the commissioning of inter-agency training is to be found in Chapter 4.

A TRAINING NEEDS ANALYSIS: WHAT IS IT AND WHY DO IT?

What is it?

The commissioning of training requires a mechanism to enable the commissioner to identify the training needs of the workforce, and to prioritise the training that should be provided. A training needs analysis offers such a mechanism. It describes the collation of the organisational, professional and individual training needs of the workforce, enabling the commissioner, ideally in consultation with managers, practitioners and service users, to identify and plan for the appropriate delivery of training to meet those needs. The analysis should include an assessment and process for prioritising the needs in line with organisational aims and objectives, and for filtering out needs that are unlikely to be met effectively through training.

Why do it?

A training needs analysis is important for a number of reasons. First, training needs are not static, as organisational, legislative and professional requirements are continuously changing. Second, different members of the workforce will have different perceptions of these needs. Finally, members of the workforce need to be consulted regarding their perceptions of these changing needs. These are considered below.

Training needs are not static

The purpose of training and development alters with changes in the focus of social care organisations. A study of the literature demonstrates this. Warren-Piper and Glatter (1979) viewed staff development as 'a systematic attempt to harmonise individuals' interests and wishes and their carefully assessed requirements for furthering their careers, with the forthcoming requirements of the organisation within which they are expected to work' (Warren-Piper and Glatter 1979, quoted in Watts *et al.* 1993).

In this definition the purpose of training and development is to meet the needs of individual staff members, focusing on their future needs and, almost as a bonus, meeting future organisational needs. There is no consideration of current organisational needs, training being perceived as an investment in individual staff that will give long-term rewards.

In contrast, fifteen years later the SSI Report (Department of Health 1995) states that the role of training and staff development is to ensure that the workforce has the appropriate skills to deliver high-quality services reliably and efficiently. This reinforces the three elements of staff development advocated by Bell (1993), and described in Chapter 1; that is, that training should meet the needs of service users and carers, contribute to the goals of the organisation and meet the developmental needs of individuals. Thus the focus has shifted from staff development as a method for enhancement of individual skills, with potential future benefits for the organisation, to staff development as instrumental in meeting the current needs of service users and organisational goals. The emphasis is on employers identifying the training needs of the workforce. Individuals in the organisation are perceived as a resource to achieve these objectives. However, more recently still it seems that perceptions are changing again to take account of future needs. This is highlighted in the following quotation: 'commissioners are likely to be responsible for ensuring all contracts provide for an adequate investment in individual and organisational learning so that long term plans for a skilled and committed workforce can be realised' (LGMB and CCETSW 1997: 30).

This implies that consideration should not only be given to responding strategically to the current requirements of the organisation but also to identification in a planned rather than *ad hoc* way the future learning requirements of the organisation.

In addition to changing perceptions of training needs, changes within organisations will result in continual shifts in emphasis in terms of training needs. This will be influenced by such factors as staff turnover, new legislation and guidance, critical incidents and changes in organisational goals and structures. Not only are there shifting perceptions of the role and purpose of training in social care organisations, there are also continual changes in the professional requirements of training. This can be demonstrated by the introduction of national vocational qualifications (NVQs), and of post-qualifying and advanced awards which are increasingly providing the framework for establishing training needs.

Different perspectives, different needs

As outlined above, managers, practitioners and service users should be consulted regarding training needs. Each will have a different perspective; these may be grouped under three headings:

1   Training needs required to enable the workforce to achieve organisational goals.
2   Professional and occupational training needs ensuring that each worker is able to complete their particular role effectively.
3   Individual training needs.

Each of these will be considered in detail.

Organisational goals and training needs

One of the primary functions of training is to equip staff with the relevant knowledge, skills and values to be able to contribute towards the organisational goals. Boydell (1976) describes three situations when organisational training needs are likely to exist and there is a need for a training needs analysis.

- A 'block' exists which prevents the achievement of current organisational objectives. For example, members of the workforce misunderstand or fail to follow the procedures.
- Training is likely to enable the workforce to respond effectively to organisational change. For example, if restructuring is being planned, training should prepare staff for their new roles and responsibilities.
- Training is likely to lead to more desirable organisational objectives being achieved. For example, by considering children in need, in a broad context, through training, it may be possible to promote and develop skills enabling a more preventive approach to practice.

Professional and occupational training needs

Trainers have a role in partnership with managers in ensuring that the workforce is prepared and equipped to undertake its particular roles and responsibilities. This requires an acknowledgement that any job involves the following training needs:

- understanding of the task;
- acquisition of the knowledge, values and skills to undertake the task;
- an opportunity to develop these to a proficient level;
- an ability to apply this in a more general or specialist way;
- an ability to learn how to learn, enabling the worker to adapt to new tasks;
- an ability to apply knowledge, values and skills in the light of new legislation and changes in practice.

As can be seen, a training needs analysis has a function at three levels in terms of professional training needs. These can be linked to the CCETSW levels of competence (CCETSW 1993). First, there is a need to identify those new to a job and consider what training is required for them and their managers in enabling them to begin to develop the relevant skills and to integrate them into their job, the qualifying level. Second, a training needs analysis should identify training needs enabling workers and their managers to consolidate their learning and develop a level of expertise, the post-qualifying level. Finally, a training needs analysis should include training needs that enable the workforce to adapt their skills to undertake new tasks that link to the advanced level.

Individual training needs

Although employers have a central role in determining training needs, ensuring that the workforce is able to meet organisational goals, individuals within an organisation will also identify their own training needs. These may be motivated by such factors as:

- their desire to meet the organisational objectives – for example, staff may identify training issues that have not been considered by managers or trainers;
- their personal development – they may have clear ideas about what they want to achieve which may or may not fit with the organisational objectives;
- a consideration of career progression – as was indicated at the beginning of this chapter staff will want to consider their future needs and work towards them;
- current problems and stresses resulting from the nature of the workload and the particular demands of the job.

As can be seen, an individual's identification of their own training needs may reflect a much wider range of needs and wants that may not be congruent with organisational or professional requirements. In addition, there can be a tension between the identified professional needs and the organisational training needs. The issue for the organisation is to balance the individual's needs with a consideration of future workforce planning. For example, managers may agree to individual requests for qualification training on the basis that the monitoring of staffing levels indicate a need for more newly qualified staff in two years' time.

The consultation process

As can be seen from the above, within any organisation there are likely to be a range of perceptions of training needs. If an analysis of these needs is to be viable and acceptable to the workforce, then it is crucial that all levels of the workforce are engaged in the identification of training needs. Thus the importance of careful consultation throughout the training needs analysis is essential. The trainer undertaking a training needs analysis needs to consult with different tiers within the organisation to gain different perspectives of the training needs. In addition, the trainer should consider factors, outside the organisation that can influence training needs – for example, inter-agency practice, legislation, Department of Health guidelines, research and national professional developments. The views of service users are frequently not taken into account in a training needs analysis. Yet service users have a major contribution to make to a training needs analysis. This was highlighted by a young woman who had been in foster care and was involved in the assessment of training needs for foster carers. She stated:

> 'all those working in social services may think they know what a foster carer needs to know and I'm sure they have some important things to say, but that is not enough. Unless you listen to those who have been foster children you will miss a whole lot of things that are important to us.'
>
> (Ex-foster care user)

It is apparent that to gain an overview of the workforce and users' perceptions of training needs it is important to consult with them. However, this is not always an easy process, as a number of factors will influence the consultation process. These are considered below.

Factors that impact on training needs analysis

Identifying training needs and consulting with the workforce cannot be done in isolation. The training needs analysis has to be done in a way that takes into account the unique features of each individual organisation. These features are:

- the organisational philosophy towards training and development;
- the contract culture;
- the workforce and their perception of training and training needs;
- the motivation of staff and their access to training;
- the boundaries between training and other organisational needs;
- the use of competencies.

Each one of these factors will be considered in more detail.

THE ORGANISATIONAL PHILOSOPHY TOWARDS TRAINING AND STAFF DEVELOPMENT

The organisation's culture will influence the way in which staff development is perceived. This in turn will impact on the consultation process. Stickland (1992) analyses the organisational philosophy towards training and development departments using a continuum model. At the one extreme there is confluence where the training and development department's 'way of working, its internal processes and procedures and most importantly, its stance to the rest of the organisation becomes indistinguishable' (1992: 310).

In these kinds of organisations, trainers absorb and respond to the organisational perception of training with little opportunity to challenge or control. For example, there is concern within an agency about intimate care within a unit for people with physical disabilities. The immediate organisational response is to commission training as the solution. The training section accepts the analysis and does not question the commission, undertaking the task as a reactive response. In these organisations the philosophy towards training and development is 'do as we say'.

At the other end of the spectrum are training and development sections which have become marginalised. These are isolated from the organisation and trainers are detached and removed from the organisational perspective. The culture towards training in this context is 'let them get on with it'. In these settings trainers create their own agenda. For example, the trainer may attend a conference on brief therapy and decide to deliver courses on this topic, feeling that it will benefit staff, with little consultation as to whether it meets an organisational need.

In conclusion, Stickland states that the extremes of confluence and marginality should be avoided, as they can result in situations which prevent active discussion and debate regarding the role of training and can suppress the potential for change. Although many training and development sections seem to fall between the two extremes, this does not mean that there will be a positive approach towards training. The training unit is not necessarily a homogenous unit, so cultures towards training may vary depending on the particular area of work. Training may also be dispersed across organisations, with certain areas of training being perceived as the responsibility of the senior operational managers (for instance, high-profile services or services dominated by specific guidance), while in other service areas trainers have more control. Individual personalities can also impact on the philosophy towards training. If senior managers have a controlling style, a confluence model is likely to exist in their areas of responsibility, with the contact flowing in one direction only, from organisation to training. Alternatively, a trainer who is charismatic and individualistic may reinforce a marginal approach to training. The position of the head of the training section within the organisation will also impact on the approach. If she is part of the senior management team and is involved in operational and policy decision making, the team is more likely to reflect the organisational needs, than a section whose head has little influence at this level. Thus it can be seen that the organisational culture towards training influences the approach to and outcomes of the training needs analysis in terms of who defines whose needs.

THE CONTRACT CULTURE

The philosophy towards training, within the organisation, is not the only organisational factor that can impact on training needs analysis. As outlined at the beginning of this chapter, the introduction of the contract culture into the training world has resulted in a range of arrangements for commissioning and provision of training. These are:

- in-house training unit providing all training;
- in-house training unit providing and commissioning training;
- in-house commissioning unit for training;
- training commissioners attached to operational units;
- operational managers commissioning all training;
- individuals commissioning their own training.

The type of arrangement will influence the focus of the training needs analysis. Each different response has strengths and weaknesses in terms of undertaking an effective training needs analysis. These are outlined in Table 3.1.

As can be seen from the table, at one end of the continuum are the in-house training units which enable a strategic approach to focuses of training needs on organisational needs. As one moves along the continuum the training needs analysis is increasingly defined within immediate operational and individual terms, which is likely to result in a less strategic approach.

Table 3.1 The impact of commissioning and provision of training arrangements on training needs analysis

Focus	Strengths	Weaknesses
In-house training unit providing all training (1) The focus will be on establishing what are the training needs for staff and how the training team can meet those needs.	The training needs analysis will be undertaken by staff who will have a knowledge of the organisation and know exactly what training has been delivered in the past. They will also have some understanding of the strengths and weaknesses of the organisation. Future developments can then build on previous training and staff developments. Staff will have been specifically recruited to meet the training needs of the organisation. As the trainers are in secure positions they can afford to be critical. Equality of access to training is easier to achieve, as trainers will be aware of ways in which the needs of minority groups within the organisation can be met. Regular trainers enable links to be developed with users, facilitating involvement in assessing training needs.	Training can become very insular. The trainers are an integral part of the organisation and consequently may accept the culture and be uncritical. Identified training needs will be assessed in terms of the skills of the available trainers to meet those needs. Needs that cannot be met may be ignored. Trainers may become complacent and the focus on outcomes and clear specifications may get lost. Specific costs are not identified, which creates problems in terms of establishing that training gives value for money.

Focus	Strengths	Weaknesses
In-house training unit providing and commissioning training (2) The focus of the training needs analysis will be on establishing the training needs of staff in the organisation. Consideration will be given as to whether their needs can be met in-house or by commissioning training.	A flexible response is possible. The training needs which require a knowledge and understanding of the organisation can be delivered in-house, while other needs which require specialised skills or a perspective from outside the agency can also be met. Training courses delivered in-house can build on previous training. The needs of minority groups can be met in a flexible way either through in-house programmes or where specialist knowledge is required through commissioning. Links can be established with service users.	The targeting of what training needs should be met internally and which should be commissioned may not be done purely on assessment of need but on the availability of the in-house trainers or cost.
In-house commissioning unit for training (3) The training section undertakes a training needs analysis to establish what are the training needs of staff. They then assess the needs and commission external trainers to meet the needs.	Training can be commissioned from external trainers to meet specifically identified needs. Consideration can be given to the specific skills required of the trainer to meet the needs. The actual cost of training is made explicit. A flexible approach can be utilised as trainers can be selected in response to the needs of the organisation.	External trainers may not have the knowledge of the organisational culture to meet the needs. Quality assurance mechanisms for external trainers are undeveloped. A training strategy can become disjointed. It is difficult to establish and build on previous training, if a series of trainers are commissioned over time.

Table 3.1 Continued

Focus	Strengths	Weaknesses
		A developmental relationship between trainer and operational staff will not exist.

Equality of access to training and uneven development of skills can occur, as the focus for commissioning can be on high-profile training. |
| *Training commissioners attached to operational units (4)*

In these settings the training needs analysis is undertaken by a trainer who is based in an operational unit. The analysis will focus on the needs of the staff in that particular unit. | The trainer is likely to have a clear understanding of the local operational issues and the training needs of the staff group.

They should be able to gain the views of service users.

They will also have a very clear idea from an operational perspective of what is required when commissioning training.

They will be aware of the specific needs of staff who may not always be considered in large-scale training needs analysis.

They may also have an idea of the most effective way of meeting these needs. | As in (3). The trainer may find it difficult gaining an objective overview of the unit needs as they are an integral part of the unit.

The training needs analysis may focus on the micro issues within the unit rather than contextualising them in terms of the organisation.

Without a central reference point for training, different units could interpret policy and practice in different ways. Training to those interpretations can result in a lack of standardisation and at the worst dangerous practice.

Training may deepen organisational splits and parochialism. |

Focus	Strengths	Weaknesses
Operational managers commissioning training (5) This is an extreme form of commissioning, where the training needs analysis is undertaken by operational managers who are unlikely to have a training background.	The managers are likely to have a good understanding of the operational training needs. They may have established links with service users that can be utilised for the training needs analysis.	As in (3). Managers are unlikely to have a training background and consequently may lack the knowledge to undertake a comprehensive training needs analysis. As their work focus is operations this may result in a blinkered approach, other training needs being ignored.
Individual commissioning (6) An individual is required to find their own training to meet the requirements of remaining registered with their professional body.	The individual is motivated to assess their training needs continuously. They can select training on the basis that it will meet their needs in terms of learning and convenience.	Individuals may not always be aware of their needs. Methods of quality assurance are limited as training is contracted by the individual. It can be difficult for supervisors, etc. to support the transfer of learning into practice.

THE WORKFORCE – PERCEPTIONS OF TRAINING NEEDS

Employees within the organisation may well have very different perceptions of what constitutes a training need. This is demonstrated in research undertaken by Campenelli *et al.* (1994) which highlighted that 'training' means different things to different people. In general, 'training' was used to refer to formal courses and did not include the idea of on-the-job learning or informal learning. For some people the concept 'training' implied the presence of a qualified trainer, with hands-on practice of skills being seen as a prerequisite for 'proper' training. Such interpretations of training will impact on the training needs analysis. Staff consulted may be selective, their identification of needs being limited to those that they perceive can be met by the formal 'going on a course' training. Other needs that could be met through worksite-based training may therefore be ignored – for example, skill development through work shadowing or co-working.

Workers will also have different individual perceptions of their training and development needs. These are likely to be influenced by views of their role and the role of others. Banks (1995), as described in Chapter 1, considers three broad models of social work practice, which could equally be applied to health-related professionals, and highlight the different emphasis that workers may place on their role. The first model is the professional one, which focuses on the worker as an independent professional working to a professional code of ethics, using the knowledge, skills and values gained through education. The priority in this model is meeting the needs of the service user, and the primary allegiance is the profession. The second model regards the worker as an organisational employee who has a duty to undertake the roles and responsibilities defined by the organisation; the priority is adhering to bureaucratic procedures. The final model is the committed/radical model where the worker is ideologically and personally motivated to create change through social action and environmental changes.

The primary focus here can vary from individual empowerment to societal change. Our analysis of the organisational context of social care agencies, as outlined in Chapter 1, indicates that a bureaucratic model is dominant in statutory agencies. However, this can create tensions with the professional and radical models which cannot be ignored. As stated by Biggs, 'the rhetoric of "contract culture" and purchaser roles has under-emphasised the continuing relevance of social work perspectives and values that place any model for practice within a context of culture, power and equality' (1992: 10).

The above can lead to confusion among practitioners, who are seeking to balance their professional values both with their own needs and with those of the organisation. It also raises issues for those undertaking a training needs analysis as the workforce and those commissioning training may have very different perceptions of the value base and models of good practice. Thus a training needs analysis may result in needs being identified that are in conflict with organisational goals and priorities – for example, a clash between organisational and professional training needs. If this is not resolved at the commissioning stage then the training itself may be resisted or discredited.

Staff perception of training needs raises another issue, and that is the problem of not knowing what one does not know. Watts *et al.* (1993) consider that there are four different areas of training needs:

1 Being aware of what one knows. As a result of this the individual is confident in certain areas and able to determine areas that need developing.

2 Being aware of what one does not know. The individual in this position is aware of what they need to develop but may not recognise their strengths and current skills.

3 Being unaware of what one knows. This person does not recognise their skills and may feel they are lacking in these skills and request inappropriate training.

4 Being unaware of what one does not know. This person is in the least favourable position for identifying their training needs as they may feel competent or may blame external factors for their inability to perform the task.

Individual members of staff are likely to have training needs in all areas. Consideration should consequently be given to methods of assessment that are not totally dependent on the individual's perception of their own needs – for example, involving managers in the assessment of staff training needs.

ACCESSING STAFF AND STAFF MOTIVATION

A training needs analysis, as described above, presumes that the workforce are prepared to acknowledge a need for training. However, Argyris (in Senge 1990) notes that education systems do not encourage individuals to admit that they do not know something. Past educational experiences may also influence individuals' ability to acknowledge training needs. For example, training can conjure up images of going back to school for talk and chalk. This was very clearly stated on an evaluation form by a domestic worker:

'I was so scared about coming on this course I had sleepless nights. I was scared I would be put on the spot and made to look a fool. I cannot read and write very well and was frightened everyone would know. This course has made me see training very differently. I can't wait for another course.'

(A course participant)

Others may have had previous negative experiences of training and be reluctant to place themselves in positions where this could be repeated.

This is discussed in detail in Chapter 5. As a result of these experiences individuals often learn to manage areas of ignorance.

In addition, the culture of the organisation may discourage individuals admitting to learning needs. For example, some members of the workforce may feel that stating they have training needs may be perceived by managers as an inability to do their job properly. Cultures can also develop within organisations that can result in some managers or very experienced practitioners feeling unable to admit to personal training needs since this may be seen as a weakness. For example, there is often an unspoken assumption that once an individual has moved from practice to management they do not require professional training; rather, that the focus should be on managerial development.

Minority groups may also be reluctant to express training needs. This may be for a number of reasons. First, this may result from their past negative experiences of training and education. For example, they may have been the only representative from their minority group on previous training courses and have been expected to act as the expert. Alternatively, they may have experienced discrimination on a course or they may have found that their experiences have been marginalised. Third, they may consider that the conventional methods of training do not meet their needs – for instance, staff with dyslexia may be reluctant to attend training which involves writing.

TRAINING IN A VACUUM: BOUNDARIES BETWEEN TRAINING AND ORGANISATIONAL NEEDS

Not only must trainers consider the distinctions between organisational, professional and individual training needs, they also need to distinguish training needs from the other factors that impact on workforce effectiveness. It is very common for training to be seen as the panacea for all ills, or as Senge (1990) puts it, the 'quick fix' solution, when what is actually required is organisational change or development, such as in the case of the death of an older person through neglect, it may well be that the review into the circumstances identifies poor communication between agencies, lack of resources, non-specific guidelines and procedures as issues. In this situation training may have a part to play, but there are clearly other organisational factors that need to be addressed. As Smith states:

> Training is not the only answer. Whilst it may form part of a wider strategy to promote change and increase knowledge and expertise

in a field, if it is isolated and disconnected from the contextual issues – such as the wider political perspective at the macro level but also the specific work experience at the micro level – it may fail to achieve any of its original aims.

(1993: 8)

When an organisation does not achieve its goals or deliver the required quality of service to users, it is important to see training in the context of other factors that influence effectiveness. These include the following:

- the political agenda at a local and national level;
- clear goals, values and roles;
- leadership;
- planning processes;
- adequate staffing;
- resources;
- relevant policies and procedures;
- support and supervision;
- an appropriate working environment;
- a positive working climate;
- user involvement.

These all affect the ability of the workforce to achieve the organisational goals. If the impact of these factors on the organisation are not considered, training will not be effective in playing its part and bridging the gap from the actual to the required levels of performance, as shown in Figure 3.2.

However, while clear boundaries are important, some flexibility and creativity are necessary. The commissioners and providers of training cannot demand an optimum organisational environment before agreeing to act; rather, they need to consider the constraints placed upon them and make an assessment as to whether there are ways of addressing the issues or whether they have to accept these as immovable blocks that will unavoidably impact on the training.

It may well be that training needs analysis has a role in identifying what is required and what changes need to be made to build the different sections of the bridge between actual and desired standards of performance. For example, in the case of the older person who died from neglect, training of senior managers may facilitate a consideration of the relevance of current policies and procedures. Similarly, inter-agency training between the health and social work professions may

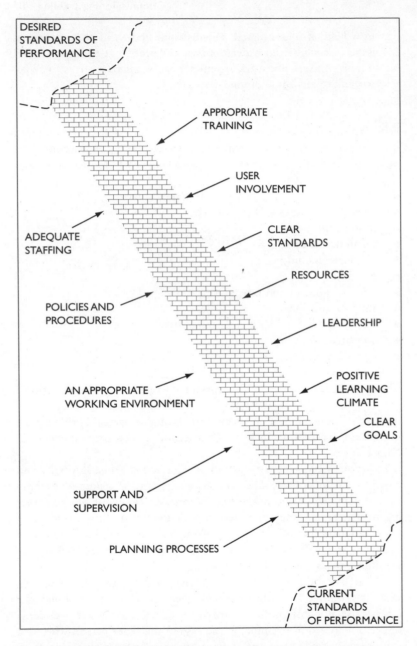

Figure 3.2 Bridging the gap between desired and current standards of performance

Source: Based on Horwath (1996)

raise issues around resource allocation. It is to enable the organisation to build the bridge that a strategic approach towards training and development is required. Thus it is important that the training needs analysis should consider whether all expressed needs or demands are in fact training needs. Moreover, training needs analysis, if done well, is an important communication exercise which can inform the organisation about much more than training needs.

A further consideration in the construction of training needs analysis is the role that a competence-based system of performance management can play. A strong competence-based system has specific and clearly defined standards, and enables all those in the organisation to have a common understanding of what is expected of various members of the workforce in terms of levels of competence. However, this model has disadvantages in terms of identifying training needs. The complex nature of a national system of agreed competences, such as NVQs, means that the system lacks flexibility and cannot respond easily to the rapid change that is taking place in social care organisations at a local level.

As can be seen, a range of factors influence perceptions of training needs. The task of the training commissioner is to establish and collate these needs and then assess which are indeed training needs and how they relate to organisational priorities. The commissioner has at hand a range of techniques to enable them to achieve this task.

TECHNIQUES FOR UNDERTAKING A TRAINING NEEDS ANALYSIS

As has been described above, undertaking a training needs analysis cannot be undertaken in isolation. In this section consideration will be given to techniques for assessing training needs. These can be divided into two groups. First, there are those geared to identifying training needs at a macro level, where the aim is to establish the training needs of the workforce in general and then to develop a training strategy. Second, there are techniques designed for a micro level where the aim is to identify the training needs of individual members of staff. Needs identified at the micro level can be added to the macro-level analysis. Each technique will be considered in terms of its advantages and limitations, bearing in mind the other factors that impact on the process of the training needs analysis.

Identifying agency training needs: the macro or strategic level

Feedback from training courses

Participants on training courses often identify training needs as they become aware of gaps in knowledge, values and skills during a training programme. These needs can be collated throughout the training – for example, by having a piece of flip-chart paper on the wall that is utilised to record further training requirements. These can be combined with feedback at the end of the course, using the course evaluation form which can include a section asking participants to identify further training needs.

Advantages

● This method enables training providers to identify training needs and wants, which can be forwarded to commissioners.
● It is a helpful way of identifying ongoing training needs, ensuring that training is a continual process of staff development.

Limitations

● The assessment may well reflect the issues of those already committed to training.
● Training needs may be very specific and focused, as they result from one area of training.
● When people are in 'training mode' they may consider problem resolution purely in terms of training, when that may not be the most appropriate intervention.
● The needs identified may focus on the individual needs of the staff concerned rather than focusing on the organisational needs and the needs of the service user.

Questionnaires

These can be distributed to staff at various levels within the organisation and to service users in order to establish their views of the training needs of the organisation and individuals within the organisation.

Advantages

- This is a useful interactive method, enabling a training needs analysis that reflects an overview of the organisational training needs from a variety of perspectives, including those of service users.
- As they can be anonymous, responses are likely to be honest.
- It can be utilised in assessment along the whole continuum, from provider to commissioner.

Limitations

- There may be a low response to the questionnaire, particularly among staff groups who feel marginal within the organisation.
- Responses will depend on individuals' ability to be honest.
- If the questionnaire is very structured it does not allow for unanticipated responses.
- There is unlikely to be an opportunity for individuals to consider the causes of the problems rather focus on training as a solution.
- It assumes that staff know what they do not know.

Focus groups

A number of small groups are set up and individuals are asked to quickthink what they feel are the agency's training needs. These are then collated and priority given to those that are most common or urgent.

Advantages

- These can be utilised in assessment along the whole continuum from provider to commissioner.
- They enable those involved to 'own' the ensuing training needs analysis.
- They provide an overview of different perceptions of training needs at different levels, from various disciplines and service delivery areas within the organisation.
- Service users can be involved.
- They reduce personalisation of needs.
- Through discussion and clarification they can allow a more sophisticated analysis of training needs.

Limitations

- The analysis is as good as the individuals within the groups and may not be representative of the workforce.
- There is a tendency to use staff who already have a commitment to training. Minority or marginalised staff groups tend to be over-looked, hence the value of targeted focus groups.
- Training is considered in a vacuum and may be utilised inappropriately when other issues should be addressed.
- Focusing purely on training can result in a Utopian approach with unrealistic expectations of what can be achieved.

Critical incident analysis

This can be done by asking a group of staff to consider a situation when the workforce did not function well where it was suspected that this was as a result of lack of knowledge and skills. The group then analyse what went wrong, and try and identify the lack of knowledge and skills that led to that incident.

Advantages

- The focus is an identified incident when required standards were not achieved, which provide a concrete example of what is required, in terms of training, to meet those standards.
- The analysis can be undertaken by providers or commissioners to ensure that training specifically addresses the issues.
- Service users can be involved in the process.

Limitations

- It is a reactive response to what may be an isolated incident – for example, the result of a review into a child's death – and can result in unnecessary training or training that does not address more general issues.
- There may be training issues that are not acknowledged by those undertaking the analysis.

Interviews

The trainer consults with personnel at various levels within the organisation, either individually or in groups, to identify what they feel are the training needs for all the different staff groups.

Advantages

- This is a very effective way of obtaining different perspectives on the knowledge, values and skills required by the different groups of staff.
- The interview process enables the trainer to explore exactly what those interviewed mean when identifying training needs.

Limitations

- Interviewing can be very time consuming and consequently costly.
- The training needs analysis is as good as those interviewed; e.g. it is easy to ignore minority and marginal staff groups.
- The effectiveness depends on the interviewer's skills.
- It can be difficult collating the results as interviewees may use the same terminology but mean different things.
- If the trainer is marginalised within the organisation those interviewed may be the trainer's allies and not a cross section of staff at different levels.
- If training is seen as the responsibility of senior managers the target for interviewing may be the managers, providing a distorted analysis.

Staff demands for training

This occurs when staff identify a need and are proactive in bringing it to the trainer's attention. (This is a macro form of analysis if a group of staff make the request and micro if the request is made by individuals.)

Advantages

- Training can respond to a current need identified by staff, who will be motivated and committed to the training as they have a sense of ownership.
- Both commissioners and providers can respond to the issue.

Limitations

- It could be a reactive response responding to a crisis.
- Training strategies need to have sufficient flexibility to respond to the demand. If not, by the time the training is provided the urgency may have passed.
- The demand may be a distorted response from one section of the workforce and needs to be contextualised.
- Some groups may become very greedy, requesting a disproportionate share of the training budget.

Development groups

A development group consists of staff at all levels in the organisation who focus on identifying training needs in a very specific area.

Advantages

- This approach can reinforce the connectedness of each tier in the organisation and ensure that training addresses the needs of staff at all levels.
- The approach is an effective method for commissioning and negotiating the provision of training.

Limitations

- The group may be too focused, and overall training can become compartmentalised and disjointed.

Workforce data

This describes the information regarding the workforce that is held on a database. It may include such training information as levels of competence, prior training, qualifications of staff and more general information regarding numbers of staff employed in different sections of the organisation.

Advantages

- It provides qualitative data.
- The system can be adapted to meet the requirements of the training

section in terms of collecting data that can be utilised for the identification of training needs.

Limitations

● The database needs to be continually updated. If this does not occur then a distorted perception of current and future training needs may be obtained.

Identifying individual training needs: the micro level

In addition to identifying the training needs of the organisation as a whole, consideration has to be given to individual training needs, focusing on the needs of individual members of the workforce in terms of knowledge, values and skills to meet the organisational goals. This information can then be incorporated into the macro analysis to provide a profile of the workforce.

Job description and specification

One method of identifying need is to consider what is required of an individual and how they and or their manager rate their ability to undertake the job.

Advantages

● This can identify training needs at a variety of levels from basic acquisition to development of specialist skills.
● It can be used effectively if linked to practice competence as described above.
● The approach can provide a systematic overview of needs of groups of staff having the same job description.

Limitations

● It is not an objective method of assessment, as it is undertaken by the individual and their manager who may have their own views on the way the job should be undertaken. This can be avoided through the use of practice competencies.

Personal profiling

This involves ongoing monitoring of an individual's development, taking into account their job, their own developmental needs and their career ambitions. It can be incorporated into supervision.

Advantages

● It is a tool for considering the needs of an individual as a whole and provides a framework for taking a strategic approach incorporating training, supervision and work experience.
● As the profile is regularly revisited and updated during supervision it reinforces a commitment to an ongoing process of staff development.
● It has the additional benefit of enabling all those involved in the organisation to take a systematic approach towards learning and development and emphasises the connectedness between tiers in the organisation, reminding both the individual and their manager of their roles and responsibility towards staff development.

Limitations

● The system is dependent on individual commitment and on provision of regular and effective supervision.
● It is a difficult process for managers responsible for supervising large numbers of staff whom they may see infrequently.
● It requires comprehensive recording, which can be time consuming.
● It can be difficult collating the personal profiles across the workforce in order to identify training needs.

Staff appraisal

This is a system for monitoring the development of staff members by assessing what they have achieved and identifying areas for further development in terms of agency, job and individual needs. It is usually undertaken by a superior, frequently the individual's manager.

Advantages

● It enables an all-encompassing approach to staff development and is linked to goal setting.

Limitations

- Perceptions of performance of tasks can be subjective.
- It may have negative connotation and be treated with suspicion, if it is felt training is to be utilised only in areas of poor performance, not as a positive model for development.

Supervision

Part of the supervisor's role is to take responsibility for supervisees' development. They should be continually identifying training needs and prioritising them with their staff.

Advantages

- This approach integrates training and staff development. It can maximise learning opportunities by advocating that staff needs be met when identified.

Limitations

- Subjectivity regarding the perception of needs or the role of training may impact on the process.
- When supervisory time is limited, staff development may fall off the agenda.
- Some staff get very limited supervision that may not focus on staff development but be managerial in approach.

The methods described above are ways of collecting data to assist in the identification of training needs. However, the effectiveness of the commissioning process will be determined by the way in which the information is collated and the principles on which a training strategy is devised.

COMMISSIONING TRAINING: THE KEY PRINCIPLES

Once training needs have been identified and collated, using a selection of the techniques described above, consideration needs to be given to the expectation of the commissioner and provider regarding the meeting of these needs. Bell (1993) states that training is most likely to contribute to the achievement of organisational goals if human resources and training are managed together and training is seen as being of strategic importance. This has implications for commissioning training in terms of a strategic and integrated approach towards training that should reflect the aims and objectives of staff training and development as described in Chapter 1.

There are a number of principles which should facilitate this strategic approach:

- The identification and implementation of training, resulting from the training needs analysis, should be planned and delivered as part of an organisationally owned, integrated training strategy which in turn should be linked to the achievement of organisational goals.
- The strategy should be underpinned by a commitment to equal opportunities.

Each of these principles will be considered in detail.

A training strategy

A training strategy can be defined as 'a planned response to the identification of training needs'. The strategy is the vehicle for deciding how, which and when different training needs will be met. The training strategy should focus on meeting the training needs of the whole workforce. It is important that the training needs of senior and middle managers are not ignored, as the Department of Health states: 'managers need regular updating on developments in knowledge and skills to ensure they are not divorced from the work of their staff' (1991b: 25). This should help managers provide appropriate supervision and support for practitioners. It should ensure that the training of front-line staff is not occurring in a vacuum but will enable learning to continue in the work place, supported by informed managers, appropriate structures and resources.

However, in the same way as the commissioning process is influenced by the remit of the training unit, both the process of establishing and delivering a training strategy will be influenced by approaches to learning within the organisation. Four different approaches to learning are described by the Local Government Management Board and CCETSW (1997), each of which will influence the training strategy and subsequent commissioning process. These are listed below.

Ad hoc *approaches to learning*

- There is likely to be a separate training and personnel section with few links to operational management and quality assurance.
- Training management is not seen as the responsibility of senior managers.
- There is likely to be no strategy for the management of change; staff supervision is erratic.
- No systems of staff appraisal or performance review exist.
- There are no personal development plans.

In this climate, undertaking a training needs analysis will be difficult as many of the mechanisms for gaining information do not exist. As a result of this there is unlikely to be a coherent training strategy and there will be no specification of organisational training requirements.

'Hot' and 'cold' approaches to learning and development

- There is an integrated personnel and training function but erratic links to operational management.
- Human resource management is not seen as the responsibility of senior managers.
- Past problems with human resources are addressed but with no follow through, so that the solutions of yesterday become the current problems.
- Personal supervision is available but not structured
- The use of personal development plans is erratic.

In this environment, the establishment of training needs will vary depending on the commitment of the managers and workforce. The subsequent training strategy may result in priorities and plans being agreed and published but the delivery and commitment may be erratic.

Planned learning and development programmes

- Senior management take active responsibility for training and equal opportunities.
- Specific competencies and staff development requirements are intrinsic to all service contracts and plans.
- Personal supervision is routinely provided.

- There is a comprehensive system for appraisal and personal development plans for all salaried staff.
- There is a systematic approach to workforce development.

In this culture, establishing training needs is seen as the responsibility of both operational and training staff and information can be obtained in a systematic way. There is likely to be a strategy for staff development. The training requirements are clearly specified and provision contracted in advance with external or internal providers.

Learning and development culturally valued and a top priority

- Human resource management and financial management are seen as of equal importance, led from the top but also allowing for control at lower levels within the organisation. Specific competencies and staff development requirements are intrinsic to all service contracts and plans.
- Workforce development and equal opportunities are central to strategic planning for the organisation and those delivering social care in the area.
- Mentor systems are in place for all staff with new responsibilities.
- Coaching, performance review and appraisal exists for all.
- There is widespread use of feedback and personal development plans, linked to service development.

In this culture, training needs are perceived in a broad context including both formal and work-based training and development. Systems and attitudes enable a comprehensive approach towards training needs analysis, resulting in a training strategy where learning is legitimised and linked directly to quality. Learning is related to assessment of competence and standards of service delivery. Joint collaborative training and development programmes with other organisations are encouraged (LGMB and CCETSW 1997: 146–8).

The ability of the training commissioner to develop a comprehensive training strategy will be affected by the organisation's particular approaches to learning. Clearly, the latter two approaches are likely to result in a more comprehensive and strategic approach to training with a clear commitment from senior managers. However, if this commitment does not exist the training commissioner needs to consider this in the planning of the training strategy, first, by taking an integrated approach towards commissioning training and, second, by negotiating viable contracts between commissioner and provider that take into account the approach to learning.

An integrated approach towards commissioning training

Hay (1992) considers the consequences for relations between providers, commissioners of training and learners if each group has different perceptions, agendas or anxieties about the role of training. She depicts these interactions as a series of triangles. Each shows a different set of perceptions and potential tensions and distortions in relation to other parties, which can fuel a mutual suspicion of hidden agendas, insecurity and mistrust that may undermine the prospects for effective training. However, if all three have a common understanding of the aims and objectives of the training strategy and appreciate how it will enable learners to meet the needs of the organisation in a realistic and achievable way, then congruence exists (see Figure 3.3).

However, unhealthy alliances can form if a common understanding does not exist. For example, a trainer may be commissioned to undertake supervisory skills training for first-line managers, on the basis that senior managers feel they are not supervising staff effectively. As shown below, when the training provider meets the learners it very quickly becomes apparent that the staff have the skills to undertake the supervisory task but are not given an appropriate workload to undertake the task effectively. In this situation both the provider and learners may feel resentful towards the commissioner and project all their concerns regarding supervision onto the organisation, ignoring the possibility that, despite other issues, they may be able to offer a more effective

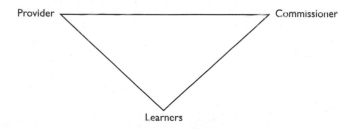

Figure 3.3 Interactions on training: congruence between parties
Source: Hay (1992)

supervisory service as a result of training. This is represented by the triangle shown in Figure 3.4.

Alternatively, the commissioner and training provider may form an alliance against the learners. For instance, the organisation wants to expand services for those with drug dependency issues. It is agreed that front-line staff will require training in this area and the training is provided. The learners are resistant stating that they need additional resourcing as training alone is insufficient. The commissioner and provider may form an alliance believing that the workforce are raising unreasonable objections (see Figure 3.5).

In the final scenario the commissioner and the learner may form an alliance against the training provider. This approach can be seen as

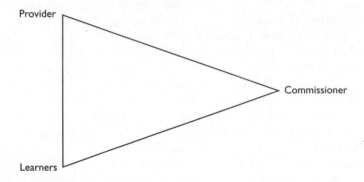

Figure 3.4 Unhealthy alliance between provider and learners
Source: Hay (1992)

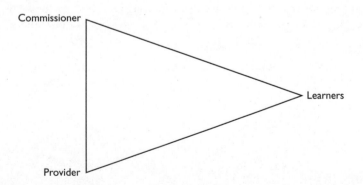

Figure 3.5 Unhealthy alliance between commissioner and provider
Source: Hay (1992)

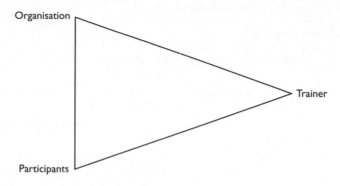

Figure 3.6 Unhealthy alliance between organisation and learners
Source: Hay (1992)

'shooting the messenger', for example, the trainer is asked to undertake training around new central government legislation and guidance. Both the commissioner and learners may be resistant to change and consequently blame the trainer, stating that the training is inadequate and does not equip them to undertake the task (see Figure 3.6).

In the scenarios described above, some of the consequences of distorted perceptions and hidden agendas are highlighted. There is a real danger that this may occur during the commissioning process if commissioner and provider allow their own agendas to dominate. For example, the commissioner wants to be seen to be doing something and the provider wants the work. This can result in collusion, with organisational, learners' or users' issues being minimised or denied and the overall credibility of training being damaged.

Negotiating a viable contract between the commissioner and provider of training

As a result of the contract culture, contracting of training has become more formalised. This may occur within the organisation, as a service level agreement between operational managers and the training section, or between commissioner and provider of training.

Hope (1992) identifies two levels of contracting: the process contract, which focuses on what the commissioner and provider expect of each other, and ways in which they will work together; and the administrative contract, which focuses on the practicalities, such as costings, dates and length and number of courses.

Table 3.2 Agendas for the process contract

Commissioner's agenda	Provider's agenda
How can training address the needs identified?	Are all the needs training needs?
How will the trainer work towards the desired outcomes?	Are the desired outcomes realistic and explicit?
Are the training programmes linked to systems of accreditation?	How will the training be evaluated?
How can we ensure high-quality training?	What is the standard required? Are standards made explicit in policy documents?
What is the trainer's value base? How does it reflect the values of the organisation?	Is the organisation prepared to accept the value base of training, i.e. enable participants to apply their learning in supported practice?
How will an anti-oppressive framework be incorporated into the training?	What is the commitment to anti-oppressive practice in terms of service delivery and targeting staff?
How will the user perspective be incorporated into the design, delivery and evaluation of the training?	Is the organisation committed to involving service users in the design, delivery and evaluation of the training?
How will the training address the organisational requirements?	What are the issues in the organisation that may impact on the commitment and appropriateness of the training?
What if the training does not meet the organisational needs?	What if there is a hidden agenda that will affect the training?
Who will work together with the provider?	Who will work together with the commissioner?
How will they do it?	How will they do it?
How do we evaluate?	Who is accountable for this training?

Tables 3.2 and 3.3 outline the agendas for commissioners and providers when negotiating a training contract. In order for training to be a means of achieving organisational objectives the commissioner and provider of the training need to reach a common understanding in terms of contracting on both process and administration issues.

As can be seen from these tables, those commissioning will view

Table 3.3 Agendas for an administrative training contract

Commissioner's agenda	Provider's agenda
How much is it going to cost and what will be provided?	What can I charge for the work, bearing in mind planning time and other hidden costs?
When will the work start and when will it be completed?	What is a realistic time-scale?
How do we ensure the work is completed on schedule, and are there cancellation fees?	What if there are unanticipated problems?
What will be the methods of delivery?	How do they want the training delivered?
Who owns the material?	Who owns the material?
What resources do we need to provide?	What resources can I expect and what do I need to supply?
What is our come-back if we are not satisfied?	What if I have been misinformed of the needs? Have I any come-back?

training from a different perspective from that of the provider. Training contracts provide an opportunity to negotiate and seek clarification, with the aim of gaining a common understanding of what the training is and how it is to be delivered. If there is a lack of congruence between the expectations of the provider and the commissioner, then training cannot be an effective tool towards achieving the goals of the organisation.

To ensure that training is effectively and appropriately commissioned, the commissioner needs to enter dialogue with the provider during the commissioning process regarding the context for training and the organisational issues that can impact on the training. The provider in turn needs to be realistic about what can be achieved. Both of them should be clear about areas that can be negotiated and those where compromise is inappropriate.

Equal opportunities and the commissioning process

Those undertaking training needs analysis should also consider the 'hidden staff groups'. These tend to be low-paid, unqualified staff who are on the periphery of the organisation and may get infrequent supervision – for example, domestic staff, home-care workers, supply staff. These staff groups are rarely consulted about their training needs and decisions regarding their training requirements are often made by their managers. This can result in a very unbalanced training needs analysis which gives no consideration to the professional needs of the individual and removes any sense of personal accountability for identifying training needs.

Emphasis has been placed in this and other chapters on the importance of consultation with the workforce to identify and address training needs. Balloch found that certain staff groups received little if any personal information regarding training opportunities. The groups of staff most commonly affected were home-care and residential staff (Balloch 1996). The information they received was often generalised and came via managers, rendering them part of an invisible workforce.

Research has also shown that older workers, particularly women, tend to be excluded from training programmes (Balloch 1996). This is occurring among a workforce that is relatively mature with 40 per cent of home-care staff aged 50 or over and a high proportion of staff in residential services being older workers. The social care workforce is also predominantly female. In addition, a high proportion of the close to 1 million people employed in personal social services are in part-time employment (Social Services Inspectorate 1997), and a minority are black staff. Earlier on in this chapter we considered some of the issues concerned with identifying training needs to ensure an equal opportunities perspective. However, as part of the commissioning process the specific requirements of these groups need to be identified and addressed. For example, consideration should be given to training strategies that enable part-time staff to participate readily in the training. In Chapter 5 we consider in detail factors that should be considered to ensure that equal opportunities are addressed.

SUMMARY

Commissioning of training combines marketing skills with the strategic management of human resources (LGMB and CCETSW 1997: 289) enabling the training needs of the workforce to be identified and addressed in a way which promotes organisational goals. In this chapter we considered this task in the context of the structures and learning philosophies of social care organisations.

Key points

Different organisational structures exist for the commissioning and provision of training which will influence the remit of the trainer within the commissioning process.

The training needs analysis is a useful mechanism which enables commissioners of training to

- consult with managers, practitioners and service users to identify deficits in the knowledge, values and skills of the workforce;
- identify the role that training can play in meeting these deficits;
- identify developmental training needs that would enhance the workforce's ability to contribute to the current and future goals of the organisation.

A number of factors, such as organisational philosophy, the contract culture, staff motivation and perceptions of training needs, will influence the training needs analysis.

A range of techniques exist for establishing training needs at both a macro and micro levels.

Effective identification of training needs and the implementation of a comprehensive training strategy will be determined by the level of integration between training commissioners, providers and the operational workforce.

Chapter 4

Inter-agency training

Possibilities, pitfalls and strategies

This chapter explores:

- current context of inter-agency working;
- definitions of inter-agency training;
- challenges and barriers in inter-agency training;
- frameworks for effective inter-agency training.

In any contest to identify buzzwords for social care work in the 1990s 'collaboration', 'co-ordination', 'inter-agency' and 'multi-disciplinary' would surely be safe bets. Indeed, exhortations for different agencies and professions to collaborate in the social care field have been unceasing over the past twenty years. And yet, as Aiken has described, 'co-ordination' is a word which is 'over-worked, under-achieved and seldom defined' (Aiken 1975). Hence it is not surprising that for many trainers, the experience of planning and delivering inter-agency training is one of the most demanding and complex processes in which they can be involved. Apparently basic forms of foundation training can become fraught with anxieties, conflicts and complications when it is delivered in an inter-professional group. While many of the issues confronted in inter-agency training are similar to those encountered in single discipline training, their intensity is much greater. Simply putting different professionals together in one room for training is no guarantee that mutual understanding and respect for each other's role will be enhanced. Indeed, it may even serve to consolidate pre-existing power differences, occupational stereotypes and prejudices. This area of training may therefore stretch even the most experienced trainers to their intellectual, emotional and facilitative limits.

This chapter will explore contexts, key concepts and frameworks relevant to inter-agency training in social care. By this we refer to the activities involved in the planning and delivery of training specifically targeted on groups made up of different disciplines and/or agencies. The different discipline groups will usually, but not always, be employed by different agencies – for example, NHS Trusts employ a range of professions. Although later in the chapter we shall explore definitional issues surrounding the terms 'inter-agency', 'multi-disciplinary' and 'inter-professional', *inter-agency training* will be used as a generic term in this book because of its stress on agencies, not just individuals being involved in shared learning.

The principal context for the inter-agency training described here is service development and delivery, as opposed to shared learning in the higher educational sector. The focus is on in-service, rather than qualification or post-qualification inter-agency training. Nevertheless, references will be made to and from the higher education field, as there are many shared challenges and much that each can learn from the other about inter-agency training.

First, however, by way of setting the scene some brief discussion of issues concerning inter-agency working is necessary before inter-agency training is explored. The reason for doing this is that the vast majority of difficulties arising in inter-agency training have their origins in unresolved issues over inter-agency working.

INTER-AGENCY WORK: DEFINITIONS AND CONTEXT

It has become almost an article of faith that good practice is inter-agency practice, although experience and research teaches that the road to co-ordination has been an exacting and sometimes illusory one, paved with more promises than firm outcomes. Moreover, as an article of faith, it can become a dangerous assumption that professionals all share a common understanding as to what is really meant, or required by, a commitment to working and learning together. Definitions of words like 'co-ordination' and 'collaboration' vary hugely both within disciplines and agencies as well as between them. One professional's co-ordination is another's collusion. While there are many different approaches to definition, Davidson offers this practical typology of terms:

- *Communication*: talking together, sharing information.
- *Co-operation*: suggestions of small-scale collaboration, *ad hoc*, dependent on individuals, not formalised.
- *Confederation*: more formalised working together, but no sanctions for non-compliance.
- *Federation*: joint structures, agencies cede some autonomy in defining shared goals and tasks.
- *Merger*: individual agency identities merged within formation of new organisation.

(Davidson 1976)

However, this definition does not include two other frequently applied terms 'co-ordination' and 'collaboration', which are often used inter-changeably. Hallett and Birchall, drawing on a range of definitions, suggest that 'co-ordination' refers to a looser, less formalised and more practitioner-based working together between individuals from different disciplines (Hallett and Birchall 1992a: 8). In contrast, 'co-ordination' refers to a more formalised relationship involving specific agreements, protocols and structures to underpin inter-agency working. (We shall follow these distinctions when using these terms.) They conclude that the purposes of both are that the 'combination of skills produces an outcome which could not be achieved as effectively or efficiently by other co-operative ways of working'. However, Hallett and Birchall also note the need for both formal and informal relationships between agencies, and that the best forms of co-ordination tend to occur where inter-agency working is embedded in strong networks of informal relationships.

Finally under definitions, there is a crucial distinction to be made between 'inter-agency' and 'multi-disciplinary' co-ordination. Multi-disciplinary co-ordination refers to individuals from different agencies and disciplines working together, in contrast to inter-agency co-ordination, which refers to agencies or disciplines working together at an organisational level. The importance of this distinction lies in the fact that co-ordination can only be limited if it is multi-disciplinary for it relies on individuals', rather than agencies' commitment to working together.

The current context for inter-agency work is both an exciting and an ambiguous one. Government guidance, and recent legislation across adult and children's services, have increasingly emphasised the importance of inter-agency working. Service users too have demanded improved co-ordination between services. However, on the other side, many of the reforms described in the opening chapter, such as the

(10) Staff care
(9) Quality assurance
(8) Supervision
(7) Service provision
(6) Training
(5) Policies and procedures
(4) Philosophy of intervention
(3) Collaborative structures, leadership
(2) Mandate for co-ordination
(1) Recognition and definition

Figure 4.1 Inter-agency framework for co-ordination
Source: Morrison (1996)

purchaser–provider separation and the development of the mixed
economy of welfare, fly in the face of collaborative working. Resource
constraints and competition have forced all agencies to rationalise their
priorities, as a result of which time and funding for inter-agency work
has been pared back. It may be that this context presents inter-agency
working with one of the greatest opportunities since its importance was
first recognised. Equally, some would speculate that it is facing its
greatest threat. What may be said with more certainty is that the unrealistic expectations being placed on inter-agency training alone to ensure
the safe delivery of the potential fruits of co-ordination are greater than
ever. This must be guarded against at all costs. While inter-agency
training can play a vital role in facilitating co-ordination, it can only
do this within a robust and clear framework for inter-agency working.
Such a framework is presented in Figure 4.1.

● *Definition.* There must be a shared recognition, and definition, of the
  need for co-ordination in any particular service delivery area. This
  should clarify the goals and intended outcomes of co-ordination.
● *Mandate.* The mandate for co-ordination must be specified, in
  terms of legislative and/or professional grounds. Unless this is
  done, some agencies will opt out.
● *Structures.* Formal structures at both strategic and operational
  levels are required to underpin co-ordination. However, formal
  administrative linkages are fragile unless they are embedded in a
  network of effective informal relationships. Thus there is a need for
  complementary *informal* local networking structures, to address
  issues such as developing trust, sharing anxieties, conflict resolution,
  and identifying local resources and needs (McFarlane and Morrison

1994). Too often, without such networks, negative experiences of the formal structures such as case conferences go uncorrected, undermining future collaboration.

- *Philosophy of intervention.* Attention to role and structure will be of limited effect if there is no shared value base. In a climate of rapid change, attention to values and rationale is easily lost. But neither legislation nor inter-agency procedures can work if they are interpreted differentially by different professional groups according to their own value system.

- *Policies and procedures.* Once underlying principles are established, inter-agency procedures are essential, which should complement internal agency policies. Role clarity is a prerequisite to effective inter-agency working. Staff must know both what is expected by their own agency in terms of working with other agencies, as well as what they can expect from other agencies. Accountabilities must be unambiguous, so that inter-agency procedures need to be clear, credible, congruent, resourced, monitored and owned at a senior inter-agency level.

- *Training.* Inter-agency training is potentially one of the most powerful catalysts for co-ordination. But to be effective, it needs to be owned by management, and located within a explicit framework, such as this, of inter-agency goals, structures, values and policies.

- *Service provision.* The aim of co-ordination is to improve and expand the range of services. However, this requires shared assessments of need, and prioritisation of services to be delivered on an inter-agency basis.

- *Supervision.* Inadequate supervision results in role confusion, which becomes highly problematic in an inter-agency context. Deficits in supervision have also been a persistent theme in child protection and mental health inquiries. While the concept of supervision is mainly associated with the social work profession, all those involved in social care would recognise the need for structured opportunities to reflect on practice, judgements, feelings, roles and the experience of working together.

- *Quality assurance/monitoring.* Clear standards and quality assurance processes for inter-agency work are required. This should include the provision of management information that can monitor service demands, provision, costs and outcomes in order to see whether co-ordination really is benefiting service users. There is also a need for conflict resolution processes for inter-agency working when it becomes badly entrenched in territorialism.

● *Staff care*. If collaboration is in part designed to share anxiety, then it follows that staff care should be a proper concern not just at an individual agency level, but also at an inter-agency level. This means far more than the provision of staff counselling. It starts from the premise that managers need to provide the sort of comprehensive infrastructure for inter-agency practice described here. Staff care exists when organisations working together attend to their staff's needs for identity, mutual respect, competence, role clarity, development and belonging. Without this working together may regress to a mechanical process of following procedures, rather than developing a truly co-ordinated service driven by a shared commitment to meet the user's needs.

Inter-agency training: definitions

To explore inter-agency training, we need to return to the question of definition, as commissioners, trainers and participants can each mean very different activities when using this term, thereby compounding a process that is already complex enough. Clarke (1993: 220) distinguishes between the following terms in his typology of multi-disciplinary education. Modifying Clarke's work slightly it is possible to define four key terms:

1   *Uni disciplinary training* is targeted at members of the same discipline or profession. This forms the basis of the conventional approaches to professional qualification and is reflected in academic departments that emphasise the mastery of a specific body of knowledge and skill, and socialisation into appropriate professional norms and expectations
2   *Multi-disciplinary training* brings individuals from different disciplines together to understand a particular problem or experience – for instance, the process of ageing. This affords different perspectives on the issue, physical, psychological, sociological and so on. This can be achieved through classroom activities and does not require work-based collaborative experiences. Clarke describes this type of learning as 'parallel play' because the work norm tends to be a non-interactive and non-intersecting activity, or occasionally intersecting at best. Hallett and Birchall's (1992b) research on child protection activity showed how few services were truly interdisciplinary; for example, different disciplines working together as a team, assessing, planning and delivering services jointly. Rather,

Hallett and Birchall found that different disciplines came together largely when required to exchange information or plan future work.

3   *Inter-professional training* is the level at which real integration of perspectives occur, so that modifications in one discipline take place in the light of the contributions of the other disciplines. The hallmark is a level of cognitive and behavioural change. Thus members acquire a deep understanding – a 'cognitive map' – of the other disciplines: their value base, ethical dilemmas, concepts, problem definitions, modes of inquiry, types of observation and explanation. At a behavioural level this is translated into collaborative skills and behaviours, in which members can carry out their own role while working closely with other disciplines, and using that experience, refine their own practice. An example might be team building within a primary health care team. Clearly, such inter-professional outcomes cannot be achieved solely through training courses. Those who learn together need to work closely and regularly together in order to achieve learning outcomes at the inter-professional level. This is an important distinction from multi-disciplinary training, where those who learn together may only work together infrequently, and even then, not necessarily in a face-to-face mode with service users.

4   *Inter-agency training* targets participating agencies/services as a whole learning system, as opposed to selected individuals. Its aim is to ensure that all members of the relevant agencies are trained together, from senior managers to practitioners, with the aims of improving co-ordination not only at the practice level, but also at the strategic, policy and service development levels. Thus one of the critical differences between this and multi-disciplinary or inter-professional training would be the involvement of senior managers as well as practitioners, and the close linkage between inter-agency training, policy and service development work. The outcome of inter-agency training should thus be an improved inter-organisational response to the problem. An example might be shared training, not necessarily all at the same time, involving strategic and operational managers as well as practitioners from police, social services, housing and voluntary sector agencies to improve awareness and co-ordination in the management of domestic violence.

Building on these definitions, and the earlier distinction between inter-agency and multi-disciplinary, it is possible to create a development matrix as shown in Figure 4.2. On the horizontal axis, there is a continuum from strategic to responsive training. 'Strategic' refers to training based on an analysis of training needs, planned within an overall training strategy, and evaluated not only on learning outcomes, but also on implications for policies and services. In contrast, 'responsive' means training that at best is responsive to fairly immediate needs, but which more often can be a knee-jerk reaction, or simply bowing reactively to demands. It is not part of an overall strategy, and has no real linkage with management processes, policy or service development planning. The matrix can be used either to analyse either a specific training activity, or undertake a broader strategic overview of training provision. The matrix positions indicated by the numbers describe different types of training activities, which in turn generate different learning outcomes.

To illustrate the way the matrix can be used, each of the four matrix positions will be examined.

1   *Strategic inter-agency training.* This would indicate a carefully planned and evaluated inter-organisational development programme. An example might be the management of Munchausen Syndrome by Proxy, involving staff from senior managers to practitioners. Such training could involve the following groups: a paediatric ward, relevant managers, consultants, doctors, paramedics and nurses; community nursing, local SSD children's services; police; teachers; and legal advisers. Although they might not all attend together, the aim would be for them all to have been

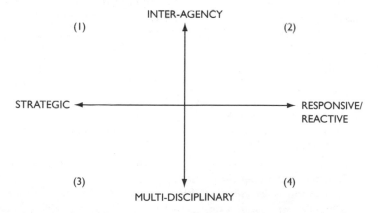

Figure 4.2 Development matrix

involved in a planned programme of inter-agency training. The aim would be to improve inter-agency policies, relations and practices throughout the agencies involved (Horwath and Lawson 1996).

2   *Reactive inter-agency training.* This can often be triggered after a local inter-agency crisis, or failure leading to an inquiry and public exposure. The most obvious examples occur following the death of a child who was on a child protection register. Such blanket training for all staff is usually ordered by senior managers from the agencies involved, and invariably targeted primarily at front-line staff, and seen as a highly visible, fast and achievable means of 'putting their house in order'. Unfortunately, there are real dangers that such training can be used as a 'quick fix' in place of examining contentious inter-agency issues, and to avoid looking upwards at the role of more senior managers.

3   *Strategic multi-disciplinary training.* Here, although the target group is still individuals from different disciplines, training needs have been carefully assessed in relation to service development and policy needs. There is therefore a much stronger linkage between training and management, and a specific emphasis on achieving clear and measurable outcomes that relate to service development. Thus this type of training may be closer to the inter-professional level described by Clarke (1993). An example of this might be the ENB/CCETSW joint training for nurses and social workers working with people with learning disabilities. An important factor as to the degree to which such training has a strategic focus is how far participants share a working context in terms of service delivery in a specified geographical area. If they do, then, although the participants are primarily practitioners, there can be strong links back into inter-agency management processes, perhaps through an inter-agency management board that sponsors and oversees the training. However, the more disparate the learner group – for instance, if they are drawn from a wide geographical area, and have no opportunities for shared working – the harder it becomes to maintain any real links back into the agency and inter-agency systems in which they each work.

4   *Responsive training.* An example of this might be a programme attracting individuals from different disciplinary settings, where the learning objectives have been generated either by the participants as 'wants', or in response to specific local and fairly immediate needs, demands or crises. There is little attempt to target specific

learner groups, as a result of which their composition may be very diverse, and where the connection between group members, or their agencies, are non-existent. A regional conference organised by a group of interested individuals would be an example: while serving some networking and knowledge dissemination needs, it can have little strategic or collaborative impact.

It is very important that the individual parts of this matrix should not be seen in isolation, as all the activities described above have a valid place within a spectrum of inter-agency training responses. However, a training programme in which all programmes fall within just one part of the matrix, in whichever quadrant, is unbalanced. What is crucial is how and why the training is commissioned, and that there is management ownership by the agencies involved of whatever shared training is being undertaken. We turn now to explore some of the opportunities that are presented for inter-agency training by the current context of social care work.

DEVELOPMENT OF INTER-AGENCY TRAINING

Whatever the strains upon inter-agency collaboration, the emphasis being given to inter-agency training has undoubtedly been growing in recent years, both from government guidance and from professional bodies (UKCC 1986; CCETSW 1991). The ENB/CCETSW good practice guide to shared learning states that a 'climate now exists which facilitates the development of shared learning and joint education initiatives in a more comprehensive and strategic manner' (ENB/CCETSW 1995: 1). Government funding for inter-agency training to support both community care and child protection work has been increased, through the Training Support Grant formula.

Another powerful stimulus to inter-agency training has stemmed from the development of inter-agency competences under the NVQ/ SVQ systems. Whatever the unresolved questions about NVQs, as discussed in Chapter 2, there is no doubt that the competency, as opposed to the discipline/professional-specific approach, has considerable advantages for inter-agency training. Hevey comments that the Care Sector Consortium's Integration Project has

created for the first time a generic qualification structure for all workers at the sub-professional level (NVQ levels 2 and 3) in the health and social care fields. . . . The new integrated structure provides the basis for the emergence of a truly integrated, inter-agency occupational group which can work across a wide variety of settings.

(Hevey 1992: 216–17)

He concludes that the NVQ and SVQ systems 'hold out the promise of a common inter-agency basis of competence which will enhance inter-professional working and encourage the emergence of new forms of inter-agency training' (1992: 220).

Other positive developments include the establishment of CAIPE, Centre for the Advancement of Interprofessional Education in Health and Community Care, the *Journal of Interprofessional Care*, and PIAT: Promoting Inter-Agency Training.

However the extent, focus and quality of inter-agency training remains extremely hard to quantify. For instance in 1996 CAIPE pub-lished the results of the first national survey of what was described as 'inter-professional' education and training in community-based health and social in the UK (Barr and Waterton 1996). A total of 455 valid initiatives were reported in which two or more disciplines came together for shared training. However, given that there was only a 20 per-cent response to the questionnaire, any generalisation from these results should be treated with caution. It is almost certainly the case therefore that the true extent and growth of inter-agency training in the UK remains uncharted.

Glennie, reflecting on the rapid growth of inter-agency training since the early 1980s, observes that it has gone through three stages:

1   1980s – asking the questions: what is inter-agency training, what are the expectations, what structures and processes should underpin it?
2   Early 1990s – acts of faith or believing before knowing: emergence of frameworks, objectives, models for inter-agency training, both in community care and children's services.
3   Mid-1990s – consolidation and sophistication: proliferation of training technologies, increased credibility, first standards estab-lished, emergence of networks amongst trainers.

(Glennie 1996)

Obviously there remains extensive variation in the sophistication of inter-agency training, and in some fields of practice people are only beginning to ask the question: should we train together? In many areas inter-agency management and support structures are still embryonic.

For Glennie (1996), the fourth and next stage will concern the capacity of inter-agency training to accept the challenge of further political and structural change without losing some of the expertise that has been developed.

Potential benefits of inter-agency training

Much is claimed on behalf of inter-agency training, so much that at times it is discussed as if it is the universal panacea. However, the danger is that it becomes overloaded with expectations, despite the fact that in terms of outcome research, many of the actual benefits have yet to be demonstrated. Glennie's (1996) phrase that we commit many acts of faith in this field of training is very apt.

The ENB/CCETSW shared practice learning guide lists a wide range of potential outcomes, both for professionals and service users from inter-agency training. They include:

● increasing understanding of, and skills to work in, inter-agency teams;
● providing an understanding of, and context for, the roles, cultures and values of different professions;
● addressing the perceptions, stereotypes and 'professional protectionism' that impede inter-professional work;
● developing a common language between health, social care, education and criminal justice professionals which is also easier for service users to understand;
● facilitating the delivery of a more co-ordinated service to users;
● ensuring a more comprehensive knowledge of current practice, research and theoretical developments;
● facilitating a more effective response to government policy and local needs/user groups via the development of local policies and inter-agency services;
● generating a shared learning culture to foster reflection, analysis and evaluation by focusing on interactive learning.

(ENB/CCETSW 1995)

The big question then is, how much is actually achieved? Certainly staff, with occasional exceptions, perceive such training as very important, and identify a need for more shared learning opportunities.

Inter-agency training at a local level provides a vital opportunity to find out who is in the network, clarify mutual roles and begin to forge personal links. Subjectively, then, staff report considerable benefits. However, many gaps in access to inter-agency training remain. For instance, Hallett and Birchall (1992b) found that 41 per cent of a sample of staff involved in child protection had had no post-qualifying inter-agency training, with the proportion in some groups being much higher – for example, class teachers at 80 per cent. Burton (1996), in her study of GPs' involvement in inter-agency child protection training in Essex, found both resistance and poor rates of attendance. The SSI Inspection of Training (1996a) noted variable successes across the board with inter-agency training, with more progress in mental health and children's services than in community care, where some of the initial momentum was reported to have been lost.

Unfortunately, only a very limited number of longer-term evaluations of inter-agency training have been published. A number of commentators (Goble 1994; Clarke 1993; Leathard 1994; Baldwin 1996) have observed that there is a lack of clear evaluative frameworks. One of the more robust studies, by Shaw (1994), followed up health and social care participants who had completed an extended course on learning disabilities. Unfortunately, he found that the short-term knowledge gains made had not been retained after five months. This was attributed to the lack of organisational and management support for inter-agency training. Thus gains were not maintained in practice once the support of the course structure had been removed, a feature which has been noted following some joint police–social worker training on the Memorandum of Good Practice.

The CAIPE survey of UK inter-professional training found that, while 90 per cent of the 455 programmes reported had been evaluated, the evaluation's focus was mainly on participant satisfaction, learner knowledge and course process (Barr and Waterton 1996). Half of the programmes longer than two days offered learning credits towards qualifications or awards. However, only 61 of the 455 programmes reported that attempts had been made to evaluate observed impact on collaborative practice. Overall, only a quarter of the total evaluations had been written up, and far fewer published. The result is that tangible evidence of longer-term impact from inter-agency training is very difficult to obtain.

A growing investment in inter-agency training is being made, with little hard evidence about the nature and processes through which its potential benefits might be achieved. We know far more about the negative consequences of the lack of inter-agency training than the precise means by which its positive potential can be achieved. Nevertheless the absence of empirical proof of its effectiveness does not mean that it does not exist, but rather that more time and resources are required to research this as yet relatively young area of training and development. An analogy might be drawn with aspirin, which millions of people were taking long before its clinical efficacy was demonstrated. Finding methods to evaluate the complexity and variables involved in such training is one of its most urgent challenges, and is considered further in Chapter 11.

BARRIERS TO INTER-AGENCY TRAINING

The few studies that have been undertaken point to substantial complexities and barriers that must be addressed if inter-agency training is to be effective in the longer term. These barriers can be divided into three groups: structural, professional and psychological. In each, it will become quickly apparent that the issues arising in inter-agency training are but a mirror, and sometimes an intensification, of the very same processes occurring between disciplines and agencies in their day-to day attempts to collaborate with each other over practice.

Structural barriers

At the outset of professional training, the separate discipline and departmental structures in higher education serve to socialise new professionals within a non-collaborative teaching environment. In Burton's study it was found that GPs reported that they had had little or no experience of working in a collaborative way with other professionals during their undergraduate or postgraduate training (Burton 1996). Tempkin-Greener, writing about teamwork within the health services, considered that the professional school and the structure of health service organisation lay at the heart of inter-professional struggles (1983). Baldwin noted a number of structural barriers in higher education settings:

- limitations on the amount and timing of multi-disciplinary training in the curriculum which do not provide the necessary continuity of learning;
- insular certification and accreditation arrangements;

- traditional linear models of professional education;
- lack of multi-disciplinary clinical role models in teaching staff;
- administrative resistance to new ways of organising education;
- difficulties in matching academic schedules and student levels;
- initial expense of new programmes.

(Baldwin 1996: 182)

CAIPE concluded that it was not clear who has responsibility for developing or funding inter-professional education across service areas, and that responsibility for it was being pushed down to too low a level (Horder 1993). As a result of this fragmentary approach to post-qualifying inter-professional training, sufficient critical mass to enable such training to become truly influential has not been achieved. Margrab (1997), conducting an international review of policies for inter-agency training for children and youth at risk, concluded that there was a lack of national policies promoting such training, and that therefore the training was idiosyncratic, locally based and lacking in standardisation.

These factors, together with organisational changes and different training structures across agencies, all conspire to place considerable practical obstacles in the way of in-service inter-agency training. These include:

- finding a mutually suitable venue and time;
- obtaining funding;
- getting service managers to attend;
- recruiting sufficient students;
- obtaining supply cover while staff are on training;
- obtaining an even mix of disciplines;
- identifying suitable placements and appropriate supervisors;
- ensuring compatible levels of knowledge.

Professional barriers

Definitional confusions arising from the different languages used to describe both inter-agency working and training abound. These reflect the wide range of meanings, activities and outcomes that may be attributed to inter-agency training, explored earlier. The consequences of this are that in setting up inter-agency training, different professionals will bring a very wide spectrum of expectations. The lack of research on outcomes means that we lack a precise understanding about how inter-agency training affects changes in values, knowledge and skills, and how these in turn have a sustained impact on collaborative practice. Clarke, commenting on the field of gerontology, concludes:

> if we are serious about developing multi- or interdisciplinary experiences we must become much more sophisticated about precisely what kind of integrative understanding we want to achieve, how it will be attained, and the implications for how we train health professionals in general.

> (1993: 218)

The lack of national co-ordination between professional and academic bodies (Horder 1993) in creating shared values, practice standards and competences for inter-agency work is a major obstacle. An encouraging development, which may point the way for other areas of practice, has been the publication by PIAT (Hendry and Glennie 1996) of standards for inter-agency training in child protection work. This occurred as a 'bottom-up' initiative when inter-agency trainers from around the country came together to produce these standards. However, there is a limit as to how far such ground-level initiatives can go without a national framework of multi-disciplinary competences, integrating academic, vocational and professional criteria.

Psychological barriers

In Chapter 1 reference was made to the impact of rapid change and professional insecurity on levels of anxiety both individually and institutionally. Vince and Martin's (1993) models of Functional and Dysfunctional Learning Cycles were used to describe the consequences for training. However, in an inter-agency setting these anxieties can quickly become intensified. In part this is due to the natural cautiousness that occurs simply as a result of coming away from one's professional enclave, where culture, roles and rules are clear, into a forum in which other disciplines may be dominant, or where the trainer may not be from one's own discipline. On top of this there may be other factors.

Organisational changes and perceived threats to professional identity mean that learners can be preoccupied with their own survival, and have little emotional capacity or willingness to engage in collaborative activity. Power, status, gender and knowledge differentials can interact powerfully to raise anxiety and generate defensive behaviours. Differences in values, understandings about the nature and origins of power relations, and commitment to anti-oppressive principles underpin many of the tensions that arise in inter-agency training. Additionally, there can be heavy displacement onto the training course and the trainers of negative experiences arising from previous collaborative encounters, or from current, unresolved issues. This can be heightened where the focus is on the management of risk, such as the management of dangerous and mentally disordered offenders, or abuse of the elderly. The emotiveness and impact of the subject material, combined with the fears and fantasies about getting it 'wrong', can lead to denial and projection of responsibility, blaming, dependency behaviours, and negative stereotyping of other agencies. Unfortunately, inter-agency training may be one of the only opportunities different disciplines have to process their day-to-day difficulties. Thus while such processes can become fruitful sources of learning, they demand a high level of skills and organisational awareness from trainers, which if not handled effectively, can lead to training programmes losing their focus and occasionally being totally derailed.

ISSUES FOR INTER-AGENCY TRAINERS

It is hardly surprising in the light of all these issues that there is an insufficient supply of experienced inter-agency trainers. Although there are a growing number of specific inter-agency training posts, particularly in the child protection field, the majority of inter-agency training is undertaken by single-discipline trainers who are simply expected to bolt this training onto their existing workload. As a result, the time and resources for them to develop expertise in inter-agency training is severely limited. At present, with the exception of CAIPE and PIAT, development and networking structures for such trainers are few and far between. Trainers are simply expected to pick up the additional skills, sometimes without a full appreciation of the different skills required.

Inter-agency trainers in this area are faced with an array of additional factors and demands. They bear a double burden, to address both practice-specific knowledge and skills elements, as well as to facilitate collaborative working. In doing so, inter-agency trainers encounter participants who have been socialised into radically different training traditions, ranging from 'chalk and talk' to T-groups. The specific issues facing inter-agency trainers fall into six main areas, all of which, although familiar to single-discipline trainers, take on additional complexity in inter-agency contexts. These concern problems about:

- mandate and accountability;
- role expectancy;
- strategy;
- values and anti-discriminatory principles;
- delivery;
- evaluation;
- transfer of learning;
- support and supervision.

Mandate

Even for trainers employed specifically to undertake inter-agency training, job description, accountability, funding and supervisory arrangements are frequently complex and often confused. For instance, whereas funding for such posts may be drawn from a range of agencies, administration may be based in one agency, while reporting requirements may be split between the line manager within that agency and other agencies. Job descriptions are often unspecified, with few performance measurement standards. Appraisal and performance review processes can also be weak, and in practice left to a line manager within one agency, who may feel ill equipped to manage such work. Maintaining clear communication with all the funding agencies can be difficult as personnel and structures change. Finally, confusion about the trainer's mandate and accountability makes the management of any complaints about the inter-agency trainer very difficult.

Role expectancies

A central question for inter-agency trainers is how to define and clarify their role. Poor job descriptions and the uniqueness of such posts combine with conflicting and excessive expectations as to what a single trainer can achieve, to make it very difficult to clarify the role. Inter-agency training can too often be seen as a panacea for a range of problems only some of which can be solved through training. These can include gaps in inter-agency policies, services, structures, staffing or uni-disciplinary training, none of which inter-agency training can resolve. There may also be unspecified and irrational expectations that inter-agency training will, for instance, resolve conflict between agencies, or manage unspoken anxieties that each agency may have about areas of practice, or ensure that inter-agency procedures are complied with! Thus the trainer may be faced with knowledge about dangerous practice and be unclear what their responsibilities are, who should be notified and how another agency or discipline might respond. One example of how difficult this situation can be occurred following a social worker and police training course when the inter-agency trainers expressed concern about the behaviour of one police participant which, it was suggested, might have originated in personal difficulties. The response from the senior officer was that the participant would be withdrawn forthwith.

Strategy

As Chapter 3 has already indicated, undertaking a training needs analysis and formulating a training strategy is hard enough within agencies, but as an inter-agency exercise it represents a major challenge. There are potentially vast numbers of staff, in different agencies, each of which have totally different structures for identifying training needs and organising training delivery. The result is that commissioning such an analysis consumes considerable time and resources, and can end up raising expectations about inter-agency training to a yet more unrealistic level. This is compounded by the fact that many professionals will inappropriately look to inter-agency training programmes to meet training needs that have not been addressed within their own agency. Inter-agency training strategies must guard against this, by insisting that inter-agency programmes run in parallel with, not instead of, uni-disciplinary training. Nevertheless, an inter-agency training strategy is vital, if management ownership is to be achieved, and to ensure that the programme works to clear policy and service development objectives agreed by the constituent agencies, which are intended to develop inter-agency working practice. The development of an inter-agency strategy is also essential to ensure that the programme is not perceived as a social services programme.

Delivery

While inter-agency trainers provide an immense boost to the visibility and range of training, it is important that delivery is shared by trainers representing the different disciplines. Not only is this required to ensure that discipline-specific knowledge is included, but also because it acts as a powerful model of co-ordination in action. Moreover, the sheer weight of demand makes the use of a pool approach necessary. The inter-agency trainer cannot be an expert across such a wide group of disciplines and subject areas. Therefore, in addition to delivering some training, a very significant part of her role must be to act as a facilitator in bringing other expertise into the training programme. However, this requires careful preparation and training of a wider group of staff from different agencies to deliver these programmes. In a number of areas this has been facilitated successfully through the establishment, and training, of a pool of trainers who service the inter-agency training programme. However, for a pool to work effectively, there is also the need to establish clear standards for inter-agency training; for instance, drawing on work such as that done by PIAT (Hendry and Glennie 1996). Standards are important if levels of trainer competence are to be established and assessed, so that eventually inter-agency trainers are properly accredited. Thus, far from inter-agency training being a quick way of targeting a wide range of professionals, the process of design and delivery is usually more time consuming. The absence of inter-professional frameworks of competence, values, knowledge and skills makes the design stage doubly demanding, as different trainers seek to reach consensus about the programme.

Values and anti-discriminatory practice

One of the most difficult aspects is how values and anti oppressive issues should be addressed, as disciplines and agencies are at very different points on this. Some agencies may have equal opportunities policies whereas others have anti-oppressive policies. In general, social work based agencies will have a more detailed and challenging approach. However, given that power and status differentials are extremely significant in how different professionals work, or fail to work, together, and considering the subsequent impact on service users, this is a central area. Inter agency training is, however, likely to be one of the first opportunities that different disciplines have had to address these issues together for the first time. As a result, the trainer can anticipate a degree of apprehension about this area, not just within the participants, but also among trainers from different disciplines working together. What is vital is that time is given to developing a clear statement of what anti-discriminatory practice means in the context of inter-agency training, and that this is worked out, not just by the inter-agency trainer alone, but with commissioning managers and inter-agency training committees. These should address the practical expression of anti-discriminatory principles, such as:

- ensuring openness of recruitment and equality of access to training;
- training being delivered by a multi-agency training team;
- attending to individuals' needs – for instance, diet and timing;
- establishing learning agreements that value difference and challenge stereotypes;
- explicit inclusion of anti-discriminatory content on courses;
- focusing on needs of service users in training;
- inclusion of users' views and experiences in content of training;
- addressing the sources and impact of professional's power on users;
- seeking to involve users in planning, delivery or evaluation of training.

Evaluation

For the reasons discussed earlier, evaluation of outcomes in this area of training is extremely difficult. Methods and resources to do so are woefully under-developed. Thus in trying to measure the success of a training strategy, or even of a single inter-agency course, there are large hurdles. Once again, it is totally unrealistic to expect this to happen if some of the mechanisms (described in Chapter 11) for evaluating outcomes within individual agency's own training programmes are not present.

Learning transfer

The absence of supervisory systems in some disciplines and a lack of management ownership of inter-agency programmes can also leave the trainer feeling immense responsibility for ensuring that the learning is translated into practice. The reality is that the prospects for successful transfer depend largely on factors beyond the inter-agency trainer's control. These include inter-agency policies; how far services are based on single or multi-disciplinary delivery structures; and the quality of inter-agency working relationships. Undoubtedly, increased transfer occurs if participants who work together learn together, and the inter-agency training acts to forge positive relationships between local professionals who discover through exploration of roles, services and skills what they can offer each other.

Support and supervision

For many trainers inter-agency training is an exciting and stimulating challenge. However, their often ill-defined role, combined with the inadequacy of supervisory and support systems, can lead to immobilisation and isolation. The basics of having an office, administrative support and appropriate letterheads – for example, not using stationery representing a single agency – can often be a problem. This can lead to the trainer feeling as if her role, identity and contribution are unrecognised. Often the post is a new one, and while there is considerable freedom to develop the role, no groundwork has been done, so it can be daunting simply to know where to start. Supervision may be provided by a senior trainer within one agency, who may or may not have a real appreciation of the challenges facing the inter-agency trainer, or who may want to poach some of the inter-agency trainer's time and resources for their own agency's training. Experienced supervisors and mentors for inter-agency trainers are not in plentiful supply.

FRAMEWORKS FOR EFFECTIVE INTER-AGENCY TRAINING

It is plain from the above that a precise and reliable map to guide those involved in inter-agency training is not as yet available. However, much has been learnt about those factors that are likely to facilitate effective inter-agency training, and these are now presented in this final section. This does not seek to specify how any particular inter-agency training session should be run, but rather to offer a framework, not just for identified 'inter-agency trainers' but to all involved in inter-agency training, as to what ingredients are essential in maximising the potential benefits of this type of training.

Whatever the quality of inter-agency training, it is important to recall the message at the start of this chapter, about the critical need for an effective inter-agency management structure. Inter-agency training can only be fully effective if it is embedded within the inter-agency framework described in Figure 4.3, which ensures that there are shared structures, policies, goals, planning processes, standards, values and quality assurance processes underpinning inter-agency working.

8 Evaluation and feedback to inter-agency management group
7 Transfer and reinforcement of inter-agency training
6 Skilled and safe facilitation
5 Planning of inter-agency training
4 Inter-agency training values, principles and standards
3 Inter-agency training strategy
2 Inter-agency training needs analysis
1 Inter-agency training management group

Figure 4.3 Framework for inter-agency training

Inter-agency training management group

The establishment of this group is the single most essential feature if there is to be a real integration between inter-agency management and training processes. For this to work the inter-agency training group, whose role is to take overall responsibility for the management of an inter-agency training programme, needs to have clear terms of reference and a mandate from the constituent agencies. The membership should involve representatives from all the main stakeholders, including commissioners, service managers, trainers and service users (where possible and appropriate), so that members can feed back to their respective agencies at a senior level. Inter-agency training frequently highlights not only further training needs, but significant intra and inter-agency management issues as well. Thus training group members should be those who have been given clear responsibility within their own agency/ discipline for the development of inter-agency training, in addition to any role they may have for uni-disciplinary training. Although this does not imply that all members should have experience of delivering inter-agency training, it should mean that they are able to:

● speak for their agency/discipline on inter-agency training matters;
● have a commitment to, and understanding of, inter-agency training;
● undertake a training needs analysis within their agency/discipline;
● obtain workforce information such as numbers of staff, disciplines, previous training, competency levels;
● identify current training requirements at national and local levels within the agency/discipline;
● identify potential trainers/contributors to the inter-agency training programme;
● negotiate time and resources to support, train and evaluate those contributing to the inter-agency training programme;

● undertake/commission an evaluation within their agency/discipline of the outcomes of inter-agency training.

   A further important role for the training management group is to support and work with specialist inter-agency trainers, acting as an inter-agency reference and management group to facilitate their work. At a practical level there are also some key logistical areas for the group to address, which, like the previous list, cannot simply be left to an inter-agency trainer even where one exists. These include:

● obtaining shared funding and identifying an inter-agency training budget;
● exploring the potential appointment of a full-time inter-agency trainer (if one does not exist);
● arranging administrative resources for the planning, publicising and organisation of training;
● negotiating work release and developmental support for those delivering inter-agency training;
● negotiating work release time to ensure full attendance of participants,
● timing the course to facilitate the members' attendance;
● identifying appropriate training venues; e.g., not located in a single agency;
● determining a charging policy for training.

Inter-agency training needs analysis

It will be clear from the above that, even where an inter-agency trainer exists, it is neither appropriate nor realistic for this to be undertaken by a single trainer. The framework for an inter-agency training needs analysis depends on each agency having its own internal training needs analysis system through which the training needs of different parts of, or disciplines within, the workforce are identified. The elements of such a framework were described in detail in Chapter 3. Through each agency's training needs analysis system, both single and inter-agency training needs should be identified. By doing this in tandem, it should be possible to ensure that inter-agency training programmes can avoid picking up responsibility for uni-disciplinary training needs. It should also provide the opportunity within each agency for their service users to be consulted. Rather, inter-agency training needs should be based on the requirements and standards of inter-agency working specified in inter-agency protocols, or procedures, and in specifications for inter-agency service delivery. The above represents the ideal, and it should be acknowledged that inter-agency training needs analysis will remain one of the most challenging areas. Systems for training needs analysis within different agencies vary greatly, and priorities for inter-agency training can be so easily distorted by changing priorities, structures and problems within each agency.

Inter-agency training strategy

This should flow from the training needs analysis, but it is important to establish a strategy even if significant gaps remain in the needs analysis. It establishes a rationale and benchmark against which inter-agency training programmes can be evaluated. A clear strategy, agreed by the training management group and disseminated throughout the inter-agency network, helps greatly to identify, validate and promote inter-agency training, not only to potential participants but also to senior managers who may have limited awareness of, or sometimes commitment to inter-agency training. It may also be used for wider circulation to service user groups, or local politicians.

The strategy is the basis from which the required budget is worked out, and thus become a basis for negotiation with managers. For the strategy to be persuasive, however, the programme must relate to local service development and inter-agency management priorities. As Druce puts it: 'Even well formulated training will not achieve its aims unless it is internally consistent and externally compatible with organisational context' (Druce, in Weinstein 1994). There is therefore a need for a flexible, bottom-up approach encompassing local needs within broad national and strategic guidelines (ENB/CCETSW 1995). A further strand to any comprehensive strategy will be the need to recruit, develop, support and evaluate a pool of trainers from different agencies and disciplines who will deliver the programme.

Inter-agency training values, principles and standards

Differences in values, especially around anti-discriminatory principles, as well as around standards of practice, present one of the biggest obstacles for inter-agency training, not least because of the paucity of nationally agreed frameworks. Leathard sees inter-agency training as key to the elimination of discrimination in social care, but comments, 'The challenge is . . . how far going inter professional either perpetuates discrimination or to see whether collaborative working can act as a lever to eliminate discrimination in health and social care' (Leathard 1994: 222).

It is vital to allow sufficient time to work these issues through. The training management group's capacity to do this is in itself a model of collaboration that involves a willingness to share power, explore difference and be open in front of other disciplines. If attention is not paid to this by the training management group, individual trainers will be left in a very exposed and difficult position. It is highly unlikely that such work can be done properly without the group, committing themselves to undertaking some additional development work together. The outcomes of this could, for instance, include:

- a statement of rationale, principles and purposes of inter-agency training;
- key values underpinning the inter-agency training programme – for instance, focus on user needs, user involvement, openness about power relations;
- defining what anti-discriminatory practices will mean in terms of training needs assessment, access to training, planning, content and delivery of the programme;
- rights and responsibilities of commissioners, trainers and learners, including how any feedback to individuals or agencies would be given.

If the members of the training pool have not been included in this important exercise, it would be necessary for them to be involved in working through and taking ownership of these standards before being expected to deliver training programmes.

Planning of inter-agency training

As we saw earlier, the list of potential benefits from inter-agency training is very wide, and for that very reason learning objectives and outcomes should be carefully specified. Much will depend on the level of joint working that is actually required in practice and at which agencies are actually involved. For instance, the learning objectives for multi-disciplinary working might be significantly different than for inter-professional or inter-agency working (see Figure 4.2). Thus the selection of learning objectives should match the collaborative task level. The participants need to be recruited carefully so that the right disciplines are present, and properly represented. Nevertheless, experience suggests that there are some common objectives that inter-agency training should seek to achieve, including the following:

● reaching a shared understanding of the overall purpose of the service;
● clarifying roles;
● identifying each agency's values;
● identifying common and complementary knowledge and skills;
● providing a core common knowledge base for a specific service area;
● explaining relevant policies and clarifying mutual responsibilities;
● sharing experiences of working together and identifying strengths, constraints and weaknesses;
● generating strategies for improved communication;
● stimulating the capacity for managing and making the most of differences;
● promoting shared learning around real practice problems.

It can be seen from this list that there are strong arguments in favour of starting with senior managers, who need to be clear on issues such as role, values and purposes of shared working. Although senior managers may not require detailed training about day-to-day practice in order to manage an inter-agency process well, they do need to understand the business they are engaged in sufficiently.

What is also necessary is to maintain the right balance between attention to task (delivery of services) and process (how agencies work together). An exclusive focus on task may prevent members from exploring process issues, and thereby deny the underlying feelings, anxieties and value differences that affect collaborative work. Conversely, an over-focus on process may leave members with a lack of basic task clarity, and an overly inter-personally focused understanding of complex inter-agency processes. Finally, there are significant advantages in recruiting course members from local networks of professionals so that those who are working together can learn together. This considerably enhances the potential for transfer of learning into daily collaborative practice, and for using training to facilitate problem solving on shared issues.

Skilled and safe facilitation of inter-agency training

As the management of group learning processes is presented in detail in Chapters 6 to 9, this discussion will be confined to some overview points. In Chapter 2, Kolb's Experiential Learning Model was described. This can be extended to conceptualise the process of inter-agency training (see Figure 4.4).

Applying Kolb's model in this way shows how inter-agency training provides the opportunity, which the rush of operational life does not permit, to reflect on the myriad daily experiences of collaborative effort. Without the opportunity to step back together and reflect on these collaborative experiences, we too often fail to identify and make use of good examples of collaboration, or to resolve and learn from negative ones. It is this shared reflection, analysis, problem solving and planning away from operational situations which makes inter-agency training such a valuable action learning tool.

However, unless a secure training environment, which is safe enough to contain anxiety, difference and potential conflict, can be established, groups will not feel confident to reflect on real practice problems. Indeed there can even be a danger that harmful stereotypes and dysfunctional processes between disciplines will simply be re-enacted. A safe structure is created when the trainers are perceived to carry sufficient authority and sensitivity to demonstrate that no single discipline will dominate, and that everyone's perceptions, difficulties

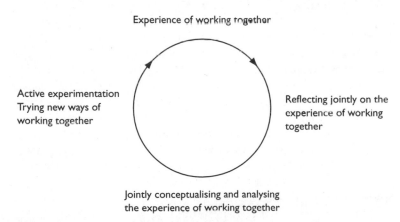

Experience of working together

Active experimentation
Trying new ways of
working together

Reflecting jointly on the
experience of working
together

Jointly conceptualising and analysing
the experience of working together

Figure 4.4 Process of inter-agency development
Source: McFarlane and Morrison (1994)

and contributions will be valued. Careful use of language is required, with a visible understanding of different agencies, so that trainers are not seen to impose their own discipline's culture and jargon on others. This enables the trainer to retain a 'discipline neutral' and facilitative role in the group.

This is done most effectively, and the programme enriched considerably, where the training is delivered by a inter-agency trainer group, as long as the co-trainers are providing a positive model of how they work together. (Chapter 7 discusses co-training in detail.) An inter-agency training team enables each discipline to identify with one trainer, and should ensure that the knowledge base and case material are inclusive of all the agencies represented.

One of the most important skills is the ability to draw out difference, conflict and commonality, especially in relation to values, status and power issues. Once again, this cannot be done if the atmosphere is not reasonably secure, and if programmes do not clarify that this will be an objective. Finally in exploring these issues, trainers also need to be able to recognise wider organisational sources of collaborative tension, so that these can be separated from the 'here and now' process in the room.

Transfer and reinforcement of learning

Finally, it is essential that consideration is given as to how the learning can be consolidated in the day-to-day realities and pressures which affect collaborative working. The responsibility for learning transfer can only in part belong to the trainers. Successful transfer, as Chapter 10 discusses, depends on agency support and reinforcement, which should be shared between the learner and their manager. In the context of inter-agency training, however, this responsibility must be extended to the inter-agency management system. In contrast to uni-disciplinary learning, transferring learning gains from inter-agency training – which tends to be in areas such as role clarification, rather than specific skills – is less dependent on individuals and far more dependent on inter-group processes. Inter-agency training frequently throws up policy, practice and communication issues which need to be resolved for collaborative practice to move forward. Hence the importance of the training management group acting as the vehicle for transfer issues to be fed back to inter-agency management forums.

Evaluation

The evaluation of inter-agency training is still at an embryonic stage. It presents more complex challenges than single-discipline training because of the multiple variables in different agencies that can effect outcomes, which are discussed in detail in Chapter 11. However, this does not mean that nothing can be done, but rather that the focus of evaluation may need to be simple and short term, rather then complex and long term. In the context of the training strategy, numbers and discipline representation are important. Thus an analysis by agency and discipline of invitees and attendances should be undertaken, which can reveal gaps in, or resistance to, the training programme. Beyond that, individual follow-up and agency-based evaluations as to the longer-term effects, despite their being subjective, are also worthwhile. Finally, some of the most valuable action learning evaluations can come from programmes targeted on local groups or multi-disciplinary teams who are actually working together, and who are in a position to report how they have translated their learning into action.

SUMMARY

- Concepts of collaboration are ill defined and mean very different things to different disciplines.
- Multi-disciplinary work/training has been defined in terms of individuals from different disciplines working/learning together, in contrast to inter-agency work/training, where agencies work/learn together.
- Clarke's typology was used to distinguish between multi-disciplinary training, in which individuals learn how to co-operate on an occasional basis while essentially working within their discipline, and inter-professional training, where the tasks are shared on a much wider basis, requiring a much deeper level knowledge and experience of collaborative work.
- It was seen how in the present climate, opportunities and barriers to collaborative working and training are finely balanced.
- There is little research to guide trainers on the precise mechanisms through which inter-agency training effects positive changes in collaboration in practice.
- Inter-agency training is still largely driven by local rather than national funding, standards or needs. There is an urgent need to

develop inter-professional competences, and the NVQ/SVQ may assist in this.

● Inter-agency training will be much more effective where it is linked closely into local service development priorities, so that it engages management commitment.

● The facilitation of inter-agency training requires the establishment of a safe climate in which difference, disagreement and common ground can be drawn out and utilised.

CONCLUSION

Inter-agency training cannot be a panacea for deficits of collaborative frameworks or will. Nor can it be the life-raft on which the whole burden of future inter-agency working rests. However, inter-agency training is brimming with potential and promise if we can learn how to use it wisely and effectively.

Chapter 5

Creating an environment for learning

This chapter explores:

- organisational conditions required for adult learning;
- blocks to learning;
- the notion of a 'learning organisation' and a 'learning team';
- the learner as a reflective professional;
- the role of the supervisor in creating an environment for learning;
- creating a learning environment within the training context.

The broad framework of social care training has been explored in previous chapters. In this chapter we begin to look at more specific issues related to training practice, paying particular attention to the interplay between training and the wider organisational framework. This connection becomes most evident when considering factors that contribute to an environment for learning. The following comments must be familiar to many trainers.

'I can't concentrate I had to do a visit after the course last night and I'm really worried about the client.'

'I'm not doing role play. I had a terrible experience on another course.'

'I feel very uncomfortable on this course as there are no other district nurses.'

'This training is all very well but there is no way I've got the time or support to think this through when I'm back at the worksite.'

(Participants in training courses)

These quotations reflect some of the personal, professional and orga-nisational concerns that encroach on learning in the context of social care training. They highlight the impossibility for a trainer of deliver-ing training that leads to learning by focusing merely on course con-tent. The trainer must consider the possible past and present experiences that participants bring with them to the training event and the potential impact of these on learning. To do this the trainer, and managers within the organisation, have to understand how, why and when adults learn and how learning is experienced by the learner (Rogers 1993). This should include organisational and professional factors that impinge on learning as well as personal experiences. These factors have to be identified and, where necessary, addressed to enable an adult to learn. In the training context, then, the aim of creating an organisational climate or environment for learning can be seen as the process of facilitation whereby a member of the workforce becomes a learner. As this book focuses on group learning, we will consider this process in terms of maximising the learning opportunities provided by training courses.

Learning can be perceived by the learner as a threatening and chal-lenging process. Claxton believes that this is the case because learning threatens the four beliefs that individuals tend to hold about themselves. They are:

1   I believe that my personal worth depends on the success of my actions. Therefore I must be competent.
2   I believe that my personal identity depends on being predictable to myself – that I am what I think I am. Therefore I must be con-sistent.
3   I believe that my survival and/or my sanity depends on my being able to understand, explain and predict what is happening in my world at all times. Therefore I must be in control.
4   I believe that it is possible and desirable to go through life without feeling bad – getting upset, anxious or guilty. Therefore I must feel comfortable.

(Claxton 1984: 145)

While a learner's personal and professional experiences can serve to undermine some of these beliefs, Claxton argues that the process of learning itself requires the learner to accept the very antitheses of these beliefs and it is this that makes learning an anxiety-provoking process. This means that:

- learning is what happens when we take the risk of not being competent;
- the learning process can involve the chance of finding out that we are not consistent;
- learning may mean that at times we are out of control;
- the risk of taking on new learning is not always a comfortable feeling.

Within this chapter we explore ways in which a climate for learning needs to exist at an organisational, professional and personal level. This is required in order to enable a learner to take the risk of learning something new and applying this learning to their work practice. We consider some of the factors that are likely to act as blocks to learning and explore the crucial role of the learner themselves, their supervisor and the trainer in terms of managing these blocks and creating a learning environment that promotes functional learning.

CONDITIONS FOR AND BLOCKS TO LEARNING

There is a joke that is heard in many school playgrounds of two men having a conversation.

One man says:
'I taught my dog to whistle.'
The second man replies:
'I don't hear him.'
The first man responds:
'I never said he learnt.'

(Anonymous)

The joke encapsulates one of the common misunderstandings about training: because someone attends a training course it does not mean they will learn. Certain conditions need to exist to enable a training environment to be conducive for learning. Knowles identified conditions that facilitate adult learning, and believed that one of the fundamental elements for engaging learners is setting a climate conducive to adult learning. This should be both physically and psychologically conducive, to ensure that the learner feels 'accepted, respected and supported; in which there exists a spirit of mutuality between teachers and students as joint inquirers; in which there is freedom of expression without fear of punishment or ridicule' (Knowles 1972: 41).

However, a criticism that can be made of Knowles is that he tends to assume that adults have a positive approach towards learning. Yet in Chapter 2 we identified that we do not always respond to experience by learning; we can reject experiences with non-learning responses. Knowles fails to recognise the negative impact of adults' previous learning experiences and the influence that race, gender and culture may have on learning. Consideration needs to be given to these negative experiences, as they can become the blocks and barriers that prevent an adult maximising a learning opportunity such as a training course. There are four types of block:

1   Personal
2   Professional
3   Trainer
4   Organisational.

BLOCKS TO LEARNING

Personal blocks

These can be defined as previous and current personal life experiences that impact negatively on the motivation of the learner. Experiences of difference, especially in terms of power relationships and experiences of authority, may have a negative impact on the development of a positive identity, which in turn can undermine confidence to engage in learning (Brummer and Simmonds 1992). Personal blocks can also be related to negative childhood experiences of education or feelings of worthlessness resulting from deficits or difficulties in early relationships in the family. Current personal experiences also impact on learning. For example, disabilities, physical health, emotional problems or changes in personal situations can all affect a learner's sense of self-esteem, level of confidence and motivation to learn.

Trainers and managers, responsible for facilitating learning, need to be aware that learners may bring with them a range of negative experiences which act as blocks to learning. Jarvis and other educationists (Brookfield 1996; Rogers 1993) identified a number of key conditions required for adult learning. These conditions need to be considered when assessing an individual's learning needs and the organisational context in which learning occurs, so that potential blocks to learning can be identified and addressed. Table 5.1, based on Jarvis's work (1995), identifies the types of past and current personal negative learning and life experiences that may impact on the different learning conditions.

Table 5.1 highlights the range of experiences that can have a negative effect on learning and can become blocks to learning experiences. Unless these are addressed at both an organisational and an individual level, it is unlikely that the learner will be able to engage in functional learning.

Professional blocks

These can be seen as barriers to learning resulting from experiences in professional practice. Social care professions are in a state of continual change, which means that staff are working with uncertainty, unpredictability and conflicting professional expectations. They are continually making professional judgements, on the basis of limited information and resources and frequently cannot achieve the ideal that they believe professionally would meet the needs of service users.

The way that individuals manage these professional dilemmas, especially in the early stages of their professional career, can act as blocks to later learning. Marsh and Triseliotis (1996) studied the professional experiences of newly qualified social workers and noted after a year in practice that they described experiencing an 'increased bureaucratisation of social work'. They found this to be alien to their motives and values and to their qualification training. In this situation the newly qualified worker is likely to feel confusion regarding their role. They may feel they are having to compromise in terms of their professional values and guilty that they have not delivered the appropriate professional service. This can impact on their ability to learn. For example, there may be a reluctance to attend training courses as the training unit is perceived as reflecting organisational rather than professional values.

As practitioners become more experienced, one would anticipate that they would learn to manage professional conflicts. However, Banks (1995) describes how even the most experienced social care practitioners find themselves encountering ethical dilemmas and feelings of guilt about the choices they make. This is often a result of defensive practice, decisions which feel morally wrong or that result in negative outcomes which the worker feels could have been avoided with more time or resources. Within the current social care climate

Table 5.1 Negative experiences that may affect different learning conditions

Conditions of adult learning	Potential sources of learner's negative experiences
Learning is a basic need.	The term 'learning' may have negative connotations.
Learning is especially motivated when there is disharmony between an individual's experience and perception of the world.	A learner may respond adversely to the anxiety associated with learning, as described in Chapter 6. This may be a result of previous experiences of disharmony. Or they may have had their experience of disharmony invalidated or supressed.
Adult learners like to participate in the learning process.	Autocratic cultures and totalitarian regimes enforce a didactic, paternalistic, non-participatory approach to learning which will influence attitudes to learning. Learners may fear the consequences of raising issues or challenging what is taught. They may not trust their own judgements. Individuals who were belittled during participation in previous learning settings may resist participative methods.
Adult learners bring their own experiences, meanings and needs to the learning situation.	These can be negative life and learning experiences; e.g. a black learner who has been confronted with Eurocentric models experiences racism; female learners' experiences of teaching situations dominated by male students; negative reinforcement with comments like 'You are stupid'.
Adult learners bring to the learning situation their own self-confidence, self-esteem, self-perception.	Negative experiences resulting from disability, race, gender, sexuality, class, level of education and literacy will have an impact. Current experiences of feeling devalued or discriminated at work, in relationships, etc., will have an effect.
Adults learn best when the self is not under threat.	Seemingly non-threatening methods of learning may be threatening as a result of previous experiences.

Conditions of adult learning	Potential sources of learner's negative experiences
Adult learners need to feel they are treated as adults.	Learners may have experiences when aspects of their adult identity have been ignored; e.g. their race, gender, disability, sexuality or class. They may have experienced education or training which was competitive, involved humiliating the learner or was delivered in a patronising manner.
Adult learners have developed their own learning styles.	These may not always be the most appropriate styles but a response to negative experiences; e.g. the learner with literacy difficulties who ensures they are never in a situation where they need to read or write.
Adult learners have had different educational biographies so they may learn at different speeds.	A learner who left school at an early age may feel anxious that they take a longer time to read and write than others.
Adults have their own perceptions of their level of intelligence; e.g. they failed the 11-plus therefore they are stupid.	Learners will be influenced by their past experiences. Failure within the education system may be equated with the view that they lack intelligence.
Adults bring different physiological conditions to the learning situation.	Learners often find the process of ageing difficult to manage and become frustrated at a failing memory. Visual and hearing impairments can result in lack of confidence about participating; e.g. will there be a loop system? The use of certain forms of medication will all affect the ability to learn.

other professionals are likely to feel similar tensions between what they consider to be high-quality professional practice and the actual services provided. This has been noted by Appleton (1996) in relation to health visitors. She states that there is a danger of health visitors losing sight of their professional goals and boundaries as they become lured into providing services that are no longer available from other professionals. This can impact on inter-agency training as learners are likely to share feelings of inadequacy and compromise.

These experiences can act as blocks to learning. For example, the learner may avoid training events as they do not want to reinforce their own feelings of guilt about what they should be doing. Scepticism and cynicism may be expressed during training, with a resistance to considering new ideas. Staff who feel that they were responsible for negative outcomes with service users may lack confidence in exploring professional issues in training and can become very defensive.

Trainer blocks

A trainer is as likely to experience blocks to learning at a personal, professional and organisational level as are learners. These can act as barriers to learning for the learning group. For example, a trainer known to us was facilitating a training course on bereavement and loss in old age. The evaluation forms at the end of the course indicated that learners had felt that the focus of the course had centred on knowledge and had ignored values and feelings. It was only after reading these forms that the trainer realised that her own feelings about her partner's impending retirement had impacted on the way she facilitated group learning. She had blocked any discussion on feelings because she could not manage her own feelings of loss.

Effective training should facilitate learning. There are four basic elements of effective training – discrimination, modelling, practice and feedback – according to Cross (as referred to in Heron 1989). The trainer's ability to train effectively will be influenced by their own learning blocks. These in turn will affect learning opportunities for the learning group. The impact of these blocks on learners will be explored, using Cross's four elements:

1 Discrimination
2 Modelling
3 Practice
4 Feedback.

Discrimination

The focus of this chapter is on creating a climate for learning. This requires the trainer to discriminate between different strategies in order to promote learning. This should be before, during and after the training event. Trainer blocks can distort the trainer's perceptions of what learners require in order to learn effectively. For example, if the trainer believes that they survived negative experiences of the education system unscathed, they may have difficulty appreciating the impact that poor educative experiences can have on learners and consequently dismiss learners' anxieties and concerns. This in turn can reinforce the negative experiences for the learner, who, as a consequence, may be reluctant to risk placing themselves in a group learning situation again.

Modelling

A trainer is required to model good training practice that facilitates learning, uses authority appropriately and addresses issues of oppression. This provides learners with a role model to emulate in their own practice with service users. In some situations trainers may model poor practice as a result of their own blocks. For example, a trainer who feels de-skilled and of low status within the organisation may become very controlling in the planning and delivery of training as a way of exerting some power and control. This provides a dysfunctional learning experience and a poor role model for learners.

Practice

Training can be a way in which learners gain new knowledge, values and skills, which can be applied to improve the quality of service provision to users. However, this partly depends on the approach of the trainer. For example, if the trainer disagrees professionally with the content of a training course, they may well provide a very subjective learning experience for learners, discrediting the value of the learning or distorting the content to meet the trainer's own needs, rather than the needs of service users.

Feedback

Feedback and opportunities to reflect critically on practice are required as part of the learning process. The trainer's blocks can impact negatively on this process. For example, a trainer who has difficulty in managing their own personal feelings towards HIV may avoid providing opportunities for learners to reflect on the impact of HIV on practice. This can occur if the trainer is unable to manage their own feelings resulting from such discussions.

The ways in which trainers can block learning are often carried out subconsciously. One of the advantages of co-facilitation, as outlined in Chapter 7, is that the co-trainer may identify the impact on learners of the other trainer's blocks. But this alone is not sufficient. The influence of the trainer on the learning group and their responsibility for creating a climate for learning makes it crucial that trainers, like learners, receive regular supervision. This should provide opportunities to recognise their blocks and identify the impact these can have on learners. The supervisory framework identified to meet learners' developmental needs applies equally to meeting the needs of trainers.

ORGANISATIONAL BLOCKS

These can be seen as the inhibitors to learning resulting from the agency context. Hughes and Pengelly (1995), with reference to social work but of relevance to other social care workers, comment that no training event that focuses on practice can avoid the powerful impact of the organisational context on the workers. They argue that the worker's approach to the whole training process is affected by their experiences within the worksite and in particular by their relationship with their managers and their attitude towards managerial authority.

The range of approaches within organisations towards the use of managerial authority will impact on the learning environment in different ways. In addition, in an organisational climate of limited resources and increased workloads, staff may feel overworked, stressed and consequently too exhausted and demotivated to learn. Pearn *et al.* (1995) consider how these factors – the organisational environment, the relationships between managers and staff and the motivation of the workforce – interact to create different kinds of organisations. They identify three different types of organisational environments that are unconducive to learning:

1   Stagnated
2   Frustrated
3   Frustrating.

The characteristics of these organisations are described below.

A stagnated organisation

In these organisations past experience is relied on for resolving current problems. Decisions are made by senior managers; the workforce is likely to be passive and detached. There is no incentive for individual or staff development.

In this type of organisation the remit of the training unit is largely determined by senior managers. There is little incentive to promote and develop new courses or learning initiatives. Courses are likely to be repeated annually and remain unchanged. Staff attendance on training will be poor, and those attending training courses want affirmation of their current practice and come with an approach, 'It has worked so far, so why change?' The consequence of all these factors is a resistance to change and new learning.

A frustrating organisation

The senior managers fails to recognise the potential to promote and develop the workforce and provide few opportunities for learning. There is a gulf between the management and the front-line workforce.

In these organisations the training unit will have little status and will form alliances with front-line staff rather than managers. There is unlikely to be a strategic approach towards learning, with *ad hoc* courses and localised, practitioner-based learning initiatives. Learners on training courses may be motivated but feel frustrated at their ability to apply their learning to practice. This will be reflected in comments like 'We don't have opportunities to develop these ideas'. Learners may disengage from the learning process and there will be a resistance to transferring learning to practice.

A frustrated organisation

Senior managers take a controlling approach to learning in this kind of organisation. All the right things are being done by senior management to encourage learning but this is done without staff consultation. Consequently the fears and needs of the workforce are rarely recognised. In this type of organisation the training unit is likely to have a stronger alliance with the managers than the workforce. Training becomes paternalistic; it is perceived as something that is done to the workforce on the basis of 'We know what you need'. Innovative initiatives towards learning may be introduced but will be unsuccessful, or effective only at a token level, as the workforce have not been involved in the developments and will feel that their needs are not being met. In a similar vein, training courses may be creative and of a high quality but will feel inappropriate to the participants, with responses like 'Get real, this is ivory tower stuff'.

Learners are likely to be defensive, resisting new learning, or may disengage from the learning process perceiving the learning to be irrelevant. Organisations are unlikely to fall neatly into one category or another and will have components of all three different types of organisation. In addition, perceptions of the organisation will also vary depending on the position in the organisation. For example, the senior management team may well feel that they are creating a positive climate for learning which is not experienced as such by the workforce. All these organisations are likely to offer training to the workforce. However, as can be seen, each type of organisation has features that are likely to block a staff member from becoming a learner. However, as we shall describe below, some organisations have achieved a positive culture towards learning. We will now consider organisational factors that are likely to maximise the learning potential of the workforce and create a positive environment for learning.

A POSITIVE ORGANISATIONAL LEARNING ENVIRONMENT

The term 'learning organisation', as described by Garrett (1990) and Senge (1990b), is much used at present as a buzzword to describe an organisation in which learning is integrated and supported throughout the organisation. Although it can be seen as the Utopian learning environment in which learning is integrated and supported throughout the organisation, Pearn et al. (1995) argue that the notion of 'the' learning organisation does not exist. The LGMB and CCETSW (1997) also recognises that there can be no blueprint for ways in which organisations promote a climate of learning; what may be appropriate at a specific time in one organisation may be inappropriate in another. They draw attention to work developed by the Tavistock Institute, which evaluated the Training Support Programme for staff working with elderly people. This survey provides some indication of factors that are likely to promote a positive organisational learning climate. On the basis of their findings they hypothesise that the following are likely to promote organisational learning and have a positive impact on the quality of service provided to service users.

Training targeted at particular groups

- Training that focuses on the enhancement of the status of basic grade staff will have a direct impact on the quality of service provision.
- First-line managers require training enabling them to facilitate the transfer of learning to practice for front-line staff.
- Management level staff should be trained in supervisory and training skills. This will have a direct impact on the quality of practice irrespective of the training offered directly to the staff they manage.
- Training should be targeted at all incoming staff. This is likely to be more effective than training staff who have been in post for a number of years.

Training related to organisational and cultural objectives

- Training should focus on overall cultural changes – for example, attitudes and values rather than training that is skill based.
- An emphasis on recognised professional qualifications makes a direct contribution to improvements in service quality.
- Basic grade staff should receive race and cultural awareness training. This is likely to improve service delivery to black and ethnic minority communities.

They conclude that there is likely to be a continuous focus on individual and organisational learning if performance management and workforce development are brought together and are linked to service developments. They also agree that if staff have had opportunities to learn within a positive environment, this should continue to impact positively on the quality of care provided to service users even if the training is discontinued. Finally, they conclude that trainers can learn from their experiences of training and that these experiences should enhance the capacity of organisations to plan for and implement further training.

As identified above, managers have a crucial role to play in creating an organisational climate for learning. It is therefore imperative that there should be a strong, strategic framework underpinning all training, as described in Chapters 1 and 3. This will enable a climate to be created that supports the learner, ensuring that the learning is relevant and is applied appropriately to practice not merely for the benefit of the learner, but also to improve service delivery and meet the organisational goals. However, these strategic developments are dependent on the training unit acting corporately with a strong, team-based approach, rather than as individual trainers who develop their own strategies with discrete groups of staff. The introduction of service-level agreements between the training unit and commissioners of training provides a vehicle enabling these issues to be identified and strategies to be developed to promote learning within the organisation. The value of this is reinforced by the SSI, which noted that, where links had been made between policy making, service development and training, staff and their managers were able to see how training contributed to their work. This resulted in a better fit between staff work practice and training activity which should promote learning (SSI 1996a: 291).

THE ROLE OF THE TRAINER IN MANAGING ORGANISATIONAL BLOCKS TO LEARNING

Learners are likely to bring organisational concerns into the training arena. This can occur for a number of reasons. First, current organisational issues are so interlinked with practice that they are likely to be on participants' minds during any training event. Second, course participants' negative experiences of the organisation can be reflected in the training room, the feelings they have towards managers being directed at the trainer, who is seen as the organisational representative. Hughes and Pengelly (1995) outline participant behaviours that manifest these feelings on the course. They include:

- mirroring their experiences of management and the organisation;
- acting out the victim/persecutor/rescuer triangle, placing themselves in the role of victim and putting the trainer in the role of persecutor or rescuer;
- projection and projective identification: feelings of anxiety, anger and vulnerability towards managers are managed by attributing them to the trainer or other participants.

The trainer has to acknowledge the strength of the feelings yet balance this with the need to confront the feelings interfering with the learning process. This can be done by avoiding responses that collude with the feelings which would place the trainer in the role of rescuer, or blame the participants, thereby becoming the prosecutor.

The trainer should reflect back on the process to the group, getting them to separate individual from organisational issues and asking them to consider how these processes interfere with their ability to learn. In this way the trainer empowers learners by enabling them to look realistically at the situation. The ability of the trainer to do this will depend on their own perceptions of the organisation. This will be determined by:

- their attitude to managerial authority;
- the influence of their work setting;
- their support and supervision.

In the same way that learners are expected to take some responsibility for managing the organisational climate and the impact this can have on their learning, trainers need to make an assessment of the factors outlined above and identify what impacts on their perception of management and how this affects their ability to manage their organisational role within the training room (Hughes and Pengelly 1995).

Team learning

The discussion above has largely focused on organisations which still retain a traditional central management structure, such as the probation service and social services. However, the introduction of devolved budgets and a more decentralised approach to management, in a number of social care organisations, means that within these settings the emphasis must be on the ability of smaller teams to create a climate for learning. This depends crucially on the attitude and ability of the manager to work positively with the team to create a learning environment. For example, a community health team known to one of us analysed, as a team, the areas of control that they had over their learning and development and their learning resources – for example, supervision, experience within the team and team meetings. They developed a strategy that raised the profile of staff development in supervision; utilised the knowledge and skills of the team by introducing training and development into team meetings, and established a system whereby more experienced staff took some responsibility for the development of other team members. Staff development needs that could not be met by the team were prioritised for training, utilising the limited budget available. This demonstrates that the concept of a learning team is often more viable than that of a learning organisation, because an organisation is often dogged by bureaucracy and political unpredictability, whereas a team, or smaller working unit, may be more in control of its destiny and much clearer about its learning needs.

If teams are unable to develop the kind of strategy described above, there is still great value in teams undertaking training courses together. This enables team members to support each other in transferring the learning from the training to practice. Team learning provides opportunities for developing team cohesion, promoting openness, establishing common values and attitudes and clarifying team goals and standards of practice.

WHO IS RESPONSIBLE FOR CREATING A CLIMATE OF LEARNING FOR INDIVIDUAL LEARNERS?

The focus of the first part of this chapter has been on a strategic approach towards creating a learning environment. The rest of the chapter considers ways of creating learning climates for individual learners. In this regard there are three key players who influence and contribute to the learning experience:

1   The learner
2   The trainer
3   The supervisor.

Each of the roles will be considered in more detail, focusing particularly on responsibilities for trainers and managers in maximising the contribution of these players.

The role of the learner in creating a learning environment: the learning professional

Trainers, supervisors, managers and colleagues can all endeavour to create an environment for learning. However, all these efforts depend on the willingness of the learner to take some responsibility and accountability for their own learning. This responsibility relates to five areas:

1   A willingness to explore previous and current experience because experience is the door to learning.

2   Acknowledgement of the need to balance personal learning needs with professional and organisational needs.
3   Active commitment to and engagement in the learning process.
4   Willingness to evaluate and reflect on learning.
5   Commitment to transfer learning to practice.

(Stephenson and Weil 1992)

Each of these raises issues for trainers and managers in terms of creating a climate that encourages the learner to engage in the learning process. Each area will be considered in detail, with a particular focus on the role of the trainer and manager.

Reflection of previous experience

This requires the learner to reflect on their past and current personal experiences in terms of inhibitors and enhancers to learning. The first task for the learner is to become self-aware, understanding the impact of past experiences on their motivation. But 'Self-awareness . . . cannot be taught in lectures. It can grow in the course of structured experience' (Stevenson and Parsloe 1993).

The role of the trainer and manager is to facilitate this process by being aware of factors that can act as potential sources of negative learning experiences, as described in Table 5.1 (pages 144–145). The trainer and manager need to ensure that the learner understands the rationale for reflection on past experiences as part of the learning process. If the learner is supported through this process, they should develop confidence in their ability to assess their strengths and weaknesses and begin to appreciate the value of their experience (Stephenson and Weil 1992).

Acknowledgement of the need to balance personal learning needs with professional and organisational needs

A learner, within a social care setting, cannot utilise staff training purely to meet their own developmental needs. They need to be accountable to the organisation and service users as well as responsible to themselves for what they learn. A climate for learning is most likely to exist if the learner is clear about their roles and responsibilities to learn, as a means of enhancing the quality of service provision for users and meeting organisational goals. This enables the learner to identify their individual learning needs in this broader context.

The trainer and manager need to ensure that learners are clear about the goals of the service, the learner's own role and responsibilities in meeting these goals, the knowledge, values and skills required to meet service requirements, the changes that the service may be going through and any standards and competences that apply.

Active commitment to and engagement in the learning process

Although every effort can be made to support the learner through the development of a learning environment, this can only provide conditions conducive to learning; the learner themselves must be committed to the experience of learning. This is the third task for the learner: 'being willing to try something is a condition for acquiring an ability to do it' (Schon 1987: 120).

Schon indicates what is required of the learner at this stage:

● Trust in those supporting the learning. In the context of training this would be in the supervisor and the manager.
● Accepting a temporary dependence on the trainer and supervisor. New experiences require taking steps into the unknown. When taking these steps the learner has to become dependent, and accept that their 'guide', the trainer or supervisor, has some idea of where they are going. Until the learner has got their bearings they are dependent on their guide.
● Retaining a responsibility for their learning and education. The learner, although supported, needs to make sense of the new learning.

The trainer and manager need to adopt an approach that enables the learner to risk dependence without feeling that this will result in criticism or be seen as a sign of weakness.

Willingness to evaluate and reflect on learning

The learner needs to be willing to evaluate their learning critically. As Jarvis (1983) states, the acquisition of knowledge, values and skills does not necessarily mean that the individual has developed as a learning professional. To do this they require the critical ability to determine what is good practice and assess their practice accordingly. If this does not occur, the learner is likely to have learnt only at an intellectual level or is merely trained to follow very specific instructions. Jarvis goes on to state that the art of assessing and judging what is appropriate is an element of education and is required for innovative practice and lifelong learning. The trainer and manager have a role in facilitating this evaluating process, providing the learner with opportunities to assess and critically reflect on their learning before expecting the learner to put the learning into practice – that is, provide opportunities to reflect before doing.

Commitment to transfer learning to practice

The learner must be willing to explore and integrate the learning into practice, in the light of their own past and present personal, professional and organisational experiences. Trainers and managers can support this transfer by providing feedback on the development of knowledge, values and skills in practice and by providing learners with a framework to monitor their progress. This is discussed in detail in Chapter 10.

THE ROLE OF THE SUPERVISOR IN CREATING A CLIMATE FOR LEARNING

Successful and innovative managers respect and value learning as the key to change, while generating some excitement and uncertainty that encourages others to develop and learn. They are able to hold the fine line between chaos and control, recognising the paradox that each is needed and managing the tension between them.

(LGMB and CCETSW 1997: 31)

This quotation clearly describes the responsibility of the manager, as supervisor, to create a learning environment enabling the supervisee to maximise their learning opportunities. It is useful inasmuch as the focus is on the supervisor as a facilitator and enabler of learning, rather than that the supervisor should be seen as an expert in the particular practice area. This distinction is important, as many supervisors, in our experience, say they are unable to address the developmental needs of staff as they feel they are no longer experts and familiar with current developments in particular areas of practice. It is not so much the practice expertise of the supervisor, rather, it is their supervisory skills that are crucial for creating and sustaining a climate for learning. As a facilitator of adult learning the supervisor has five tasks. These are based on Morrison's (1993) three tasks for staff development. The way in which these tasks are managed will influence the creation and sustainment of the learning environment. The supervisor should:

- enable the supervisee to reflect honestly on their performance in identifying their professional competence. This should include a consideration of the supervisee's theoretical perspectives, their skills, values and knowledge and their contribution to the organisation;
- assist the learner in setting relevant professional goals by identifying gaps in knowledge, values and skills between what is expected and the supervisee's actual performance;
- help the supervisee to identify the appropriate sources of professional development available to them. This should include a consideration of the impact of past personal, professional and organisational experiences on their approach to training. Opportunities should be made available in supervision to enable the supervisee to identify their learning style and develop effective and efficient approaches to learning;
- support the learner through the learning experience, ensuring that the supervisee is able to maximise the learning potential of the training course and other developmental opportunities;
- provide opportunities and practical support to enable the supervisee to reflect and apply the learning from training to practice, continuing to provide opportunities to learn from this application. (This final task is explored in detail in Chapter 10.)

The quotation at the start of this section refers to the difficulty of maintaining that fine line between chaos and control. First, changes that are occurring within social care organisations frequently make it hard for managers to maintain this line and effectively undertake the tasks described above. The de-layering and restructuring that has occurred in many organisations means that teams are increasing in size so that managers are now expected to balance staff supervision with many other managerial functions. Second, supervisors managing very large teams have difficulty spending sufficient time in meeting with staff to discuss their development. This can be particularly difficult for those, such as home care managers, who manage large numbers of staff who rarely use an office base. In addition, supervisors often undertake the tasks described above with no opportunity, through training and their own supervision, to gain knowledge and understanding of adult learning and to develop skills in facilitating reflective practice. Against this backcloth it is not surprising that in our experience of supervisory skills training, the supervisors have difficulty addressing the staff development function.

Establishing a climate for learning utilising the supervisory agreement

The ability of the supervisor to create a learning environment for their supervisee depends not only on organisational and professional influences but also on the relationship with the supervisee. Both the supervisor and the supervisee approach learning with their own personal agendas. For example, the supervisor may resent discussing the supervisee's training needs as they feel their own learning needs are never addressed by their supervisor; alternatively, the supervisee may feel intimidated, fearing that an acknowledgement of need will be perceived as an inability to do the job.

In addition, there are power issues that impact on the supervisory relationship. Personal, cultural, structural and institutional inequalities of power can have a profound effect on the supervisory relationship. This will be in addition to and linked to, the power issues associated with the relationship of supervisor and a supervisee. To create a positive learning environment, the supervisor and supervisee need to relate in an open and honest way that acknowledges these power differences. A supervisory contract is a useful tool for achieving this. It is a means of making power relationships and aims explicit, and identifying the ways in which both parties will work together towards achieving their goals. Contracting is particularly important at the start of the supervisory relationship as it clarifies the boundaries and sets the scene of the working relationship (Brown and Bourne 1996). Although a supervisory contract should cover all aspects of the supervisory task, the focus here will be on the way it can be used to create a learning environment.

When beginning the contracting process it is helpful if the supervisor and supervisee share past learning experiences. It is particularly important to explore the way that negative personal, professional and organisational experiences and experiences of power and oppression could impact on training and staff development. The positive learning experiences should not be ignored. Consideration needs to be given to ways in which lessons can be learnt from both these positive and negative experiences. Both the supervisor and supervisee should be prepared to discuss their experiences, as those of the supervisor can block the learning of the supervisee as much as the supervisee's own experiences. For example, a young female supervisor blocked learning opportunities for older team members as she felt very insecure in her managerial role and felt she lacked practice knowledge. The experience reminded her of her past social work training, when she had been younger than others on the course and lacked social work experience in comparison to the other students. Until she explored her attitude to learning with a supervisee, she did not appreciate that she had not encouraged older members in the team to attend training as she feared that she would feel disempowered if they developed further.

In this situation the supervisor had felt safe enough to discuss her experiences with a new, younger member of the team. She realised that she had not even approached contracting about learning with the older team members. This indicates the need for both supervisor and supervisee to work on establishing an open and honest relationship to enable the supervisory agreement to be a meaningful tool. It also highlights the need for supervision to take place at all levels in the organisation. If this supervisor had been given the opportunity to discuss her negative learning experiences in a safe supervisory setting, she could have begun working on these issues before it affected the team.

Maintaining a climate of learning through supervision

In busy social care organisations it is very easy to set out with good intentions and try and establish a climate for learning at the contracting stage. However, it is important that the climate is maintained. Current experience of supervisors and supervisees in social care organisations indicates that supervision is often cancelled or curtailed as other demands are made on staff; or the focus is on cases in crisis, and staff development falls off the agenda or is adjourned to the next session when, once again, events overtake both supervisor and supervisee.

Use of staff profiles

Tools are required to ensure that staff development remains permanently on the agenda and is given priority. One way of achieving this is through staff personal profiles. This is a tool for assessing the developmental needs of the individual, and provides a framework for a strategic approach incorporating training, supervision and work experience. Sheffield Family and Community Services has used this system for a number of years. Every member of staff is issued with a profile on appointment, from the Director to front-line staff. The profile provides a framework for monitoring the learning needs of an individual; identifying appropriate methods of meeting these needs; considering ways of transferring learning to the worksite; and evaluating effectiveness through supervision. The profile is an ongoing document, for staff members' use throughout their time in the organisation. If a worker changes their job their learning needs can be reassessed on the basis of their prior learning. There is an organisational expectation that the profile is regularly revisited and updated, which encourages the supervisee and supervisor to have regular supervision sessions where the primary focus is staff development (Horwath 1996). This system is a useful way of maintaining a climate of learning for a number of reasons:

1   It recognises the importance of learning at all levels within the organisation.
2   The learner is engaged throughout the learning process.
3   A systematic approach to learning, endorsed by senior managers, means that staff education and development is seen as an important supervisory function and consequently is less likely to be ignored. The information gained from the profile contributes to a comprehensive overview of the training need of the organisation.
4   The supervisor is provided with a very clear framework for managing staff development and is likely to feel more confident about discussing learning needs than a supervisor working in a vacuum.
5   The supervisee also has a framework which makes clear their responsibilities and that of their supervisor, which can be utilised to challenge their supervisor if they feel their needs are not being met.

Although personal profiles are an effective tool to maintain a climate of learning, they do not lend themselves to all social care settings. The process is time consuming, reliant on frequent supervision sessions and works best when regular supervision is provided and there is a commitment to training and development throughout the organisation. Another tool that can be utilised is to include an individual professional development planner in staff appraisal schemes. This provides opportunities to identify learning needs, consider appropriate methods for meeting those needs and opportunities to evaluate effectiveness (Miller 1990).

THE TRAINER'S ROLE IN PREPARING A CLIMATE OF LEARNING

'I wish I had your job. Read a few books stand up and talk for a bit, do a few exercises and then go home.'

(Course participant)

How many times have course participants come out with these comments without appreciating the work that the trainer does to make it seem so easy? It is only when things go wrong that participants begin to become aware of the issues and the tasks facing the trainer. At the beginning of the chapter consideration was given to the strategic responsibilities of the trainer in terms of creating a climate for learning. This section focuses on the operational role of the trainer in terms of creating a climate of learning for individual learners. Responsibilities start well before a learner enters the training room and their role continues once the learner is back in their worksite. Within this chapter the focus will be on the trainer's role before the training event. The role of the trainer in terms of creating a climate for learning during a learning event is described in Chapter 6, and their role in transferring learning back to the worksite is explored in Chapter 10.

Recruitment

A number of years ago one of us attended a training course which was advertised at a team meeting. This was done by the manager waving a leaflet about regarding the course on risk assessment, and asking if anyone was interested in a two-day event where lunch would be provided. There was no information regarding aims, objectives or target group. The course itself was a frustrating, poor learning experience. Participants attended with very different agendas, varying levels of experience and diverse hopes and expectations that could not possibly be met; indeed it was presumed that the course was on risk assessment in child protection when in fact the focus was mental health assessment! This is an extreme example but similar confusion still occurs, with participants arriving for courses very unclear about the aims and objectives or not sure why they were recruited to the course. This kind of experience is not conducive to learning. With this in mind, careful consideration needs to be given to the kind of information that is sent out to recruit to courses. Information regarding training courses are usually distributed in two stages:

1   The annual training brochure
2   Targeted circulation.

Annual training brochures

It is becoming increasingly common for training units to produce a brochure that indicates the courses that will be provided for the year. This enables managers and their teams to plan training strategically and to utilise the training provided in a way that promotes the learning of individual members of staff. The type of information that the workforce will require are these:

● aims of the course;
● objectives, a clarification of the way in which the aims will be achieved;
● brief summary of likely course content;
● level of knowledge, values and skills required to undertake the course;
● indication of other courses that should have been attended before this course;
● training techniques that are likely to be utilised;
● group size and balance – for example, an indication as to whether participants will be informed if they were likely to be the only black participant;
● venue – an indication as to whether the needs of people with disabilities or dietary requirements can be met;
● length of course;
● course dates;
● brief particulars of course leader.

Targeted circulation

As the date for the training course draws near further information is required by targeted groups. More specific information on aims and objectives, course content and training approaches will be required, as well as details of any particularly emotive content. This allows the learner and their manager to ascertain whether the course will actually meet the needs of the learner at the time.

Selection

The needs of learners, within a group context, must be a primary consideration when selecting participants for a particular learning group. Learning in a group depends on people having a sense of identity and security and belonging to a 'safe base' from which they can be receptive to learning. In training groups this comes from individuals recognising that they share at least some similarities with others (Brummer and Simmonds 1992). However, difference is also important, and little learning will take place if the group is homogeneous and all group members hold similar views. The trainer consequently is aiming at a balance so that individuals are not isolated in terms of race, gender or work discipline but that there is sufficient range to ensure different perspectives. Selection is consequently a two-way process. Potential course participants need to make informed choices, in conjunction with their manager, as to whether the training is appropriate to meet their needs, but trainers also require information enabling them to select participants.

The trainer should consider similarities and differences at both a personal and professional level. Professionally, individuals can feel very vulnerable if they are unable to identify with others within the group or if they consider other course members are more experienced and knowledgeable in the particular practice area. This can be a particular issue on inter-agency training when an isolated professional from one agency may feel overwhelmed by representatives from other agencies whom they perceive as being more powerful and having more status. At a personal level it is important that the course does not become a microcosm of wider society, mirroring gender and racial imbalance. Trainers, when selecting for training courses, need to be mindful of the likely life experiences of potential participants from minority groups and try to avoid replicating these experiences, otherwise training can exacerbate feelings of loneliness and isolation (Brummer and Simmonds 1992). Trainers need to beware of making simplistic assumptions or of utilising a hierarchy of oppression – for instance, assuming that black people will identify with each other and ignoring or playing down other differences relevant to the black person, such as gender, religion or culture. One of the most effective strategies, to ensure that learners do not feel isolated on a course, is to discuss selection with the potential participants concerned, being clear about the choices available. For example, on very specialised courses there may be little choice for a participant regarding other participants. If this is the case the trainer can negotiate with the participant what strategies can be utilised to support that individual.

CREATING A CLIMATE OF LEARNING BEFORE A TRAINING EVENT

The mind can absorb what the seat can endure.

(D. Macarov in his address 'Directions for the new millennium' delivered to a conference in Dublin, Culture and Identity: Social Work in a Changing Europe: Implications for Education and Practice, organised by the European Schools of Social Work and the European Association of Social Workers, August 1997)

If a trainer is to engage the learner during a training event they must give consideration to a number of factors over and above course content and training techniques. Maslow (1968) considered an individual's need to learn, within a hierarchy of needs, identifying the levels of need to be satisfied before a person is generally ready for learning (see Figure 5.1).

Maslow's hierarchy is based on the premise that, as one need is met, another level of need is uncovered. He believes that the lower levels of need must be satisfied before personal development can be attempted. Although there has been much debate, in the literature, regarding the positioning of the need for knowledge and development (Jarvis 1995), the model provides a useful framework to identify needs that should be satisfied to create an environment for learning. In this chapter the Maslow hierarchy will be applied at a micro level to identify the needs within the context of a specific training event. If these needs are not addressed, the learner or – on occasion, the whole group – is likely to regress to meeting more basic needs, thus failing to maximise their learning opportunities. This will strike a chord with most trainers who have learnt how obsessed a group can become with temperature, if the room is too hot or too cold, to the extent that there is little focus on learning.

Preparing the learner for the learning group

For some potential learners, levels of anxiety regarding a new learning situation can be so high that it is important to allay as many of these as

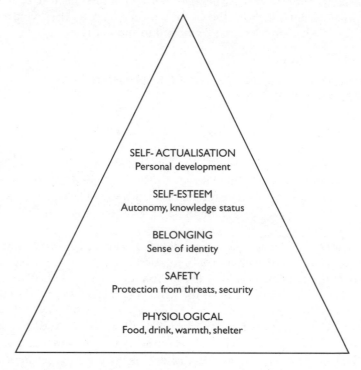

Figure 5.1 Maslow's hierarchy of needs
Source: Maslow (1968)

possible before the training event. As described at the beginning of the chapter, learning can be an uncomfortable process as it requires change. Many anxieties are linked to learners' fears that they will be placed in a position which will repeat negative past learning experiences and that the process will be destructive rather than supportively challenging. By providing them with information about ways in which the trainer intends to meet needs, the learner, on their own or in conjunction with their supervisor, can make an assessment as to whether this is an appropriate learning experience.

Figure 5.2 indicates the type of information to consider when addressing individual needs before a training event. Particular attention is paid to addressing needs at the bottom of the hierarchy. If these needs are not met they can get in the way and distract from the learning process.

Although many basic needs may be addressed through the provision of information before the course, this information may raise levels of

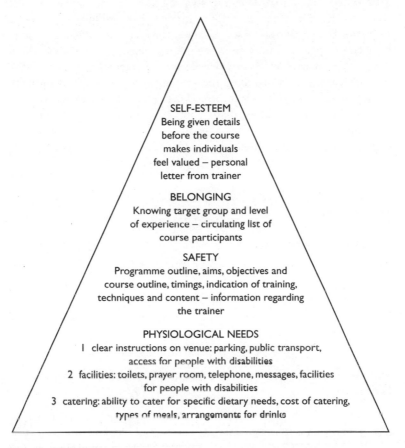

Figure 5.2 Meeting learning needs before the training course

anxiety among some learners. For example, a participant with poor literacy skills may become concerned if they note that one of the training techniques involves the use of written case studies. Others may become concerned about their ability to manage specific course content at both a professional and personal level. Therefore trainers need to consider ways in which the individual can discuss their concerns and needs without feeling threatened, while recognising individuals' ability to do this may be determined by their perception of self and that of the trainer. A trainer can facilitate this process by acknowledging in the programme some of the difficulties that participants may be encountering – such as anxiety about training techniques and course content, or isolation on the course. They can also suggest ways of managing these concerns, by, for instance, writing anonymously, ringing or meeting with the trainer. Personalised contact through individual letters to each course participant, reinforcing the above, can make it easier for the learner to contact the trainer. It is also important that learners' managers are briefed regarding the training content and training techniques so that they can have informed discussions of the issues with the learner. By acknowledging these concerns and anxieties, the trainer normalises the experience of individual participants with the aim of creating a climate where the issues can be addressed before the training course.

SUMMARY

Blocks to learning

Learners are likely to approach learning with anxiety and fear. Although learning itself can be an anxiety-provoking experience, each learner will have additional anxieties, fears and blocks to learning. These are based on their past and present organisational, professional and personal experiences.

Working together to create a climate for learning

The trainer, supervisor and learner need to identify these potential blocks and work together towards creating a climate of learning in which functional learning can take place. This can only take place if there is an integrative learning system based on open and honest communication between the trainer, the supervisor and the learner.

The organisational context

Each contributor to the system is also part of the wider organisation and none of the contributors can dissociate themselves from the organisation. The climate of learning will be influenced by the organisational culture. Organisations that are committed to promoting quality services for users by linking training, human resource development and service developments are the ones most likely to maintain a continuous focus on individual and organisational learning (LGMB and CCETSW 1997).

Creating a climate for learning

Effective learning can only take place if the learner's needs, fears and anxieties about learning are considered before the learner enters the training room. Managers, as supervisors, have a responsibility to create a learning environment in which these issues can be addressed in order to maximise learning opportunities. This can be achieved through the use of a supervisory contract. The trainer is also required to consider ways of addressing anxiety through the recruitment and selection procedures and the information provided to learners before learning events.

Chapter 6

Group dynamics
Implications for the learning group

In this chapter the following topics are covered:

- groups as a medium for learning – the learning group;
- the impact of anxiety on group process;
- theoretical models of group development;
- the impact of status, power and discrimination on group learning;
- models for managing conflict within group settings;
- a framework for assessing learning group dynamics.

Learning groups: mechanism of delivery or medium for learning?

Group learning is one of the most common forms of learning within the social care arena and can have positive benefits for the learner. These benefits include:

- providing support and reinforcement of the learning through sharing the experience with other learners;
- offering opportunities to share concerns and discuss issues which can reduce feelings of isolation, inadequacy and anxiety;
- enabling learners to listen to, evaluate and address differing viewpoints;
- a positive group learning experience can increase the learner's self-confidence, self-esteem and social skills.

(B. Taylor, n.d.)

A group setting enables the trainer to utilise a range of learning methods. The trainer can also draw on the experience and difference within the group in order to promote learning. This offers course participants a range of different applications of learning to practice.

However, not all groups provide these benefits for learners. The training is two-ways as we have already considered in Chapters 2 and 5 – 'The learner controls the switch that makes learning happen' (Sheal 1997: 15).

The task of the trainer is to create a group environment that encourages the learner to switch on and learn. If this group environment does not exist the training course is likely to remain little more than a medium for training delivery. So what is it that transforms a group from a mechanism for delivery to a medium for learning?

What is a group?

To begin to answer this question we need to consider what is meant by a group. Jaques believes a collection of individuals can be defined as and when some, or all, of the following exist:

- *Collective perception*: members are aware that they are together as an identifiable group.
- *Needs*: participants enter the group feeling it will address some of their needs.
- *Shared aims*: the focus is on meeting the common, identified aims.
- *Inter-dependence*: events that occur during the life of the group will influence and affect its members.
- *Social organisation*: the group is a unit with its own rules, relationships and power dynamics.
- *Interaction*: members communicate with each other in a variety of ways that influence and affect other group members. This interaction creates a sense of being a group even when members are not physically together.
- *Cohesiveness*: participants want to remain together in the group to achieve the aims.
- *Membership*: when two or more individuals interact for longer than a few minutes a group can be said to exist.

(Jaques 1992: 13)

A group as a medium for learning – that is, a learning group – can be said to exist, in a social care context, when some or all of these characteristics combine to provide structured opportunities for participants to acquire new knowledge, values and/or skills with a view to influencing their subsequent work practice positively. This definition shows that a learning group does not necessarily require a trainer – for example, a team could become a learning group. However, in this chapter we give consideration to how the trainer can facilitate the creation and maintenance of a learning group. Theoretical perspectives on group behaviour and group development are examined and the implications for training practice discussed. The relationship between the individual learner and the learning group are analysed in terms of managing the anxiety and conflict that can affect learning in a group context.

INDIVIDUAL NEEDS AND THE IMPACT ON GROUP PROCESS

A recurrent theme of this book is that experiential learning can be anxiety provoking because the learner is required to take responsibility for what and how they learn. As described in Chapter 5, the anxiety of learning can be influenced by past and present personal and professional experiences. This anxiety can be shaped through group processes and result either in a positive engagement or to an emotional resistance and avoidance of learning within the group setting (Vince and Martin 1993). According to Vince and Martin, when the process is managed effectively, anxiety is contained or managed in a way that promotes learning. Vince and Martin highlight this in their functional learning cycle (see Figure 6.1). This is referred to by Morrison as 'green cycle behaviour', as it should be encouraged within a group context (Morrison 1996). Vince and Martin believe that anxiety about engaging in learning gives rise to uncertainty. For example, will the course be OK? Will I feel able to contribute what I know? If this is acknowledged by the trainer, the learner contains their feelings of anxiety and are enabled to start taking risks – for instance, 'I don't know how anyone else feels but I can really identify with what is being said and I am going to tell the group about my feelings.' Learners then struggle with the consequences of having taken a risk – for example, 'How will others respond to what I have said?' A result of this struggle is a feeling of confidence and empowerment involving either insight or increased authority – for example, 'Others in the group disagreed with me but I was respected for sharing my feelings.'

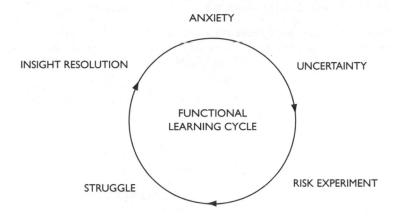

Figure 6.1 Micro model of the functional learning cycle
Source: Vince and Martin (1993)

Functional learning is likely to take place, because the trainer has contained the anxiety of learners in such a way that ensures that attention is being paid to both the group process, which contributes to developing a climate for learning, and the group task. Maintaining green cycle activity requires the trainer and group learners to utilise a range of behaviours at different times in the life of the group (Benne and Sheats 1948). It is most likely, particularly at the beginning of the group, that the trainer's behaviour will need to address both group task and maintenance issues. However, as the group engages in functional learning the group members are likely to take more responsibility for the maintenance and task roles.

The roles identified by Benne and Sheats (1948) and Taylor (n.d.) have been expanded and adapted in Table 6.1 to identify the range of behaviours that promote functional group learning. While these types of behaviour are useful throughout the life of the group, in terms of group maintenance and achieving the group task, particular behaviours are useful at certain stages of the functional learning cycle. The trainer has a major responsibility for modelling and facilitating these behaviours.

Dysfunctional learning

However, there are other times in learning groups when the risk seems too great and the learner becomes defensive and resistant. Taylor (n.d.)

Table 6.1 Green cycle behaviours that promote functional learning

Group behaviours that facilitate the management of uncertainty	*Encouraging*: responding warmly, verbally and non-verbally to others who contribute, supporting participants' contributions by acknowledgement and comment *Harmonising*: reconciling different points of view, suggesting how they may complement and inform each other *Compromising*: being prepared to admit mistakes or meet others half way *Gatekeeping*: trying to facilitate the participation of quieter members so that the group is not dominated by a forceful few *Standard setting*: expressing standards that the group can attempt to achieve in its level of operation. Referring to the learning contract *Commentating*: observing what is happening within the group and facilitating an assessment or offering an interpretation *Following*: going along with the group, encouraging and accepting the ideas of others and being a good listener, allowing the group to lead *Clarifying*: answering questions regarding the process and task
Behaviours that facilitate risk taking	*Initiating*: suggesting new ideas or a change of focus regarding the achievement of the task *Information seeking*: asking for facts *Opinion seeking*: probing and eliciting clarification of the values or attitudes pertinent to what the group is considering *Information giving*: providing relevant facts, frameworks and information or sharing pertinent, relevant personal experience *Opinion giving*: stating values and beliefs pertinent to the area the group are considering *Elaborating*: expanding on contributions, providing examples to enable the group to consider the suggestion in a broader context

	Eliciting difference: for example, 'What do the women here feel?' *Challenging*: by the trainer or setting tasks for the group to challenge itself *Drawing out emotional responses*: this includes some self-disclosure by the trainer of her own feelings
Behaviours which support struggle and encourage insight resolution	*Co-ordinating*: linking together a number of ideas and suggestions *Orientating*: defining the current positions within the group in terms of achieving the desired goal *Evaluating*: assessing where the group are at in terms of reaching a realistic solution *Energising*: attempting to stimulate the group into activity *Recording*: acts as the group memory noting what has taken place *Validating difference*: acknowledging that there are sometimes no easy solutions *Facilitating creativity*: by using metaphor or in problem solving *Summarising/feedback*: allowing groups to struggle not always reassuring. Making contradictions and ambiguities explicit

cites a number of fears that can be sources of resistance and avoidance of group-based learning. They include fear of:

- finding acceptance;
- losing face;
- discomfort;
- being ignored;
- not being influential;
- being denied privacy.

In these situations dysfunctional learning is likely to occur, as shown in Figure 6.2. This is referred to as red cycle behaviour as it blocks learning and needs to be discouraged. Anxiety is still present, but because it is not contained by the trainer results in fight or flight responses – for

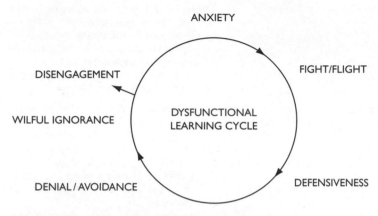

Figure 6.2 Micro model of the dysfunctional learning cycle
Source: Vince and Martin (1993)

example, 'I am sure no one can be feeling as angry as I do so I'd better keep quiet.' The learner is not ready to share, participate or question. These feelings can then turn into defensiveness and avoidance, resulting in unwillingness to undertake learning tasks during training – for instance, 'No one understands my job so this course will not meet my needs.' If these responses do not work, the learner can become openly resistant and engage in denial, about the need to learn or about what is happening in the group. For example, 'You have no idea what I have to cope with. If you did my job you would realise this is not going to work.' As these mechanisms deepen, the individual's resistance can become socially reinforced by the negative behaviour of the group as a whole, and they appear to become wilfully ignorant. For example, 'This course was irrelevant and a waste of time – we never learned a thing.' This in turn can result in disengagement from the whole learning process: 'I knew there was no point bothering with training – I'm certainly not wasting my time in this way again.'

In the same way that there are behaviours which facilitate learning, there are a range of behaviours that can result in dysfunctional learning, which are described in Table 6.2. These behaviours can often be undertaken by individual learners acting on behalf of other group members who will collude with the behaviours to avoid learning. Trainers are not removed from dysfunctional learning, they can mirror these behaviours.

Vince and Martin emphasise that these two cycles seek to identify

Table 6.2 Red cycle behaviours that promote dysfunctional learning

Behaviours that indicate fight	*Overtly aggressive*: openly and verbally hostile towards the trainer and other group members who are committed to meeting the learning objectives *Passively aggressive*: indicating reluctance to engage through the use of aggressive non-verbal cues, cynicism and sarcasm *Quarrelsome*: challenging everything that is said as a way of resisting the proposed programme *Dominating/controlling*: having their own agenda – often an area that they feel secure and knowledgeable about and continually attempt to get the group to focus on this area
Behaviours that indicate flight	*Negatively silent*: saying very little, but the non-verbal cues indicate resistance rather than the nervousness that a shy participant may exhibit *Passivity*: going along with the group programme but does not engage; or sitting outside the main group *Doodling*: this is done to avoid, for example, completing their diary or reports *Poor timekeeping* *Expressing ambivalence*: stating that they are not sure if they should be at the training
Behaviours that indicate defensiveness and avoidance	*Challenging*: confronting the trainer and resisting new learning by continually arguing or procrastinating *Clowning*: using humour as a diversionary tactic, often at the expense of others who are committed to learning. The rest of the group will frequently look to the clown to perform when the going gets tough; the clown will always rise to the occasion *Non-compliance*: failing to complete small group tasks, gossiping or moaning in the small groups

Table 6.2 Continued

Behaviours that indicate denial and avoidance	*Knowing it all*: has all the knowledge that is required and consequently can learn nothing from the course *Scepticism*: the new learning will be of little use as there will be no opportunity to apply it, or it is irrelevant to practice *Been there, done that, bought the T shirt*: seen it and done it all – there is nothing to be learnt *Joking*: lightening the atmosphere at inopportune times to avoid the task *Persistent questioning*: continually questioning and seeking clarification in an unconstructive manner which is a delaying tactic *Diverting*: questioning or making contributions that take the focus of the group away from the task in hand *Busy-beeing*: dipping in and out of the training; arriving late, leaving for meetings, rarely there and resistant to making any firm commitment to the group
Behaviours that indicate wilful ignorance	*Rebelling*: challenging and disagreeing throughout the course stating that the course was a waste of time. Drawing out delinquent responses. Creating an anti-task sub-group *Alternative leadership*: leading a group of dissidents who dissociate themselves from the learning and directly challenge the programme *Absenting*: appearing at the start of the course and attending periodically, sufficiently to be seen as a group member, but not enough to have actually completed the programme
Behaviours that indicate disengagement	*Non-completion of assignments* *Physically dissociate*: reading the paper

processes and stages in a learning group whereby an individual learner, a number of learners or the whole group move either in the direction of functional or dysfunctional approaches to learning. This process is largely unconscious and the behaviours are fluid, varying especially in response to the trainer's behaviour. During the life of the group, individuals, and indeed the whole group, may move from behaviours that encourage learning to ones that discourage learning. For example, the trainer introduces a new approach to risk assessment: a minority of participants may feel anxious about this new learning and demonstrate flight behaviours. This may give permission for other participants to express their anxiety in negative ways and they too will begin to demonstrate fight or flight behaviours. This can create a general feeling of anxiety among those who are in a functional learning cycle and are influenced by the negativity around. Detecting these shifts, the trainer engages the group in an exercise which is designed to demonstrate to the learners that they already have many of the skills and knowledge required to undertake the assessments. This can restore confidence and place the learners back on the functional learning cycle. In contrast, if the trainer introduces an exercise that reinforces their fears, the group are likely to become more entrenched in red cycle behaviours.

The demands of inter-agency training means that anxiety levels are likely to be particularly high in an inter-agency learning group. This occurs because the group will include learners who hold a range of professional values. Charles and Stevenson (1990) describe the way in which red cycle behaviour can be exhibited in inter-agency learning groups. Anxiety is likely to become manifest in fight behaviours such as competitiveness if individuals feel that their professional identity is under threat and they are struggling for professional survival within the learning group. Defensiveness may occur as participants deny the need to examine difference, particularly regarding anti-oppressive practice, or state that the trainer is not from their particular agency and is therefore unable to appreciate their particular needs. This then sets the scene to ignore the potential learning from the course by dismissing it as irrelevant.

Trainers themselves need to be very aware that they are not removed from the group process and that their own behaviour has a powerful impact in helping or hindering the maintenance of a healthy, green cycle learning process. If the trainer does not maintain a high level of self-awareness they may find themselves in some situations unwittingly engaged and modelling red cycle behaviours. This can occur for a number of reasons. The trainer may feel ambivalent about the material they are delivering or the organisation for whom they are working. They may lack confidence and consequently want to control the group – that is, fight, or collude with the group (for instance, flight from their role). There are a range of ways in which the trainer can unwittingly come to mirror the dysfunctional group processes. For example, a trainer introduces new practice guidance. The majority of participants are resistant to this as its implementation requires the acquisition of new skills and will need additional time. Participants begin to exhibit avoidance and denial behaviours, and the trainer responds with similar red cycle behaviours. As a result of this the whole group now ignore the programme content and have a diversionary discussion about imminent budget cuts. The trainer, in terms of the Hay's triangles referred to in Chapter 3, has formed an unhealthy alliance with learners against the organisation instead of maintaining their separate role. This example illustrates that the trainer is responsible for assessing not only group process behaviour but their own response to group behaviours. This can be a difficult task, particularly if one is training alone. These issues are explored in further detail in Chapter 7.

GROUP DEVELOPMENT WITHIN THE LEARNING GROUP

As described above, an individual within a learning group is unlikely to learn in isolation, and will be influenced by the feelings and responses of the other learners. The extent to which this is likely to occur will depend on the nature of the learning group. For example, learners brought together for a two-hour information session are unlikely to influence each other to the same extent as learners brought together for the lengthy mental health approved social work training. Heron explores the different ways in which groups impact on the learning process in terms of 'the combined configuration of mental, emotional and physical energy in the group at any given time; and the way this configuration undergoes change' (Heron 1989: 26).

Heron notes that there is no predictable way of determining how the dynamic will develop and unfold during the life of the group, as the positive and negative forms of energy will influence the process. These forms of energy reflect the red and green cycle behaviours described above. For example, Heron cites task-orientated, process-orientated, interactive and confronting behaviours as positive energy forms which can be seen as green cycle activities, while negative forms such as educational alienation, cultural restriction and psychological defensiveness are red cycle activities. Despite limits in the ability to predict group behaviour, Heron believes the group is likely to pass through four phases. These phases share some commonalties with other models of group development (Tuckman and Jensen 1977; Bion 1961; Napier and Gershenfeld 1985). For example, Tuckman describes groups as processing through the following phases:

- *Forming* – the first phase of the group when individuals come together to 'form' it.
- *Storming* – once the group is formed individuals test out group boundaries.
- *Norming* – this describes the stage when established patterns or 'norms' for group behaviour become established.
- *Performing* – the most productive period in the group's life when the group is working effectively towards achieving its goal.
- *Mourning* – this describes the final stage, when the group disbands.

The models highlight that groups are not static, but change over their life span, get blocked at different phases, and they can ebb and flow as they attempt to manage conflict. Heron's four phases of group development are:

1 Defensiveness
2 Working through defensiveness
3 Authentic behaviour
4 Closure.

Heron's phases are explored in detail below. Each phase in the life of the group is analysed in terms of levels of anxiety and trust and the subsequent impact on learning. The implications for the trainer, in terms of group facilitation and programme content, are also considered.

THE STAGE OF DEFENSIVENESS

This describes the very beginning of a group when it is no more than a collection of separate individuals with their own agendas. At this stage trust is low and anxiety high. Each individual will draw on previous experiences of other groups and they are likely to bring with them some of the concerns and anxieties described in Chapter 5.

As the training course commences, participants begin to check out the group at two levels: the emotional and the task. At the emotional level individuals make an assessment of others in the group and decide how much they are able to invest. For example, participants may feel reassured by the presence of certain other learners, or they may recognise others with whom they have had clashes and may feel anxious about what position this could put them in. At a task level, this is the stage when individuals make an assessment as to whether the group is going to meet their learning needs; for example, they may have misunderstood the aims of the course or the level of previous experience required.

During this phase learners look towards the trainer for leadership. The trainer may ask for views and opinions and get little response, as individuals are reluctant to engage until they have established exactly what is expected of them in terms of the group norms. Some individuals may dominate at this stage – for example, the course participant who feels confident and superior, or the individual whose own anxiety needs are so great that they cannot stop asking questions.

The tasks for the trainer

Embarking on training is like beginning a journey. It is a time of anticipation and excitement, anxiety and fearfulness (Scaife 1995).

This description emphasises both the ambivalence and anticipation which course participants experience at the start of a training course. The trainer has a crucial role as a container of anxiety. Their aim is to create a climate where anxiety is used to facilitate learning and to demonstrate that risk and uncertainty can be engaged with and lead to positive learning outcomes. What happens within the first thirty minutes of a training course is crucial, as it indicates to learners whether the trainer is likely to manage to contain the group's anxiety. The start of a training event can, consequently, be a very anxiety-provoking time for a trainer who wants the event to be a success both in terms of meeting individuals' learning needs and also as a positive, enjoyable experience. It can engender similar feelings to hosting a party. As at parties, the trainer is keen to break the ice, and 'ice breakers' are often suggested in training manuals as a tool to release tension and provide opportunities for members to introduce themselves to each other. However, this type of exercise can sometimes defeat its purpose. Individuals at the very beginning of the group do not feel confident or safe enough to challenge the trainer, and may consequently participate in an exercise that raises their levels of anxiety and reinforces feelings of isolation, believing that the rest of the group do not object to the exercise.

Because the beginning of a training event is crucial in giving this message to learners, the initial session should be designed to meet the

basic needs identified in Maslow's hierarchy, as described in
including addressing any practical concerns, enabling particip
secure and ready for learning. Figure 6.3 indicates ways o
learning needs during the first session of a training course.

Once participants are in the training room, to some extent they lose
their individual identity and become a group. One of the fundamental
issues for a trainer is to balance the range of individual needs with the
needs of the group. Exercises and discussions that take place at the
beginning of a training event provide trainers with a key opportunity
to begin to 'read' the group by asking, listening and analysing comments to assess what course participants require to ensure a climate for
learning, whether the planned programme will meet their needs, and

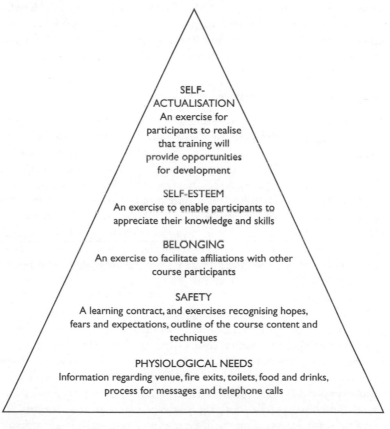

SELF-
ACTUALISATION
An exercise for
participants to realise
that training will
provide opportunities
for development

SELF-ESTEEM
An exercise to enable participants to
appreciate their knowledge and skills

BELONGING
An exercise to facilitate affiliations with other
course participants

SAFETY
A learning contract, and exercises recognising hopes,
fears and expectations, outline of the course content and
techniques

PHYSIOLOGICAL NEEDS
Information regarding venue, fire exits, toilets, food and drinks,
process for messages and telephone calls

Figure 6.3 Meeting learning needs in the first session of a training course

whether there are any issues that are likely to impinge on the learning process.

Introductions and scene setting can be seen as a form of group initiation. Brown (1996) describes this process as serving four functions in terms of engaging individuals. First, they enable the individual to identify the boundaries of the particular group; second, they help to underline the distinctiveness of the group from other groups; third, they indicate the standards, knowledge, values and skills required for effective functioning within the group; and finally, they elicit a commitment from the individual.

An assumption is often made by trainers that learners who are regular course attendees and train together on a frequent basis will feel safe and confident in the training arena and do not need this 'ritual'. This approach ignores the fact that, although the trainer may consider the group is confident that it will learn together, it fails to recognise that other things may have changed – for instance, changes within the organisation can impact on relationships within the group.

Negotiating a learning agreement

Mention ground rules to many trained in social care organisations in the late 1980s and they are likely to cringe and describe how half a day was spent on setting the ground rules; or they will be able to recite some of the standard ground rules: 'respect each other', 'one person talking at a time'. As a result of these kinds of experiences, for some trainers and learners the term has negative connotations. Participants frequently complain that the same points are made on every course and the whole process can be tokenistic. This in turn has made the whole concept of ground rules redundant in some settings. For some workers, from agencies that do not use ground rules, inter-agency training that began with this lengthy focus on ground rules was often a bewildering and confusing experience.

The phrase itself is not helpful; 'ground' implies some foundation or basis – but of what? The term 'rules' is defined as a set of standards and has negative links with rigidity, control and penalties. However, learning groups do require a framework which works towards clarifying mutual expectations and clear boundaries. This should be explicit in the terminology used, consequently the term 'learning contract', or 'agreement', would seem to be more appropriate for a number of reasons. By using the term 'learning' the focus is clear, and 'contract' or 'agreement' does not have the same rigidity as rules and is something negotiated between two parties. This is important as both trainer and participants have a responsibility to create a climate of learning.

However, the trainer and the trainee are not equal partners in the training relationship. Hughes and Pengelly (1995) consider this point, arguing that trainers are the managers of the courses. In this role they need to clarify their areas of responsibility, decide on basic standards and consider what action to take if there are problems. This recognises the authority dimension between trainer and participant. Second, a theme throughout this book is the importance of learners participating throughout the learning process. 'Participation' and 'partnership' are terms used with service users, who often expect more of an equal relationship than actually happens. The same is true of training; the trainer needs to consider what is and what is not negotiable, bearing in mind their role, so that the nature of the learning partnership becomes clear.

Many training units have learning contracts that are standardised and used on every training course. These have often resulted from consultation with the workforce, are included in the training brochure and course details, and are displayed in all training venues. These should be regularly reviewed in the light of the experiences of participants, trainers and managers. This provides the workforce with a very clear framework for a learning environment within the training room. Nevertheless, the learning agreement still needs to be explicitly discussed at the start of the course. It may be that learners felt happy with the agreement until they started the course and want to make adjustments in light of their anxieties.

There are a number of areas that need to be considered within the learning contract. These should cover the conditions required to create and maintain a learning environment. As described earlier in this chapter, the learner, their supervisor and the trainer all have some responsibilities and these should be reflected in the contract. Areas to consider are the following.

Quality control

The trainer should provide opportunities and structures for participants to gain the knowledge, values and skills that are identified within the course aims. Consideration needs to be given to ways in which the participant can express concerns if this is not taking place.

An anti-oppressive framework

Experiences of oppression within society should not be mirrored within a training course. Attention has also been paid to ways in which past and present learning and personal experiences can be oppressive. The contract should cover responsibilities of both trainer and participants to attempt actively to ensure that these experiences of oppression are not repeated within the training room by actively addressing difference and power, and challenging when appropriate.

Learning

This should cover the trainer's and participants' responsibilities if the expressed learning needs as reflected in course aims and objectives are being ignored. Consideration should also be given to the active role required of learners during a course to ensure that they maximise the learning opportunities. This should also include an acknowledgement that there are different styles and methods of learning (as described in Chapter 2), which together with anxiety about learning can influence levels of participation. However, there should be a commitment to learning, and the learning contract should state that non-participation will be challenged otherwise dysfunctional learning behaviours may become established.

Confidentiality

This is a complex area. It used to be thought that anything said in the training room should be confidential to the group. But part of learning is sharing experiences with others. Consideration should be given to defining information that can be or may have to be shared outside the learning group and information that is confidential to the group. It is important to bear in mind that training is an organisational event and both trainer and learners are attending in their organisational role and therefore are responsible if they identify poor practice. This should be channelled back to the relevant supervisor by the trainer. This responsibility to identify and respond to poor practice should be explicit.

Group process

Group process and maintenance tasks are essential if there is to be a safe climate for learning; both trainer and participants have shared responsibilities to perform this task, which is explored in detail in Chapter 6.

Time keeping

It can be very disruptive to learning if individuals arrive late and leave early or come and go throughout the course of the training event. As indicated earlier in the chapter these behaviours indicate red cycle behaviour and can have a negative impact on the rest of the group. In addition, other red cycle behaviours, such as gossiping and moaning or avoiding the task, can occur when learners are asked to complete exercises in small groups. This results in time being wasted and the task not being completed. It is for these reasons that time keeping should be part of the learning agreement.

Attention should be given to the responsibilities of both the trainer and participants in these six areas. However, contracting is of little use unless the trainer models the underpinning philosophy of the learning agreement. The trainer can feed the anxiety of the group through modelling behaviour that is oppressive and disempowering or neglects their responsibilities as a trainer. The goal of an effective learning agreement is to create a climate that provides both support and challenge.

Managing the introduction of the learning agreement or group contract requires careful handling. The trainer needs to be realistic about the ability of participants to commit themselves to a contract at this stage. If the contract is a standard one utilised on all training courses, participants may have concerns about parts of the agreement but feel too insecure and vulnerable at this stage of the process to voice their concerns. If the contract is negotiated by the group, individuals may not be sufficiently knowledgeable about each other, the trainer or the programme to be able to consider the agreement in the context of this particular group; they will be devising the terms on the basis of past experience. The trainer can address these issues by providing opportunities, during the course, to confirm that the learning agreement is meeting the needs of the group.

In conclusion, the trainer can be seen to have seven tasks that need to be completed successfully in order to promote functional learning at this stage:

1   To facilitate introductions.
2   To make clear the purpose of the group and the learning aims and objectives.
3   To clarify why individuals have attended and what they hope to achieve.

4   To negotiate and agree a group contract.
5   To consider the programme and methods to be utilised.
6   To indicate the ways in which the trainer will work with the group
     and the roles and responsibilities of the trainer and group members.
7   To begin to establish a group culture.

(Brown 1994)

THE STAGE OF WORKING THROUGH DEFENSIVENESS

The group begins to take on a life of its own. If it is operating predominantly in green cycle, learners are likely to have checked out each other and the trainer, and are now ready to begin to trust each other. Anxiety is contained and the group is committed to achieving its learning goals. At this stage the norms and patterns of behaviour of the particular group will emerge. The norms serve an important function in terms of defining the limits of acceptable and unacceptable behaviour. They enable the individual participant to predict how the group will operate and how to regulate their behaviour to conform. They also promote a sense of identity and facilitate the attainment of group goals (Brown 1996), creating an environment where it is safe to take risks.

However, all groups will have some degree of defensiveness, and working through this stage may result in some engagement in red cycle behaviours. This may become entrenched if anxiety is not contained and a culture of mistrust is established as the norm. This can manifest itself in a variety of ways – for example, as a 'flat group' which appears to be completing the tasks and engaging with the course content. However, this is done in a superficial way; learners avoid and resist opportunities for real learning by failing to ask questions, and do not engage in discussion and debate. In other groups a culture may become established where certain learners dominate the group. The anxiety becomes manifest in such fight behaviours as a struggle for domination through status, power and control. Alternatively, other learners may exhibit flight behaviours, and withdraw if they feel their needs will not be met or they have a low status position in the group (Taylor, n.d.; Bion 1961; Brown 1994).

Tasks for the trainer

● To promote functional learning by containing the anxiety of the group. This can be achieved by using the learning contract agreed at the start of the course.

● To utilise the cohesion and energy within the group to maintain a focus on the aims and objectives.

● To maintain a balance of learning through thinking, feeling and doing.

● To encourage participants to work through defensiveness in order to begin to take risks with new learning.

The trainer can achieve these tasks by behaving in ways that are likely to encourage risk taking, as described on page 174. At this stage, if the group is in green cycle, exercises can be more challenging than in the earlier phase, as learners are prepared to take more risks in assessing and analysing their work so as to accommodate new learning. Learners are ready to consider difference and are able to share feelings. Exercises can begin to focus on these aspects. Feedback can become more challenging, bringing out difference and seeking responses at both an intellectual and emotional level. At this stage the trainer should encourage group members to explore and probe each other's views and opinions.

If the group is operating in red cycle, the trainer has to work with learners to restore a green cycle culture. This requires the trainer to assess how anxiety is being manifested and to explore and make explicit the reason for this anxiety. For example, with the flat group, it may be that insufficient time was spent creating a climate of trust to meet the needs of this particular group. It could be that there is unspoken anger about the way the training was commissioned or about some other organisational changes. If this is the case, the trainer might need to alter the programme to include an exercise designed to establish trust. Without such trust, the group as a whole cannot work through defensiveness and therefore will not go on to the next stage. However, there will always be some individuals who do move on even when the group is stuck.

THE STAGE OF AUTHENTIC BEHAVIOUR

The group will only reach this stage if they are operating predominantly in green cycle. Trust is high and anxiety is being used constructively to encourage growth and change. Learners are given support, and take risks in a struggle to maximise their learning and explore some of the more difficult or unresolvable areas of practice. Learners are receptive to new ideas and to sharing views and opinions. They are prepared to move between different approaches to learning, engaging in challenging and risky exercises. Leadership and initiative become shared between the learners and the trainer; the group takes responsibility for maintaining itself. At this point the group should be working to its maximum potential harnessing energy, cohesiveness and commitment, to work towards achieving the aims and objectives.

Tasks for the trainer

- To act as facilitator rather than leader.
- To encourage the taking of risks.
- To provide opportunities for feedback and challenge.

These tasks are likely to be achieved if the trainer utilises the behaviours described on page 175 that support struggle and encourage insight resolution.

This is the stage when emotionally demanding, challenging and experiential exercises should be included. Participants are ready to take risks, therefore training techniques which require a degree of risk taking – for example, role play and video work – should be undertaken at this stage. Longer exercises, such as phased case studies, should be included in this stage, as this is the time when participants are focused on achieving the task and are working well together. This is also a good time to probe issues of anti-oppressive issues or beliefs; or on a inter-agency course to explore difference and disagreements between agencies.

CLOSURE

As the group comes to an end, the learners evaluate and review their learning and prepare to transfer it back to the worksite. This can be a time of mixed emotions. Group members and the trainer may feel a sense of achievement or frustration, sadness or relief, depending on whether the group was predominantly a functional or dysfunctional learning experience. Learners may also have mixed feelings regarding the return to their work base, and the organisational realities and cultures begin to re-enter the group's consciousness and behaviours.

This phase is characterised by individual group members withdrawing and reducing their level of commitment to the group.

Tasks for the trainer

● To enable the participant to make connections between their learning experiences on the course and their work context. (This is explored in detail in Chapter 10.)

● To provide opportunities to evaluate the learning experience and identify ways of consolidating learning back at the worksite.

● To assist the learner in assessing issues that need to be taken back to the worksite and those which remain in the training room.

● To identify organisational and managerial issues for the trainer to feed back to managers.

Course content should focus on enabling the participant to make the links between the learning on the course and its application to their work practice. As group members are beginning to separate from the group, their level of investment and the risks they are prepared to take will also reduce. However, learners need opportunities to express their views about disengaging from the group and how they feel about the learning experience. It can happen at this ending stage that some learners feel it is safe to express negative feelings towards other course members or the trainer. This may well occur if the group was operating in red cycle and no real learning took place. When this happens the group is likely to express views or demonstrate behaviours that indicate their wilful ignorance and disengagement from the learning process.

Participants are often reluctant to leave a successful training course and request recall days, often on the grounds that this will provide them with opportunities to evaluate how they applied their learning in practice. A trainer can feel flattered that participants want more, and will agree to organise a recall day without making an appropriate assessment as to whether it is relevant or whether it is a way of avoiding dealing with feelings of sadness and loss.

THE IMPACT OF STATUS, POWER AND DISCRIMINATION

Learners bring with them the norms, values and beliefs of the broader culture of the organisation and of the society in which they live and work. These can influence the way that a learner will behave and will be perceived in a group setting. For example, in a study by Tuckman and Lorge (1962) the contributions of members perceived to have low status were dismissed, when solving problems within a group. Brown (1996) argues that high status implies an ability to initiate ideas and activities and a 'consensual prestige' which affords the individual a positive ranking by other members of the group. Linked to status differentiation are processes of social comparison through which individuals assess their abilities and hierarchical position within the group. These social comparisons will reflect the inequalities that are determined and maintained by powerful groups in society. This is referred to by Shardlow and Doel (1996) as socially structured difference. For example, a sole black learner may feel disempowered in a learning group because that is their experience of the broader society. These comparisons influence self-perception and affect behaviour and task performance (Brown 1996). The comparisons can be based on a range of dimensions, from organisational position and level of experience to race, gender and disability. Heron (1989) argues that unless these forms of oppression are confronted they will become the accepted values and norms of the group and can result in dysfunctional learning. In addition, red cycle behaviour is inherently oppressive, as it invalidates difference and individual responsibility. Therefore green cycle functioning is crucial in establishing an anti-discriminatory environment.

Dysfunctional learning, or red cycle behaviour, can occur in a number of ways. For example, a situation can arise where the group is moulded around compliance rather than collaboration. This can result from an individual need to conform to the attitudes and behaviour of the majority. It can occur to the degree that individuals are prepared to deny their experience in order to go along with the majority view. For instance, if a group are talking negatively about gay men as foster carers, a gay man in the group may be resistant to any discussion of sexuality. Festinger and others (Brown 1996) suggest three reasons why this need for conformity exists. First, individuals depend on others for information and perspectives; second, the achievement of group goals requires a uniformity of purpose; and finally, individuals need to belong and not be seen as different. The need for conformity can result in participants denying some of their individuality in order to become accepted within the group. Yet in Chapter 5 we described how validating individual experiences is important if learning is to take place. This creates two dilemmas for trainers: the first is to recognise status differentiation without creating a hierarchy of oppression, and the second is to use the diversity of experience within the group as a source for learning rather than a reason for division. Difference should become an integral part of the learning experience. As Brummer and Simmonds state,

> We learn by perceiving difference. . . . Learning is the process by which these differences are perceived and become incorporated into our prior frameworks and in the process become transformed and changed by them.
>
> (1992: 57)

CONFLICT WITHIN THE GROUP SETTING

Brookfield, defining classrooms, states:

> they are not limpid tranquil ponds cut off from the river of social, cultural and political life. They are contested spaces – whirlpools containing the contradictory cross currents of struggles for material superiority and ideological legitimacy that exist in the world outside.
>
> (Brookfield 1995: 19)

Most models of group development identify a stage of conflict, disruption and challenge. This phase can be perceived as one of uncertainty and testing out. Tuckman and Jensen (1977) refer to this as 'storming', Heron (1993) as 'stormy weather', echoing the turbulence described by Brookfield. They argue that this stage is likely to occur before the group establishes its norms, or that it occurs at any time within the life of the group in response to an incident that raises anxiety and lowers trust, resulting in red cycle behaviours. However, in our experience of learning groups, not all groups go through this stage. It is dependent on the length and purpose of the group; for example, a short information-giving session is unlikely to provoke the same level of anxiety in learners as a five-day counselling course.

The word 'conflict' tends to have negative connotations. It is seen as something that is unpleasant and should be avoided. Consequently, groups tend to avoid conflict by denial, displacement, withdrawal, suppressing opinions and failing to challenge. This enables both learners and trainers to avoid some of the uncomfortable feelings that accompany disagreement.

Yet conflict can be productive and can result in the following benefits:

- an exploration of a range of ideas and views;
- an intense involvement with the task;
- a better understanding of the problem;
- active participation;
- an increase in confidence and skill to address other conflicts.

(Schultz 1989)

Within the learning group, conflict that engenders this type of response can be seen to promote learning, because participants are actively engaged in green cycle activity. It also equips learners with tools for managing conflict effectively in their working practice.

Types of conflict

It is important to differentiate between types of conflict as not all forms of conflict promote learning. The trainer needs to assess the type of conflict that is occurring within the group so that they can try to use it productively. Schultz (1989) describes four different types of conflict, which are considered in Table 6.3:

1   Productive
2   Destructive
3   Integrative
4   Distributive.

The productive and integrative types of conflict reflect learners' openness by reconsidering their positions as they listen to other perspectives. The destructive and distributive forms of conflict are not so conducive to learning as they describe situations which can be stressful. In these situations learners hold polarised views and become defensive, putting up blocks to learning (Schultz 1989).

Managing conflict

Table 6.3 describes the different forms of conflict that can occur within a learning group. The trainer has a task in managing the conflict so as to

Table 6.3 Types of conflict

Type of conflict	Definition	Indicators	Task for trainer
Productive	Promotes the finding of a positive solution based on negotiation. This can include agreeing to disagree on certain points	Participants discuss and debate the issues to resolve a problem	Ensure that the focus remains issue based and the group is working towards a problem resolution or at least a respect for and willingness to reflect on difference
Destructive	The issues are unresolved and the focus becomes person centred	Relationships become strained. Individuals are attacked and discredited for holding their views	To restore the focus on the issue. Reinforce the idea that the difference being debated is views, not individuals
Integrative	A resolution is found which is based on collaboration and integrates the various group members' perspectives. In this situation there is a sense of everyone having their needs met	Participants listen and debate to understand each other's points of view with an open mind and are prepared to reframe their perspective in the light of others' contributions	Ensure that all contributions are given a voice. That certain group members do not dominate and that the agreed solution reflects the group discussion and is based on this rather than manipulation or abuse of power by a forceful few. This method is particularly relevant to multi-disciplinary groups
Distributive	Somebody wins at someone else's expense	A sub-group are dominating and making all the decisions, ignoring or discrediting the contributions of others	In this situation some participants can feel intimidated and discredited. Trust and effective communication between group members needs to be restored

enable the group to use difference as a way of promoting learning. When a conflict situation arises the trainer needs to make an assessment as to the way in which both individual group learners and the trainer themselves are managing the conflict. Individuals will have very different styles – some will want to confront and challenge; others may be more contained. It may be that they are using a method of conflict management that promotes learning; however, at other times they may be managing conflict in a way that blocks their learning and the learning of others. For example, a learner may state that anti-oppressive practice is 'irrelevant'. The individual learner's own need to hold this view is so great that they will not take on board the views of others. Other learners in the group become so intimidated that they avoid any challenge. In this situation, unless the trainer intervenes, the course learning can be undermined. The task for the trainer, in terms of managing conflict, will also depend on the stage which the group is at, how it has been functioning and the agency or inter-agency culture of conflict management. If conflict occurs at the beginning of the group when anxiety is high, the trainer may need to emphasise collaboration while not suppressing issues of difference. As the group progresses, the levels of anxiety and trust should enable the group to manage more conflict, provided that it is utilised to facilitate learning. In every situation the trainer needs to assess what is occurring within the group, and consider methods of intervention that seek to use conflict as a productive way of exploring difference. Consideration needs to be given, when planning the programme, to ways of managing conflict, as the trainer may be required to alter the course content to address issues of difference. In this situation it may be necessary to change the programme to enable the learning agreement to be revisited or exercises introduced to reduce anxiety and increase trust or explore the area of conflict further.

The trainer can thus be seen to have a number of tasks to complete in conflict situations. These are:

- to restore green cycle activity and contain anxiety;
- to model and facilitate an expression of difference, enabling learners to model this approach in managing issues of power and conflict with service users;
- to reinforce responsibilities of individual participants for their own learning;
- to establish the learning contract as a framework for working through issues of difference;
- to demonstrate that the course will meet learning needs.

SUMMARY

The learning group

A group becomes an effective medium for learning if attention is given to both group task and group process. Consideration also needs to be given to the way that individual learners manage and contain the anxiety and uncertainty associated with learning and the influence that this has on others within the group. The trainer needs to be mindful that they are also a member of the group and that the way they manage their anxiety can influence group learning. A central task for the trainer is the containment of anxiety.

Functional/dysfunctional learning

The way in which individual learners, the group and the trainer contain their levels of anxiety during the life of the group will influence the learning process. Different behaviours give an indication as to whether the learners are operating in a functional green cycle or in the cycle of dysfunctional learning's red cycle.

The trainer needs regularly to evaluate group behaviours and their own responses. Their role is to model and maintain green cycle behaviours and address red cycle behaviours if they occur.

Group phases

Each learning group will have different dynamics that will influence the way that the group develops. The trainer should be mindful of the various phases that the group may pass through. Heron defines the four phases as:

1 Defensiveness
2 Working through defensiveness
3 Authentic behaviour
4 Closure.

Each phase requires the trainer to undertake specific tasks in order to enable the group to move successfully to the next stage.

The impact of status, power and discrimination

A learning group does not function in isolation. Learners bring with them the norms, values and beliefs of the organisation and culture in which they live and work. The trainer has a responsibility to ensure that the learning group does not mirror the broader culture, reinforcing oppression that can act as a block to learning.

Managing conflict

If issues of difference are to be addressed by the group, then situations of conflict are likely to arise. Conflict can be positive, promoting learning, or can be negative, disempowering learners and blocking learning. The trainer needs to analyse the way in which conflict is being managed by the group but also by individual learners, promoting conflict management that encourages learning.

Chapter 7

Facilitating group learning

This chapter considers:

- the impact of the training style on group learning;
- the roles and responsibilities of the trainer as facilitator of learning;
- the benefits of co-facilitation;
- promoting learning through co-facilitation;
- managing the co-facilitation partnership;
- dilemmas for visiting trainers.

'A good trainer is someone who gives you something you could never have from reading books.'

'A trainer is someone who helps you appreciate what you already know.'

'A trainer is more than a teacher. They share their knowledge and experience but also make sure that everyone else is able to share theirs.'

'A trainer is someone who makes learning fun.'

'A trainer should send me away with a thirst for more.'

(Group of social workers in Ukraine)

These comments were made by a group of social workers in Ukraine, evaluating their first experiential social work training course. Facilitation of learning is perceived by educationists to refer to the methods by which the facilitator 'assists' the learner to make sense of the learning experience (Taylor 1996; Brookfield 1996). The comments above indicate that this is also, partially, the expectation of learners. The term 'assists', used on its own, implies that the trainer is there to deliver the training package, utilise the training materials appropriately and ensure that conditions to facilitate learning are in place. Yet the Ukrainian social workers' remarks indicate training being more than this. What is it that distinguishes a 'good' trainer from the rest? Why do we get a sense on some training courses that the trainer is mechanically working their way through a programme while others make the programme come alive? These questions imply that there is another dimension to facilitating learning that is crucial and that is the relationship between the trainer or facilitator and the learning group. A good facilitator will identify the group's uniqueness and develop a rapport with the group that is designed to meet the learners' specific learning needs. This was described very clearly by one of the Ukrainian social workers, who was comparing and contrasting the experiences of different learning groups.

> 'It is bound to be different. As you have different relationships with different friends I suppose you will have different relationships with different groups. . . . Our group didn't need much to get us thinking. I suppose others may need more.'
>
> (Ukrainian social worker)

Facilitating learning is not a standardised process. It requires skill in terms of assessing the learning needs of the specific group and adapting the style of facilitation to meet these needs. In this chapter we explore the various dimensions of the relationship between the trainer and learner, identifying the challenge for the facilitator of balancing task and process issues. The roles and responsibilities of the trainer during the learning event are identified and the impact of the management of these roles on the learning process discussed. The second half of the chapter explores another dimension of facilitation – the benefits and challenges of co-facilitation – and concludes with strategies for establishing and managing a co-facilitation relationship that promotes group learning. Finally, there is a consideration of issues related to the use of visiting trainers.

The term 'facilitator' will be used, throughout this chapter, to refer to the facilitation of learning, and references to trainers will be in the context of them as facilitators of learning.

THE JUGGLING ACT: BALANCING CHALLENGE AND SUPPORT TO PROMOTE LEARNING

The key task for the trainer as a facilitator of effective learning is to create and sustain a climate that is supportive yet encourages challenge and risk taking in order to promote change. Jacobsen and McKinnon (1989) consider how challenge and support interact in the context of counselling. This has been adapted so as to consider the lessons for the trainer facilitating learning.

The way in which the trainer balances challenge and support is likely to influence the learner and can promote or discourage functional learning, as described below.

High challenge/low support

The trainer

The trainer is likely to present as the 'expert' or take a very didactic and controlling approach. They may well see training as an ego trip. The message the trainer gives is this: 'I'm the expert let's see what you're made of.' There is no responsibility for the group or acknowledgement of the personal, professional and organisational blocks that may impact on the learner's ability to learn and apply the learning to practice.

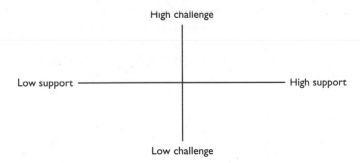

Figure 7.1 The interaction of challenge and support in facilitating training
Source: Jacobsen and McKinnon (1989)

The learner

The learner can feel anxious and under stress, as any challenge to the trainer is seen as a personal attack and dismissed, so that learners are unlikely to challenge the trainer. Learners are often pushed to take risks and placed on the spot with little warning, and this is often done in a highly competitive manner that is designed to display the trainer's expertise. The trainer may become defensive and hostile, exhibiting the fight and flight behaviours associated with anxiety. Whatever the learner attempts to learn from the training it is unlikely to result in positive change as there is no framework of support.

Low support/low challenge

The trainer

The trainer is likely to be distant from the group and uninterested. They do not bother to establish a rapport in order to engage with the group. The course content and methods of delivery will provide few new learning opportunities and there is little attention to time boundaries, absentees or specific needs raised by participants. This approach may be dressed up as self-directed learning, the trainer giving the message, 'I'm sorry but I'm not an expert – don't expect too much.'

The learner

The learner is likely to feel bored, devalued and demotivated. This may result in apathy and the learner is therefore unlikely to challenge the trainer. The learner is likely to disengage both physically, through poor attendance, and emotionally and intellectually, through lack of participation.

Low challenge/high support

The trainer

The trainer colludes with the group or encourages the group to look after the trainer; the focus is on process rather than task. The emphasis is on feeling safe and enjoying being together as a group. The message from the trainer is, 'I'm no expert, you are the real experts.' The trainer is unwilling to take any risks in terms of offering challenges. The content reinforces the learner's current practice, using familiar and safe training techniques.

The learner

The learner is likely to feel safe, secure and complacent. The lack of dissonance prevents any prospect of real learning or change. There is likely to be strong group pressure to preserve the *status quo*, and the individual learner who challenges this situation is likely to be isolated by the trainer and the rest of the group. Such groups may in fact be very insecure underneath, as the trainer may have displaced personal insecurities onto the group. They may become angry at the double bind they have been placed in as learners and protectors of the trainer.

High challenge/high support

The trainer

The trainer will provide a course that is challenging in terms of both content and methods of delivery. However, this will be delivered in an environment that feels supportive. The trainer will pay attention to both task and process, creating a climate of trust and respect, recognising the potential for learners to learn not just from the trainer but also from each other. The message from the trainer is, 'I've got expertise you've got expertise, let's make it work'.

The learner

The learner will be prepared to take risks and learn from their mistakes without fear of criticism. They are likely to feel supported in their learning by both the trainer and other learners. There will be a high level of motivation to reflect and to learn, with a willingness to reappraise values and learn new skills and knowledge. Difficult issues will be confronted and anxiety is used productively to harness energy.

The use of authority

The task, then, for the trainer is to create a high challenge, high support environment as this is the setting that is most likely to result in effective learning. However, the trainer's ability to achieve this will be influenced by their previous experiences. For example, they may lack confidence as a result of a previous learning group experience and their learned responses, especially in relation to the use of authority. For instance, in more challenging environments do we tend to become controlling and authoritarian or do we withdraw? A trainer is therefore bringing with them their own fears and anxieties – such as anxiety about losing control or of being resented by participants for having all the power and control. Reid, referring to ways in which social workers manage these anxieties in therapeutic groups, highlights issues that can apply equally to those facilitating learning groups. He states, 'The anxiety linked to these fears and fantasies lead to defensive manoeuvres and security operations by the worker as a means of maintaining control' (Reid 1988: 124).

It is helpful to consider the actual authority that the facilitator has by virtue of their role, which promotes effective learning. The main types of authority are described by Jaques (1992) as follows: 'in authority', the legitimate authority vested in the trainer by agency and learners to ensure that effective learning occurs; 'an authority', the trainer usually has some recognised expertise – knowledge, values and skills – that enables them to facilitate the learning group.

However, a trainer who is unable to contain their own anxiety while facilitating a group is likely to use authority in a dysfunctional way. Jaques describes this as follows: 'authoritarian', a directive, controlling approach towards facilitating group learning which disempowers learners.

Facilitators may adopt a high challenge, low support approach if they have anxieties about managing the legitimate forms of authority vested in them as trainers. For example, if a trainer is unsure about their ability to manage the group process, ensuring effective learning, they may become very controlling and directive, concerned that by giving up some of the leadership function the group will get out of control. Alternatively, the trainer may hand over responsibilities to the group, denying any authority and take a low challenge, low support approach. A trainer's anxiety about being an expert, constantly in the limelight and feeling the need to get everything right may result in an authoritarian style where questioning and challenging are discouraged. Alternatively, the trainer may avoid the expert role and expect the group to become the experts for each other.

THE TRAINER AS FACILITATOR OF FUNCTIONAL LEARNING: FOUR KEY ROLES

In a high support, high challenge climate there should be a shared sense of responsibility for learning and an understanding of teaching as being about listening and eliciting information as well as imparting knowledge (Jaques 1992). In this way the trainer becomes a facilitator of learning for members of a learning group. However, creating a shared sense of responsibility for learning is not a simple task. As described in Chapter 5, it requires an appropriate climate for learning, and as highlighted above the trainer also needs to pay attention to both process and task as well as self-awareness about their own ways of managing anxiety. Thus the facilitation of learning requires the trainer to take on a number of roles. These can be grouped as follows:

● leader: the trainer is responsible for the management of the training event, ensuring that the task is achieved and process issues are addressed;
● teacher: the trainer has a role in introducing new knowledge, values and skills, enabling the facilitation of learning that meets the aims and objectives of the learning programme;
● member of the group: the trainer by their very presence will influence the dynamics of the group;
● audience: the trainer provides opportunities for participants to experiment and gain feedback on their learning.

(Rogers 1996)

Facilitation is therefore multi-faceted. The relationship between trainer and participant is based on the management of these roles. The issue for the trainer is that each group needs a different balance of these roles at various stages in its life. Consequently, effective facilitation requires continual assessment and evaluation of the various roles.

The leadership role

The trainer facilitating a learning group can be compared to a conductor of an orchestra. The conductor is responsible for guiding the members of the orchestra through the piece of music. Yet, to enable this to be done effectively, the conductor needs to listen continually and assess the way in which the sections of the orchestra are working together, ensuring that certain players do not dominate, that the pace is appropriate for all sections and, when appropriate, that different sections of the orchestra are allowed to be heard above the rest. If the conductor does not pay attention to the way in which the individual players are playing together and the way they are influencing each other, the quality of sound will be affected. In the same way the trainer facilitating a learning group needs to pay attention to the task and the group atmosphere (Bion 1961; Brown 1994). This requires the facilitator to demonstrate two types of leadership style: task leadership – the focus being on achieving the learning aims and objectives; and maintenance leadership, which is concerned with the interactions of the group members, their feelings and level of participation (Brown 1994). The task for the trainer is achieving the right balance between meeting the aims and objectives of the course and maintaining a positive group atmosphere, ensuring functional learning, as described in Chapter 6. If this balance is not achieved it can reduce the potential for learning. For example, if the focus is exclusively on achieving the task, participants can feel that their individual needs are being ignored. In contrast, a trainer who is concerned with maintaining a positive group atmosphere may be reluctant to introduce controversial material or challenge group participants for fear of jeopardising the group atmosphere (Schultz 1989).

Smith, evaluating research undertaken on the interaction between group facilitator and group, concludes that 'an effective facilitator continually assesses the learning climate and takes responsibility for providing the elements, at least temporarily, that the group are unable to provide for themselves.' He concludes, 'leader skills lie in tailoring one's interventions to the emerging culture of the group' (Smith 1980: 98).

Heron reinforces this point, and describes three different modes of facilitation that are likely to be required during the life of the learning group:

- *Hierarchical mode.* This is usually required at the beginning of a group when the learners are feeling insecure and dependent on the trainer.
- *Co-operation mode.* As the group gains confidence there is potential for collaboration and negotiation. At this stage learners are able to orientate themselves and participate in decisions about the learning process.
- *Autonomy mode.* Towards the end of the life of the group learners have gained some competence in the development of their newly

acquired knowledge, values and skills and are able to take responsibility for their learning.

(Heron 1989)

Heron believes that these modes are indicators of the leadership styles likely to be utilised by the facilitator in conjunction with learners, at different stages in the life of the group. However, as described in Chapter 6, learning groups do not follow rigid rules in terms of the way in which they develop. Anxiety regarding learning and levels of trust within the group are likely to fluctuate. This in turn will influence the ability of learners to engage in the leadership tasks implied by the co-operative and autonomy modes in Heron's description. For example, if levels of anxiety are contained and trust is high, learners are likely to engage in decision making. When anxiety is high and trust low it is more likely that learners will want a leader-centred approach. Thus the trainer will need to provide for more of the decision making which the groups are unable to manage. Coulshed presents a continuum of leadership styles which demonstrates the different effects of either a leader- or group-centred approach on decision making (see Figure 7.2). She applied this to teams, but it has been adapted to apply to a learning group.

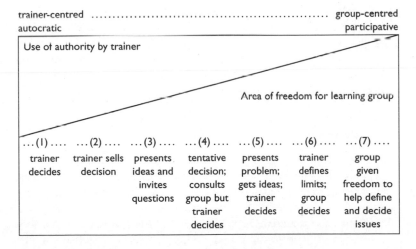

Figure 7.2 A continuum of leadership styles
Source: Coulshed (1990: 108)

Responsive leadership facilitation

As tensions and conflict arise during the life of the group the trainer may have to vary their style to address these issues. Baldwin and Williams (1988) highlight how the leadership style adopted by the trainer should be part of a continuum which responds to learner behaviour (see Figure 7.3).

Trainers need to be able to operate along all of these dimensions in response to the needs of the learning group.

The educator role

As a trainer, one needs to balance valuing participants' experience and facilitating their learning with the provision of new knowledge, values and skills. As facilitators of adult learners, one can become so determined to value the participants' experience that the focus becomes restricted solely to the sharing of past and current experiences rather than offering new knowledge, values and skills in the context of those experiences. If trainers are not prepared to act as a resource in terms of providing additional information, beyond that of the participants' own experience, then they are 'Condemning . . . adults to remaining within existing paradigms of thought and action' (Brookfield 1996: 124).

One of the roles of the trainer is therefore to act as educator to offer new information, alternative approaches and skills, and to challenge current thinking. Jarvis (1995) describes three different approaches towards the teaching or educative task. A trainer is likely to require all three approaches during the life of most training events, as the approaches can be seen to reflect the continuum from teacher- to student-centred learning, which was discussed above. However, the needs of different learning groups may require a greater emphasis on one or others of the approaches.

Didactic teaching

A trainer operating in this fashion would act as the agent of transmission of a body of knowledge. The course participant is expected to learn what is being transmitted and to be able to reproduce it when necessary. As described above, there is a positive role for clear presentations of theory and case material. The drawback to this approach is that little consideration is paid to the way in which the learner is actually understanding, analysing and evaluating the learning.

This style is often adopted in training when a significant number of

The trainer moves between being:

in the forefront	→	to being →	in the background

the learner moves between being

passive	→	to being →	active, self-directing

The trainer moves between being:

directive	→	→	non-directive
making decisions	→	to being →	enabling decisions
taking the lead	→	→	following

The learner moves between being:

dependent	→	→	planning, proactive
a follower	→	to being →	self-programming
uncommitted	→	→	committed, engaged

The trainer moves between being:

protective	→	→	challenging
sheltering	›	to being →	exposing
controlling	→	→	releasing

The learner moves between being:

unsure	→	→	taking risks, experimenting
insecure	→	to being →	secure
cautious	→	→	creative

The trainer moves between being:

energetic	→	→	quiet
controlling	→	to being →	reflective
assessing	→	→	facilitating self-evaluation

The learner moves between:

observing the rules	→	→	leading/challenging
unreflective	→	to being →	self-critical
distanced	→	→	involved

The trainer moves between:

monitoring	→	to	→ reviewing
assessing	›		→ facilitating reflection

The learner moves between:

assessed	→	to	→ valuing

Figure 7.3 Responsive leadership styles
Source: Baldwin and Williams (1988)

the workforce need to be made aware of and be able to apply new legislation, policies and procedures. This can result in what is often referred to as 'sheep-dipping exercises', where large numbers of staff are introduced to new policies and procedures through a presentation by the trainer. This may be followed by questions of clarification and an exercise that focuses on policy implementation. There is usually no opportunity to challenge, or look in depth at the implications of the policy.

Socratic teaching

This approach describes the use of reflective questioning in the teaching and learning process. The trainer asks a logically sequenced series of questions of learners, encouraging them to respond utilising their knowledge and skills. However, the questions are asked in such a way as to enable learners to make explicit learning that may have been internalised implicitly but never actually formulated or articulated. The benefit is that the learner, through reflecting as to why they work in certain ways, can begin to transfer that learning to new situations. For example, learners may have experience of undertaking needs assessments with a specific client group. Through appropriate questioning the trainer encourages learners to identify the key components for an effective assessment enabling them to generalise from their specific experience. These generalisations can, in turn, be applied to other client group assessments. This may be done by setting questions to be discussed in small groups, enabling all learners to be involved in the discussion.

Facilitative teaching

This approach centres on the trainer providing or creating a climate in which learning may occur, but the trainer does not entirely control the outcome of the learning experience. The approach seeks to create an awareness of a specific learning need among learners. Once they are aware of a learning gap, the trainer provides the participants with an experience and encourages reflection on that experience, thus facilitating learning. The participants may reach conclusions that are different from those held by the facilitator. For example, the trainer may facilitate an exercise asking participants to identify potential abusive behaviour towards vulnerable adults. The exercise may raise participants' awareness of abusive behaviour but they may employ different standards from that of the trainer. This can generate a different view of what can be perceived as abusive behaviour – an outcome which the trainer may not have anticipated and which causes the trainer to change tack and explore underlying assumptions and attitudes towards what constitutes abuse.

The facilitator as group member

The relationship between the trainer and the learning group is crucial to the learning group dynamic, as described in Chapter 6. Rogers considers this, and concludes that 'to facilitate significant learning the trainer requires certain attitudinal qualities that they should utilise in their relationship with learners' (Rogers 1993). These are set out below.

Realness

The trainer is not merely there in a neutral capacity but brings with them their own feelings, values, likes and dislikes. It is by demonstrating this realness that participants are able to relate to the trainer and begin to feel that they are sharing a real experience. For example, one of the authors is a weak speller; for many years she tried bluffing her way through training events writing on flip charts in an ambiguous way if she felt the spelling was not accurate and wondering whether participants would laugh at them. Eventually she decided to be open about this weakness and state at the beginning of the course that she cannot spell and had no objection to having spelling corrected. Group members responded positively to this approach. Participants have often commented that they felt far more relaxed once the comment about spelling was made, as it made them feel that the trainer was human and helped to break down a barrier between the trainer and participants. Others have stated that it gave them permission to make mistakes.

Realness cannot rely merely on what the trainer says; it requires congruence between verbal and non-verbal communication, between the trainer's attitudes and values and the way in which these are modelled in the trainer's behaviour. For example, the trainer sets an exercise, the group complete the task but the trainer senses a feeling of flatness among participants and finds that facilitating feedback is extremely difficult. Unless the trainer is honest and states that they sense a flatness among the group and describe how this makes them feel, they do not give the group permission to express their feelings and identify and resolve issues.

Prizing, acceptance and trust

This describes the way in which a trainer accepts each learner's right to their own views. This enables each participant to feel that they are being recognised as individuals with their own learning needs, and should promote a climate of learning. However, acceptance of learners' views and opinions does not necessarily mean agreeing with them. Prizing, acceptance and trust need to be considered within an anti-oppressive framework where difference is accepted and valued. If this is not the case, the trainer needs to challenge. Acceptance is not an excuse to ignore behaviours, views and opinions that oppress and devalue, as this will result in an atmosphere of distrust, with some learners feeling devalued.

Empathetic understanding

Rogers describes this as the way in which the trainer tries to appreciate the issues for participants struggling with learning, or with issues in their agency, from the learners' perspective. The trainer does this by observing both the group and individuals and their struggles, and perhaps approaching them individually, or acknowledging out loud difficulties facing individuals or the group as a whole – for instance, sharing concern regarding lack of management support or allowing some time for the group to process a difficult issue. In this way the learner's struggles are valued and accepted.

Power and status

It is the way in which the trainer acknowledges and manages power and authority within the learning group context that facilitates or debilitates the learning experience. Authority can be seen as the sanctioned use of power, while power is the ability to implement the rights of authority (French and Raven 1959). The way these are modelled by the trainer are particularly important in social care training, as the use of power and authority is an integral part of social care practice. The inappropriate use of authority within a learning group could be mirrored in poor practice back at the worksite.

The attitudinal qualities described above emphasise the importance of respecting and valuing the learner and should facilitate learning. However, what the trainer considers to be a respectful and democratic way of relating to learners can be experienced by learners as oppressive and restrictive. Brookfield identifies the following methods thought by trainers to be co-operative and empowering approaches but which may be perceived by some learners as oppressive:

The circle   Social care training courses are usually physically set up so that the group of learners are sitting in a semi-circle. This is designed to draw everyone into discussion and enables everyone to be seen and heard. However for some learners who are shy, or self-conscious about their appearance or have a physical disability the circle can feel very threatening. Some professionals who are used to more formal training also prefer and need to sit behind tables.

Trainers at one with learners   Some trainers emphasise that training is about co-learning and stress the equality between themselves and the learner. However a trainer cannot ignore the power and status she has within the group because of her very position as trainer. This can be particularly difficult for some trainers to accept, particularly in situations where they are paid significantly less than those who are attending the training.

The trainer as fly on the wall   As a trainer it is easy to forget that one still exerts an influence when learners are working together in small groups. The presence of the trainer in the room is likely to have an influence in as much as learners may be guarded about what they say or look to the trainer for approval or censure.

Discussion as spontaneous combustion   Trainers often regard group discussion as an effective way of engaging the group in learning, particularly when the trainer remains silent and the discussion is between learners. For some learners this can be an oppressive experience. For example, if they are too anxious to talk in a large group or are afraid of saying something that sounds stupid. Other learners need time to reflect and may find the pace of discussion intimidating.

'I want to hear your opinion not mine'   Trainers often withhold their opinions to encourage learners to express their points of view. However, this can induce mistrust and block if learners believe the trainer is tricking them into making mistakes only to then give them the 'right' answer. In these situations trainers who do not share their opinions can be seen to be playing power games.

(Brookfield 1995)

While acknowledging that the facilitator has to exercise certain forms of power and authority in order for the group to feel secure and leadership to be exercised, there are other forms of authority and power that may be inappropriate. These would include the ascribed types of power which maintain group dependency on the trainer and do not encourage experiential learning. There is also the power which is self-promoting or self-seeking in support of the trainer's own ego. The trainer needs to be clear about what are their legitimate and necessary powers to facilitate learning while rejecting sources of power which are illegitimate and can block learning. Figure 7.4 shows the interplay between legitimate and illegitimate forms of power and those that are implicitly and explicitly used by the trainer.

Burgess and Taylor (1995) suggest that the facilitator can take account of the power issues and manage them in an empowering manner if they are clear about the following:

- their roles over and above the facilitating task. For example, is the trainer there in an assessment capacity? What are the

Legitimate

POSITION, EXPERT, ASSESSOR	INFORMATION, EXPERIENCE
This provides a clear framework. Learners are aware of authority and power held by the trainer.	Both trainer and learners may be unaware of the way in which these legitimate sources of power are being used. This can lead to uncertainty and anxiety as learners are not clear as to the power and authority of trainer.

Explicit ———————————————————————— Implicit

'STAR' POWER, COERCION, SOCIAL REWARD	CONNECTION, REFERENT, GENDER, RACE
Emphasis here is on the trainer controlling the group in an overt way. This can result in fear and oppression. Learners may suppress views and opinions that do not conform to the trainer's expectations. The learners may be aware of the power being used but feel too disempowered to challenge. Alternatively, strong groups may begin a mutiny.	The group may be covertly divided between those 'favoured' and those out of favour with the trainer. Feelings of fear, anxiety and uncertainty are likely to dominate. Learners are unable to challenge as the source of the trainer's power is not clear.

Illegitimate

Figure 7.4 Interplay between legitimate and illegitimate sources of power and those explicitly and implicitly used by trainers

trainer's responsibilities if they have concerns about a participant's practice?

- what is negotiable during the life of the group and how the trainer will exercise this power. For example, is a certain level of attendance required? What will happen if participants continue to behave in an oppressive manner?

- the power relationships that exist outside the group within the context of the social care organisation, and the impact that this has on the power relationships within the group. For example, the organisation's value base, the policies and procedures on equal opportunities.

This process makes explicit the trainer's legitimate forms of power and authority.

The trainer as audience/evaluator

Critical analysis is essential during the learning process if it is to have meaning (Taylor 1996). This analysis should include an evaluation of both process and content, enabling participants to make sense of their learning experience. The trainer has a role in facilitating this analysis, but the way in which this evaluation is managed will affect the way in which it is received and acted upon. If the trainer analyses what is going on in the group or comments on an individual's contribution, this can feel very threatening and disempowering. Much of the threat can be taken out of the process if the trainer enables the group to take much of the initiative and responsibility to self-evaluate (Jaques 1992). Heron describes this approach as the co-operative mode. In this situation the trainer alerts participants to the task or process issue and asks them to comment and give their own meaning to it. Once they have done this the group will become much more receptive to the trainer's evaluative comments. The view of the trainer will be balanced by these other perceptions (Heron 1989).

Consideration also needs to be given to the timing of feedback during the course. Feedback is most constructive if given when participants have time to act on it to enhance learning, rather than at the end of the course when the potential to respond and act on the feedback is severely reduced. In this way mutual evaluation can become an integral part of the learning process that can inform both individual and group development. Jaques identifies four features of effective evaluation which are likely to promote learning (1992):

1 If it creates a climate of openness and trust rather than a sense of secrecy and mistrust.

2 If it is undertaken co-operatively.

3 Where it is organised as a process through the life of the group with a view to learning from the evaluation and opportunities to change and adapt.

4 If the evaluation is to be used for formal assessment this should be made very explicit.

The trainer has a facilitative role in assisting the group to give and receive effective feedback continually. An effective way of managing this is by acting as a role model (Burgess 1992). This can be achieved by inviting participants to comment on the way the trainer is managing their role and responsibilities and facilitating the participants' learning. Although trainers can feel very anxious about this, if group participants see that the trainer is prepared to adapt their approach, in response to feedback, the participants are more likely to respond to feedback in a similar manner (Miles 1971).

In this section we have considered the complex tasks that a trainer needs to undertake in order to facilitate group learning effectively. The learning experience can be enhanced if these tasks are shared between two trainers. In the last half of the chapter we consider the ways in which this can be achieved.

CO-TRAINING

Co-training, at its most minimal, refers to a team of two trainers who, to a greater or lesser extent, share the task of group facilitation. However, in this chapter we argue that to maximise the potential of co-training for both participants and trainers, co-training should include the joint planning, delivery and evaluation of the training course. Consideration is given to ways in which to negotiate, plan, deliver and evaluate a co-training event to ensure that it provides an appropriate learning climate for participants and a rewarding experience for the trainers. The starting point is an exploration of the potential benefits and pitfalls of co-training.

What are the benefits of co-training?

If effective, co-training, can promote functional learning because it enables trainers:

- *to share the task of preparation, course design and delivery.* This provides different perspectives and a wider knowledge and skills base, which means that a broader span of learner needs are likely to be addressed in the design and delivery of the training;
- *to divide group facilitation roles* so one trainer can focus on process issues while the other trainer focuses on task. For example, as one trainer delivers a presentation or facilitates feedback from an exercise, the other trainer can focus on the group response, identifying ways in which course participants relate to the material, each other and to the trainers. As a result, it is easier to monitor the performance of group task but also to evaluate the group process. This is likely to promote a green cycle environment and aid the identification of red cycle behaviour, as described in detail in Chapter 6;
- *to tease out issues* – for example, learners' poor practice or dysfunctional learning behaviours. Co-training enables a sharing of perspectives and observations so that the trainers can make a mutual assessment of the cause of the problem, ensuring that one trainer is not simply acting on a personal basis;
- *to offer each other support and guidance.* This support can be cognitive – for example, a trainer may be unsure of a response to a question from a learner and can check out with the other trainer. It can also be emotional. At times during a training course the trainer's energy levels are likely to fall or a trainer may be personally affected by some material that is considered. In these situations the co-trainer can provide space for the other trainer to manage their feelings. Physically, co-training means that such tasks as dividing groups up, distributing pens and flip-chart paper, using video equipment can all be shared;
- *to increase a sense of objectivity.* As a trainer it is very easy to become subjective when facilitating a learning group. This can occur in terms of feelings towards the organisation – for example, if the trainer feels personally very sceptical about new guidelines and procedures – and this can be conveyed to learners so they in turn become negative, which can block their learning. Trainers can also relate subjectively to different learners. For example, if a learner gives the trainer positive feedback, the trainer may inadvertently be

seen to 'reward' that learner by responding to their learning needs over and above those of other learners. Alternatively, a trainer may feel hostile towards a learner who continually challenges them and may respond by ignoring their learning needs. A co-trainer can restore a sense of perspective by pointing out the behaviour and analysing with the other trainer why this may be occurring and considering strategies to restore a more objective approach;

● *to utilise a range of learning methods.* Some training methods require two trainers in order to be effective – for example, demonstrations, providing feedback on small group role plays and skill development work;

● *to provide a more diverse learning experience.* Two trainers are likely to bring a broader range of experience. This can be particularly important in terms of gender, race and different disciplines for inter-agency training. Two trainers, from different backgrounds, working together in an anti-oppressive way, provide positive role models for learners;

● *to take the pressure off learners.* Learners can feel responsible for protecting a trainer facilitating a learning group on their own by, for example, being reluctant to raise issues. Co-training enables the trainers to maintain boundaries between themselves and the learners; they establish an identity that is separate from that of the learning group, which allows issues of difference and conflict within the group to be explored more readily as members do not feel the same need to look after the trainer. It also enables learners to have some choice in terms of relating to the trainers, particularly regarding personal issues that may arise as a result of the learning.

● *to pay greater attention to the needs of individual participants.* As described in Chapters 5 and 6 individual learners come to learning with their own specific needs. While the trainer attempts to create a climate of learning that will meet these needs, it is likely that some learners will have specific needs that require more individual attention. For example, it may be that most of the group are operating in green cycle but two learners are displaying flight behaviours. Co-training provides opportunities to give these learners some individual attention to restore them to green cycle, while still meeting the learning needs of the rest of the group.

Many course participants, and indeed some trainers feel that co-training is an easy option. Trainers divide up the course with your 'bit' and my 'bit', and consequently the burden of work is halved. If this minimalist approach is adopted, few of the benefits outlined above will become apparent. Indeed, it is more likely to result in dysfunctional learning. Effective co-training, like most relationships, requires continual attention to enable it to develop and grow so as to promote effective group learning opportunities.

To co-facilitate or not?

The decision as to whether a learning group requires one or two trainers should take into account the needs of the group and whether the learning is more likely to be promoted by single or co-facilitation. This can be considered in terms of the benefits of co-facilitation. If these benefits are unlikely to promote or increase the learning for the specific group, then it may be more appropriate to consider single facilitation. An assessment can be made by considering the following questions. This should be done at a very early stage in the planning of the course.

- *How many learners are there likely to be in the group?*
  Is the group so large that learners may feel a responsibility to support the trainer and consequently fail to challenge if they consider the trainer is overwhelmed by the size of the group? Is the group so small that two trainers could inhibit learners' willingness to take risks?
  What is the gender, race and status of the trainer? For example, a single, male trainer delivering a course on sexuality and older people to a female learning group may result in the learners feeling awkward and embarrassed, which could act as a block to learning.
- *What is the course content?*
  Does it include a diverse range of knowledge, values and skills that is most likely to be covered by two trainers with different areas of experience and expertise?
- *What methods of delivery are being considered?*
  Do the training methods require more than one trainer – for example, modelling and demonstrations of practice?
- *Are there likely to be very challenging process issues?*
  Is the focus of the training likely to provoke anxiety among learners, or evoke feelings of anger and anxiety towards the organisation, requiring two trainers to contain the anxiety?
- *Is the trainer on their own likely to feel threatened or vulnerable?*
  Does the trainer feels anxious or vulnerable, because of their own

past experiences or because of the training content and consequently likely to block learning?

Does the trainer feel vulnerable and anxious that they do not have sufficient knowledge and skills to manage the learning group?

● *What are the individual needs of learners likely to be?*

Are the learners likely to feel anxious about the learning experience – for example, care assistants who may not have had much formal training?

Are there individual learners who have specific needs – for example, they have a physical disability or hearing impairment which requires some individual attention from the trainer?

Promoting learning through co-training

Co-training is a difficult process that requires commitment, honesty and the valuing of difference; otherwise it can lead to situations of mistrust and competition that result in a negative learning environment – that is, both trainers and group operating in the red cycle. The major pitfalls centre on

● differences in status and power;
● conflicting approaches to training;
● different understanding of co-training;
● dysfunctional trainer behaviour.

Differences in status and power

These differences can occur in a number of arenas. We will explore this in the context of different professionals co-training, and power and status in terms of race, gender and disability. Cross (1994) highlights the issues of co-training between professionals by exploring the tensions between child protection workers, who are often perceived as of high status, and professionals working with disability, who are a group of staff often marginalised, with little or no recognition. This is especially true if the disability worker is themselves disabled. Cross states that co-training confronts the child protection worker with recognising the skills of an undervalued group of staff and facing their own attitudes towards disability. Both sets of workers need to acknowledge their ignorance of the other specialism, admit that a power imbalance exists, analyse the nature of the power differences and consider how these issues will be managed during the training course. If this does not occur, the trainers may mirror the stereotypical images that course participants hold. For example, if the child protection trainer begins the course, they may be perceived as holding more power and set a precedent whereby participants pay them more attention and direct questions to them throughout the course.

Similar differences of professional status can raise issues in inter-agency training – for example, a consultant training with a health visitor. The consultant is likely to be perceived by the group as having more power and status than the health visitor. Likewise, an external and internal trainer training together are likely to be treated in the same way, with the group and indeed the internal trainer deferring to the external trainer. Power and status can also be an issue if a trainer is training with a manager. Both the trainer and course participants may defer to the manager. If the manager has line responsibility for the trainer, the trainer may feel that they are being continually watched and evaluated and feel unable to criticise because of the managerial relationship.

Power and status are also issues in terms of gender, race and disability. Cross (1994) and Mistry and Brown (1991) identify some common problems. These include lack of awareness among the co-trainers regarding the extent to which structural racism and oppression can be mirrored by themselves or the group. For example, our experience of male/female training is that course participants tend to defer to the male trainer, directing questions and maintaining eye contact with him. Gender splitting can occur when male learners relate to the male trainer and female learners to the female trainer. In other situations the male trainer can find they are dealing with managing the task while the female trainer processes feelings. The dilemma for the female trainer is that, if the issue is not addressed, she is likely to be marginalised, and if she addresses the issue it can be perceived that she is only interested in issues that concern her. It can also be a problem for the male trainer, who may feel unable to disagree with the female trainer in front of the group.

One difficulty for co-trainers is agreeing how to manage the issues of oppression while not losing control of the training programme. As Mistry and Brown state in terms of race, white trainers tend to talk about the choice of challenging, whereas for black trainers there is no choice.

Cross highlights another issue for trainers from oppressed groups. Their potential level of internalised oppression may lead them to think that the myths and stereotypes about them are true. Consequently they can begin to take on responsibility for all the problems that arise within a group. For example, a disabled trainer with a hearing impairment may feel that the group is not engaging in debate and discussion because they think the trainer will not be able to hear and respond. The hearing-impaired trainer may suggest that their co-trainer facilitates the next session in order to promote discussion. If the co-trainer accepts this without analysing what is happening in the group, they can disempower the hearing-impaired trainer and both trainers may ignore the real reason for lack of participation.

Conflicting approaches to training

As indicated above, there are a number of different leadership styles that a trainer is required to use during the course of a training event. One of the most common pitfalls of co-training results when the trainers have different perceptions of appropriate leadership styles. This can result in situations where one trainer tends to adopt a hierarchy approach and the other trainer tends towards an autonomy approach. The consequence can be that the trainers respond to issues in different ways. For example, one trainer may want to respond to an incident by waiting to see whether the group resolves the problem before any intervention from the trainers, while the other trainer wants to be confrontational. In the same way trainers can take different approaches to learning; for example, one trainer may be didactic while the other is facilitative. In these situations learners begin to identify with, or play one trainer off against the other, and in some situations this leads to splits in the group.

Different understandings of co-training

Trainers can have different perceptions of the co-training task. Sheal outlines a range of approaches towards co-training, which are adapted and listed below:

- shared responsibility;
- turn taking;
- speak and add;
- speak and record;
- task and process;
- dominant leader;
- apprenticeship model.

(Sheal 1997)

These different approaches can be represented on a continuum, as shown in Figure 7.5.

Figure 7.5 shows that the different approaches reflect the extent to which the trainers work as equal partners within the co-training relationship. It may be that in some circumstances it is appropriate for the trainers to take an apprenticeship approach – for example, if one of the trainers is new to training and wants to learn from a more experienced trainer. However, issues can arise if trainers have not discussed and agreed on the approach for working together. The trainers also need to consider which approach is most appropriate for the particular learning situation. For example, one trainer may want to take responsibility for a certain section of the course and believes the other trainer should sit quietly and take a passive role, the turn-taking approach. They may then feel undermined if the second trainer becomes more active and responds with the speak-and-add technique and can perceive this as the second trainer taking over the session. Alternatively, a trainer may expect their co-trainer to participate, and may feel unsupported if they fail to do this. All of these responses can emphasise existing power differences.

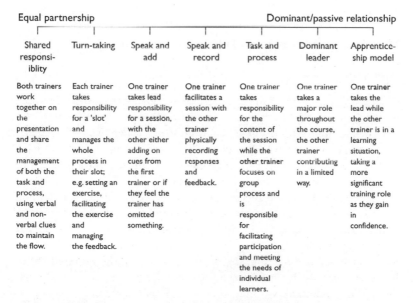

Equal partnership						Dominant/passive relationship
Shared responsiblity	Turn-taking	Speak and add	Speak and record	Task and process	Dominant leader	Apprenticeship model
Both trainers work together on the presentation and share the management of both the task and process, using verbal and non-verbal clues to maintain the flow.	Each trainer takes responsibility for a 'slot' and manages the whole process in their slot; e.g. setting an exercise, facilitating the exercise and managing the feedback.	One trainer takes lead responsibility for a session, with the other either adding on cues from the first trainer or if they feel the trainer has omitted something.	One trainer facilitates a session with the other trainer physically recording responses and feedback.	One trainer takes responsibility for the content of the session while the other trainer focuses on group process and is responsible for facilitating participation and meeting the needs of individual learners.	One trainer takes a major role throughout the course, the other trainer contributing in a limited way.	One trainer takes the lead while the other trainer is in a learning situation, taking a more significant training role as they gain in confidence.

Figure 7.5 Different approaches to the co-training relationship

Dysfunctional trainer behaviour

Early in the training, trainers may, take on roles that quickly become fixed, which results in the trainers becoming stereotyped. For example, one trainer may, early in the course, deal with a participant who is distressed. A second participant may then approach them with their problems, and very quickly that trainer is cast in the nurturing, caring role. In other groups the trainers may act out the stereotypical casting of roles in terms of race, gender and disability – for example, if the female trainer always checks on refreshment arrangements and the course domestics, modelling a negative image of a woman's role.

Learners take notice of the way in which trainers work together and will be aware of any lack of trust, openness and support for each other. This can result in the trainers modelling poor approaches to learning as they are not demonstrating the trust required to facilitate learning. For example, if one trainer continually contradicts the other trainer, and does this using put downs, the message to the learners is that it is not safe to take risks and make mistakes.

Trainers can also mirror dysfunctional group processes. For example, the trainers can get sucked into the 'flatness' or negativity of the group or its anti-management stance, or they can collude with oppressive group processes.

Managing the co-training partnership

Evaluating viability

What is apparent from the pitfalls described above is that an effective co-training partnership is dependent on trainers being prepared to work on the co-training relationship in an honest and open way. Not many trainers have the luxury of selecting a co-trainer purely on the basis that they have identified that they can train effectively together. The majority of trainers are placed in situations where they are given little choice regarding their co-trainer. For example, for inter-agency training the priority may well be two trainers who represent different disciplines rather than whether they are likely to train effectively together. Other co-training partnerships may be established on the basis that two trainers happen to be free to deliver the training on the required dates. In these situations it is easy to almost grin and bear it, and decide that there is little point considering whether their partner is the most appropriate co-trainer and that they will avoid confronting issues related to co-training. However, bearing in mind the detrimental effects that a poor co-training relationship can have on a group, co-trainers need to identify ways in which they can work together, both in the planning and delivery of the training. They need to be clear about their bottom line, beyond which either or both acknowledges that the partnership is not a viable one. There must therefore be a sharing of perceptions regarding some of the factors that contribute to the co-training relationship. These can be seen as:

- any personal experiences that the trainer feels may impact on the co-training relationship;
- their professional and training experiences of adult learning, co-training and group process;
- their knowledge, understanding and past experiences of the subject area;
- perceptions and experience of power and oppression;
- their knowledge and relationships to potential participants.

The purpose of exploring these areas is to identify:

1 Areas of congruence and potential difference and to consider whether these can be utilised to enhance the learning experience for course participants.
2 The strengths that each trainer brings to co-training and to consider how the strengths can be exploited.
3 Areas of weakness and to consider how trainers can support each other in these areas.
4 Areas of training that neither trainer feels able to fill.

Exercises designed to facilitate this process can be found in most training manuals. The exercises range from a series of questions for both trainers to consider to inventory sheets. The problem with many of these exercises is that they focus on the content – for example, 'What is your worst fear regarding co-training?' They fail to address process issues – for instance, 'We have not created a climate in which I can tell you what I fear about training with you as a result of my previous experiences.' These exercises are of little use if trainers do not feel able to be honest with each other or if differences arise which make one or both trainers feel unable to work together, and they have no strategy to manage this.

Careful consideration needs to be given to issues of power and status, and co-trainer matching, at a very early stage in the training process. One way of managing this is, at the pre-planning stage, to consider the viability of certain pairings, not in terms of individuals but on a more generalised basis. Those responsible for the management of trainers have a role in anticipating some of the problems that may arise through certain co-training matches. Consequently, processes for addressing these issues should be incorporated into training practice and planning. For example, it could be policy in a training unit that those training together for the first time meet with a consultant. The third person, acting as consultant, with the appropriate facilitation skills, can enable the co-trainers to discuss issues that may be difficult to discuss on their own (Mistry and Brown 1991).

Managing the co-training relationship needs to be an ongoing process and can be divided into three stages:

1   Planning and preparation
2   Delivery
3   Debriefing.

Planning and preparation

Assuming that the trainers feel able to work together, it can be useful to draw up a contract that covers the areas listed below. However, the trainers need to be aware that discord may only become apparent once they begin to draw up a contract and need to consider how this will be managed:

1   *Approach to planning* – this should include:

    a   a schedule and framework for planning (as described in Chapter 8);
    b   frequency, time and place of planning meetings;
    c   division of administrative tasks;
    d   process for debriefing.

2   *Approach to working together* – this should include:

    a   identifying areas of strength and weakness in terms of subject, expertise, methods of teaching and in management of group process;
    b   expectations of the co-training relationship, areas of compromise and areas of no negotiation;

c   particular needs and requirements such as, access to a flip chart
     if using a wheelchair;
d   ways in which each trainer likes and dislikes the other trainer to
     behave in terms of support and intervention;
e   identification of power issues and other factors that will
     influence the working relationship and ways of managing these.

3   *Agreed strategies towards group management* – this should include
     agreement on managing:

     a   oppressive behaviour;
     b   dangerous or poor practice;
     c   personal disclosure;
     d   conflict among participants;
     e   division of task and process.

Delivery

Co-trainers need to identify ways in which they will communicate with
each other through the life of the group. This should include evaluating:

- process issues (as described in Chapter 6);
- programme content and methods utilised (as considered in
  Chapters 8 and 9);
- working together;
- problems and issues in terms of course participants, the trainers and
  the relationship between trainers and participants.

Debriefing

At the end of the process it is important for trainers to evaluate the ways
in which they worked together and the outcomes of the course. This is
useful for a number of reasons. It enables each trainer to receive feedback on their training skills from someone who has observed their
practice, and consequently this facilitates professional development.
Second, the trainers need to evaluate the effectiveness of their co-
training relationship in order to identify strengths and weaknesses,
to consider for the future co-training as a pair, or to identify issues
to consider in new training relationships. Third, any concerns regarding learners or practice need to be considered and ways of managing
these agreed on.

The following areas should be considered, and together the trainers could identify ways of developing areas of weakness:

- the strengths and weaknesses of each trainer in terms of managing both content and process;
- the strengths and weaknesses of each trainer within the co-training relationship;
- the strengths and weaknesses of the trainers as a training pair.

Visiting trainers/speakers

Some courses involve one or two trainers taking responsibility as the anchor people on the course. However, the course may be designed with a view to other individuals attending in order to deliver certain sessions. These visiting trainers are frequently practitioners, managers, academics or professionals from outside agencies, with little training experience, who are involved in the group learning because of their organisational position or expertise. For example, a senior manager may be called upon to describe the system for implementation of new guidance. These trainers are placed in the position of a guest who arrives late to a party. The party may be in full swing, and it takes a time for the new guest to get a feel for and join in with the party mood. Likewise the visiting trainer needs an opportunity to get a feel for the group. They need to know whether the group is running as an effective learning group and if not, what are the issues and how they will impact on the visiting trainer's role. For example, the senior manager may be faced with a group who are displaying red cycle behaviours because of their anxiety regarding the new skills required to implement the guidelines. Unless this is addressed, the presentation on implementation is unlikely to result in learning and learners may displace their anxiety and anger onto the visiting trainer. The visiting trainer is likely to come with prepared material, based on the remit given to them before the course started. This can raise a number of issues – for example, the content and style of delivery may not actually meet the current needs of the learners. These are all difficult issues to address if one is a skilled trainer, but the situation presents significant problems to someone with limited training skills who is only working with the group for a very limited time.

The lead trainers have a responsibility to manage this situation. This can be done in a number of ways. First, the visiting trainer should be informed of any problems as soon as possible so that they can alter their session accordingly. Second, the visiting trainer should allow time, before the session, to meet with the lead trainers, enabling them to discuss the ways in which the learning group is functioning. It can also be helpful if the visiting trainer arrives before a lunch or drinks break and has an opportunity to meet the course participants informally.

SUMMARY

The facilitator of learning has to create an environment which is both challenging and promotes change yet is supportive and encourages risk taking in order that learning may take place. The ability of the facilitator to achieve this balance will be determined by their own levels of anxiety and ways in which these are contained and managed.

As a facilitator of learning, the trainer needs to perform a number of roles to promote functional learning. These include:

- taking responsibility for managing group learning through adopting appropriate leadership styles;
- managing the educative role by being flexible to group learning needs in terms of training style;
- being able as facilitator to act as a member of the group, acknowledging how this impacts on group functioning in terms of power and status;
- recognising that learning requires reflection and feedback, the trainer has a role in facilitating reflection and opportunities for learners to evaluate their learning.

Co-facilitation can provide potential benefits to both learners and trainers in terms of offering a richer, more diverse and varied training experience (Sheal 1997). However, these benefits will only occur if co-facilitators are able to recognise and manage difference in terms of power status and approaches to training and co-facilitation. In addition, an assessment is required as to whether the learning needs of the group are more likely to be met by single or co-facilitation.

Some trainers do brief sessions as part of a fuller training programme. Their ability to do this effectively so as to promote learning will be determined by the way in which they are briefed by the lead trainer and are able to adapt their content to meet the learning needs of the specific group.

Chapter 8

Planning training

The aims of this chapter are:

- to explore the role of the trainer as planner;
- to explore the importance of programme design;
- to present a framework for course design based on adult learning theory;
- to demonstrate through examples the application of the design framework.

Previous chapters have focused on context, learning theory and the importance of establishing a secure and positive climate for learning. In this chapter our focus returns to the content as we look at training programme design and planning. However, this is closely linked to the earlier discussions on group process and group management. Good course design, clear planning and skilled delivery of appropriate methods are essential if a secure learning environment is not only to be established but also maintained. The trainer's emotional responsiveness will not be enough if the training programme lacks direction or coherence. This requires an ability to design a training event that can translate training needs and objectives into a programme which is grounded and directed throughout by an understanding of how adults learn and a knowledge of group dynamics. The focus of this chapter is thus on the role of the trainer as planner, whose intention is to bring about learning. There are close links between this and the following chapter. However, whereas this chapter concentrates on a framework for programme design, Chapter 9 describes the variety of teaching methods available to the trainer. In this chapter, the words 'trainer' or 'facilitator' will be generally employed, in preference to 'teacher', except when work from another source is being quoted. The former terms more aptly describe the trainer's role as a facilitator of learning.

THE IMPORTANCE OF PROGRAMME DESIGN

The role of the trainer in the planning of learning is a crucial one, not because individuals always require someone else to facilitate their learning, but because where learners and trainers are engaged powerful processes are generated. As Claxton (1988) reminds us, the emotional range of experiential learning covers anxiety, fear, disappointment, surprise, shock, boredom, interest, absorption, excitement, threat, resentment, hurt, blame and comfort. These can result in both positive and negative outcomes for the learner, and indeed the teacher, but rarely result in neutral outcomes. In other words, almost everything that a trainer does, whether intentional or not, verbal or non-verbal, has an effect on learners. Thus the responsibility and the power of the trainer, which start not at the point of delivery but at the outset of planning, are considerable and sometimes underestimated. Look at the rather facetious piece quoted below, which is making a serious point about the real dangers of taking a casual approach to training.

How to create a disaster without trying hard at all

- Don't waste your time by considering the *objective* of your presentation. Get down to business immediately.
- Don't engage in futile exercises such as *analysing* your *audience's background and attitudes*.
- Don't be burdened with *strategy*. Your presentation will carry the day.
- Never lose precious time *organising* your information. No one bothers with outlines anymore.
- By all means, don't prepare a *script*; it's overkill. The important thing is to get some visuals. Some of the one's from your old presentation will do.
- If you start worrying about *physical factors* such as the room, seats, projector, you will be distracted from your main duty, being the presenter.
- Don't be too concerned with your *delivery*. You don't have to

be an actor to explain theory or research. Anyone can speak to a group of people.

- Never have a *dry run*. This wastes time, and your practice presentation is likely to be better than the real thing. So rely on spontaneity.
- Above all, don't *get ready* too soon. Stay flexible.

(Adapted from L. Meuse, 'Mastering the business and technical presentation')

The message is a simple one: a cookbook approach to training which assumes that anyone can put together and produce a programme if the ingredients and menu are available will not do. Effective training requires expertise both in the delivery and management of learning, and in its design. Careful programme planning is important for four main reasons.

First, the process of programme design should act to ensure that the sponsoring agency (or agencies) takes ownership of the programme in terms of learning objectives, and the selection, support and post-course follow-up of learners. Thus the planning process is not just about preparing for what should happen in the training room, but about establishing management commitment to, and linkage with, the development process. This linkage should also be strengthened at the planning stage by checking that there exists a framework of agency policy, standards and performance management in relation to the aspect of practice that the training addresses. Without such a framework, standards may be idiosyncratic and highly variable, so that learners can choose whether or not to apply the learning in their work. This part of the planning process, therefore, starts a long way before the design of a specific programme, and is concerned with performance management frameworks rather than delivery planning. It must also address the question of how the proposed training will assist the agency in meeting the needs of its users, and in achieving organisational goals.

Second, a programme design framework ensures that there is a rational and coherent approach to training, through which identified training needs are linked to intended outcomes. Moreover, as education has increasingly become a marketable commodity, and with the emphasis on measuring outcomes in terms of competency and credits, programme planning has assumed a much more significant role (Jarvis 1995: 228). Programme design must ensure that learners do indeed have the opportunity to obtain the agreed outcomes during the programme. Thus programme design is the key to consistency and standardisation of learning opportunities.

Third, a transparent programme design framework should reduce the danger of the agency or trainer's 'hidden curriculum' infiltrating the training process. In Chapter 3 Hay's triangles were described, showing how contracts for training could be undermined if ulterior motives existed, or were perceived to exist between the organisation, the trainer or the learners. In Chapter 5 reference was also made to situations in which the trainer may carry a hidden curriculum, in terms of personal agendas which can infiltrate the planning process. For instance, the trainer may want to use the course to attack management, or undermine an area of agency policy.

Fourth, a clear programme design process also protects learners from sloppy and ill-conceived training programmes in which, at best, little is achieved or, worse, which leave participants wary of engaging in future training activity. The experience of trainers who are neglectful, uncaring and dismissive of their audiences is probably worse than that of trainers who are too prescriptive and inflexible. Thus a programme design process should ensure that the training activity is legitimate, purposeful and ethical, because it should make explicit the values, assumptions, organisational agendas, needs, expectations, rationale and authority underpinning the training programme.

Power issues in programme design

What is apparent from all four points is that the trainer cannot plan a programme in isolation from commissioners, other managers, potential participants and service users. However, from the outset a key issue is who has what control over what parts of the programme design process. To what extent can the potential participants exercise influence or make decisions about the aims, ingredients or management of the learning process? How far will users be consulted or involved in the programme? As Bell (1993) has observed, the first aim of staff development in social services departments is to meet the needs of service users and carers, then to contribute towards organisational growth and only then to meet the development needs of individuals. In consequence, staff attending training have limited control of a number of the elements of the learning process, such as analysis of needs, setting of learning objectives, programme design, quality and choice of trainers, venue, timing, course membership and reinforcement and rehearsal opportunities.

While this may often be appropriate or inevitable, the trainer needs to be particularly alert as to how this power imbalance may impact on both trainer and course members and its implications for programme design and delivery. This is given added emphasis because power, authority, choice and negotiation are central themes in social care practice, which should be positively modelled in the planning and delivery of training. As Claxton (1988) observes, learners may lend their control to the trainer, but they never give it away. Indeed, the trainer is hired to empower the learner, not vice versa. For instance, in the case of a charismatic trainer whose agenda is self-promotion and demonstration of expertise, there is a real danger that the experience becomes disempowering or patronising for the learners, as a result of which they may disengage or become very challenging as a way of taking back their legitimate power.

In adult learning terms there is therefore a clear tension to be managed in programme design between the requirements of the organisation and the needs of the individual learner. Staff development programmes are not free to pursue a purist adult education methodology in which the needs of the learner are the sole or even paramount consideration. There must be an understanding and accommodation of agency and learner needs and goals.

This tension in the power relations between trainers, learners and agency can be represented in the cycle shown in Figure 8.1. The main parties potentially involved in the planning process are positioned around the cycle. In preparing any particular training programme, one or more, or possibly all parties may be involved in the planning process, as indicated by the arrows pointing to the circle in the middle, that represents the training planning process. The question for the trainer is, from the outset, to consider to what extent power is to be shared, with whom, in the training design process. Of course, in some situations the trainer may have little influence in such decisions.

Although a wide range of permutations exist, seven scenarios are described below to illustrate the effect of involving different parties in the planning process. They range from the most prescriptive to the most inclusive approaches.

1   Goals and objectives selected by agency, trainer carries them out, with little or no scope for negotiation. An example might be the dissemination of information about a new organisational structure.
2   Agency determines general focus. Specific goals are determined by trainers and presented to learners.

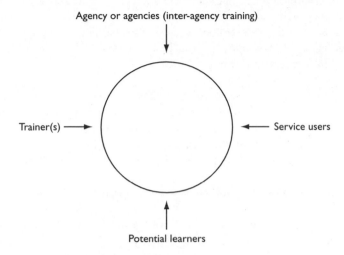

Figure 8.1 Power relations in the planning of training

3   Trainers determine general focus, and gather information from learners to help shape specific goals and programme.
4   Trainers determine general focus, gather information from learners and, in the first part of the design, present this to learners, who can modify goals and programme.
5   Trainers present broad learning aims only, and provide in the first part of the design a framework in which learners can develop their specific learning goals and programme.
6   Learners determine goals and objectives and employ a trainer to facilitate all or some of their learning.
7   Service users involved with trainers and learners in planning process. (It should also be noted that service users could equally be involved in some of the previous scenarios.)

Different contexts will require different arrangements. For instance, a trainer acting in the role of team facilitator might well be operating from position 5 or 6, in contrast to a trainer designing a competence-based course on assessment of needs which would be at position 2. Finally, where inter-agency training is concerned, the permutations become even more complex. For instance, one agency, funding the training, may exert overarching influence, so that other agencies feel that they are being invited along to someone else's party.

What is important is that agencies, trainers, learners and service users are explicit with each other about who has what power to determine which parts of the programme, for what reasons. Thus, in designing any programme, trainers must ask the basic question, 'What is the framework for partnership in this process?'

- Who are the interested parties in this programme?
- Who holds what power in relation to this training programme?
- Do they have clear and congruent expectations?
- What is my mandate to design this programme?
- What opportunities will I give, at what points, to involve others in designing this programme?
- What is negotiable and what is not negotiable, and why?

These points are important in deciding and framing learning goals, objectives and programmes, and in clarifying the trainer's role in the design process. They also have an impact on the role and authority of the trainer 'in the room' with learners, as discussed in Chapters 6 and 7.

Planning learning objectives and outcomes

By way of an introduction to this section four important terms require definition. These are:

1 Training inputs
2 Learning aims
3 Learning objectives
4 Learning outcomes.

Training inputs refers to everything the trainer does to facilitate group or individual learning. This includes planning, recruitment, delivery and evaluation. Jaques (1992) distinguishes between aims as broad directions for teaching, and objectives as describing what the learner should be able to do and know by the end of the training event. When these are transferred into job behaviour they become outcomes, which should in principle be measurable. Therefore programme objectives should differentiate being able to know or do something by the end of a course (an objective) from being able to apply knowledge and skills on the job (an outcome). For instance, a training course on needs assessment might have an objective such as 'Knowing and understanding the basis for, and elements of, a needs assessment by the end of the course', and an outcome such as 'Applying an understanding of needs assessment in work on five cases over a three month period following the course'.

Although this sounds straightforward enough, the very nature of group-based learning means that the precise dynamics and direction that a group of learners may take in experiential learning cannot be predicted, however detailed the planning process. Therefore it is not possible for anyone – commissioner, trainer or learner – to predict all the outcomes from a training event. The relationship between training inputs, learning aims, objectives and outcomes is complex, so that the setting of learning objectives and outcomes is not a simple business. Effective learning produces outcomes that

- can be both intended and unintended;
- can be behavioural, cognitive and emotional;
- concern personal and political, as well as professional domains;
- can occur both immediately and over the longer term;
- can change according to the context in which the learning is applied.

For instance, a participant on a supervision course returning for the second module reported little progress since module one. When asked about the behaviour of her supervisees she began to recall that they had become open about feelings. The supervisor was puzzled about this, until further exploration revealed that in fact the supervisor's learning had been at an unconscious level (Jarvis 1995), with the result that she had in fact changed her job behaviour, modelling clearer permission for feelings to be discussed, without being aware of it. Indeed, if she had not been returning to a second module, this deep-level, unplanned learning might never have become apparent to her. It was only through a process of facilitated critical reflection that her learning had been elicited. Had her learning outcomes been evaluated prior to this discussion, it is likely that she would have reported little or no outcome.

This raises a potential tension in competence-based training, where specific goals and outcomes are determined by lead bodies and agencies rather than learners. Competence-based training specifies outcomes in terms of what a learner will be able to do and know by the end of a programme, and be able to apply in the work place. However, for this to become real for the learner, the competence requirement needs to be translated in terms of 'what does it mean for me in my work place?'. It is this reflection that makes the vital link between an outcome that is externally prescribed and a learner's individual need. Thus outcomes, even within a competence-based training programme, will vary between learners, who will need to demonstrate the application of the knowledge, values and skills taught in training, in different ways according to their different jobs. Each unit of competence taught in training is also a unit of assessment, therefore every learning outcome ought to be measurable. Here again there is a potential tension with group-learning approaches in which some of the learning outcomes may be less predictable, behaviourally specific, more diverse and occurring over a longer time-scale than the course.

All of this does not mean that specific objectives should not be set, or outcomes sought, but rather that stated aims, objectives and outcomes should not act in a limiting way on either the trainer or the learners to prevent other, often unintended opportunities for learning that effective learning groups generate. Planning remains essential, as it provides an intentional and open framework which guides the trainers and the learners, and substantially increases the likelihood that both the objectives and the learning outcomes will be achieved. It does mean, however, that in defining learning outcomes, trainers, learners and commissioners need to take into account that these are complex and multi-faceted, and unfold over time.

PROGRAMME DESIGN PROCESS

In this chapter the focus is on designing a specific training event, rather than on the broader development of training strategy based on training needs analysis, which was described in Chapter 3. The starting point here is that a training event has been commissioned, and it is now time to design the programme. The essence of the design process is that it contains four areas which need to be integrated within the programme's design: aims and objectives; methods and organisation; subject matter and evaluation. These are depicted in Figure 8.2, by Jarvis (1995: 194).

The rest of this section of the chapter is devoted to the presentation of a ten-stage training design framework, which expands and explores in practical detail the four key areas identified by Jarvis. As each of the ten stages are described, examples are provided.

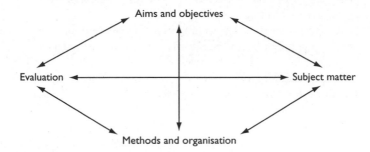

Figure 8.2 Jarvis's four design areas

Ten-stage training design model

- Define primary client aspirations and concerns.
- Assess trainer resources and skills.
- Assess needs, speculate on how the learning group may present.
- Set training goals and objectives.
- State objectives for each session.
- Select training methods, place in learning sequence, set time-scales.
- Allocate tasks within training team, preparation for co training.
- Assess and plan for logistical tasks.
- Plan learning transfer tasks and post-training learning support.
- Plan an evaluative component.

(Adapted from *50 Activities for Trainers*, University Associates)

In the section that follows, each of these elements will be explored. However, where material is discussed in depth elsewhere in the text, it will be dealt with only briefly here. This applies particularly to the following: training methods, see Chapter 9; co-training, see Chapter 7; planning learning transfer tasks, see Chapter 10; evaluation planning, see Chapter 11.

Define primary client concerns and agency/ inter-agency context

This involves consideration of questions concerning the organisational context in which a particular event is planned, and its potential viability.

- How has the need for this event arisen?
- What positive outcomes are expected by the agency/ies?

- What problem is this expected to solve for the agency/ies?
- Is the need a training need?
- Is the proposed training event part of a coherent staff or policy development strategy, or a legitimate one-off or a 'quick-fix'?
- What specific changes in knowledge, values or skills are sought?
- Who are the interested parties for this event? Who is paying?
- Which of the parties have been consulted?
- Is there a clear primary customer?
- Are expectations between commissioners, potential learners and the trainers clear and congruent? If not, is there a process by which differing expectations can be negotiated? Is there the time/permission to do this?
- Who in the agency/ies is or is not taking ownership at a management level?
- Who are the target group? How have they been selected?
- What contact will the trainer have before, during and after the training event with commissioners, learners or their managers?
- Will the agency be expected to take action as a result of the programme – for instance on policy, resources or further development of staff?
- Is there a commitment to take follow-up action?
- Does the programme design meet the commissioner's expectations?
- How realistic are the commissioner's expectations?

The purpose of these questions is for the trainer to assess whether the event is viable, and that it is likely that it will promote the development of staff. The fact that money and a group of learners are available does not mean that the proposed event is viable. For instance, one of us was invited to undertake a supervision training event in the context of there being no supervision policy, considerable anger about the lack of agency support for supervision, and confusion as to the responsibilities of supervisors! The biggest disasters in training can occur because of a failure to consider the organisational context at the commissioning stage. Often what is required is a different sort of developmental event, rather than an outright refusal. In the example above, a supervision policy development day was negotiated in place of the original event.

Thus the trainer, having established that there is a legitimate development need, must then consider from a range of options how best this need can be met. These options could include either or both on- or off-the-job development opportunities such as following:

- *Self-directed learning*
  reading
  study days
  maintaining a learning diary;
- *On the job*
  one-to-one coaching
  assignments, project work
  mentoring
  shadowing
  direct observation
  co-working
  secondments
  evaluation or survey work
  action learning
  quality circles
  interactive video
  computer-based learning;

or

- *Off the job*
  open/distance learning
  residential programme
  workshop/participative programme
  seminar/discussion
  journal club
  lecture/presentation
  observation placement
  outdoor development.

These three development pathways are visually depicted in Figure 8.3.

Assess trainer resources and skills

Clearly, whether the aims and outcomes of the course will be achieved depends not only on the abilities and motivation of the learner, but also on the skills, resources and competence of the trainer. This means, that not only must the trainer be well versed in the subject area, but equally must have the teaching and group facilitation skills to enable learning to take place. It is an old truth that good practitioners, highly knowledgeable specialists or good platform speakers do not necessarily make good trainers. Equally, an expert facilitator who has no subject-specific knowledge will only be able to elicit and help learners share

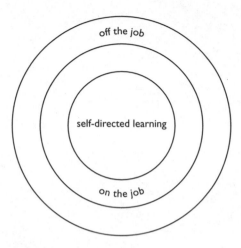

Figure 8.3 Learning development pathways

existing knowledge rather than add to it. In this regard, the use of generic trainers, with little subject-specific expertise, sometimes without any professional background in social care work, is increasingly common. Therefore before the precise learning objectives are determined, it is important to establish the following:

- What training experience do the trainers have, with what kinds of target groups?
- What is the gender/ethnic make-up of the participants, what implication does this have for trainers?
- What teaching and facilitation methods do they possess? For example, if a group sculpt is to be used, has the trainer used this method before?
- What current subject knowledge and professional experience do the trainers have?
- Have these trainers worked together before?
- Does this target group pose any particular challenges for the trainer? For example, have they had previous negative experiences working with some of the participants or the other trainers before?
- What teaching resources and expertise are required beyond the trainers' capacities, and where can these be obtained?
- What supervisory/consultancy support is available to assist the trainers in preparing/managing the course?

It is an ethical obligation for the trainer to be aware and open about the limits of their competence. In the light of these considerations, the trainer may decide that she is not competent to deliver all parts of the programme. It may be that the learner group are willing to accept limited experience in some areas, on the basis that the trainer offers other areas of expertise. However, this is not an excuse for the trainer to accept a commission on the basis that 'it will be OK as long as I can stay just one step ahead'. Neither is it acceptable for a trainer to start the course by apologising for their lack of knowledge, stating, 'I am no expert – I feel very nervous' and so on. This is certain to create immediate irritation in the audience who, after all, are entitled to believe that the trainer brings something to add to and extend their experience and knowledge.

Assess needs, speculate on how the learning group may present

Having decided that the proposal is a viable training commission, and that the trainer is competent to deliver it, the next step is to explore the nature of the target group, their work context, and their aspirations and needs in relation to this event. All of these need to be taken into account by the trainer in designing the programme. Key issues include:

- What do the participants' current jobs involve?
- How far does the proposed training fit with their current work roles and responsibilities or impending changes?
- How clearly have their training needs been identified and by whom?
- Who is likely to know whom, in what context? Will there be cliques, dominant groups, or those who might feel very isolated?
- What are their likely ages, gender, ethnicity, previous training/ qualifications?
- Are there any special needs identified regarding hearing, disability, ...c.?
- What are the identified strengths and difficulties of their work place? Have they been through major changes? Has there been a high turnover of staff? Is morale high or low?
- What positive motivation might the learners bring?
- What blockages, demotivating feelings/factors might they bring?
- Has this group worked together before?
- What are their expectations for this event? If unknown, how can the

trainer find out? Should the participants be seen, written to, phoned up?
- What information does the trainer need at the beginning of the event?

Several years ago one of us was invited to work with a residential children's unit on managing young people who sexually abuse. In the introductions it was revealed that three participants had been recruited as staff only in the past three months, without any prior social work training, whose knowledge base about sexual abuse was based simply on what they had gleaned from newspapers. The learning needs were far too wide in this instance for the group to be able to work together on the programme. If the range is too wide, there is a danger that the less able/trained members will become isolated, or that the training becomes focused at the level of the lowest common denominator.

Effective learning groups need to contain a healthy balance between commonalities and difference. A group who share a very narrow view about practice, permit little discussion about difference and depend for their cohesion on mutual agreement will be very resistant to learning. Such groups can be encountered in most organisations, particularly in very closed settings, such as secure units. They sometimes represent 'how things were in the good old days', or represent deeply entrenched groups of staff, mostly male and white, who operate like an old boys' club, for example, 'us versus the world'. Such groups are too homogeneous to contemplate change. On the other hand too great a diversity of knowledge, values and skills can seriously impede a learning group's progress. Equally, an imbalance in a group can act as a block for those who then find themselves in an isolated position – for instance, where a black member of staff is the sole member of an otherwise all white group. Thus a key role for the trainer is in defining the size and membership of the group. In Chapter 5 there is further discussion about recruitment and selection of course members.

Armed with this information the trainer can plan the programme that is relevant. They can also anticipate some of the ways in which the learners may present on day one, and consider the best way to respond to them, accepting, however, that even with careful preparation, different needs may emerge when the trainer finally meets the group. For instance, the trainer may anticipate with a particular group the need to take more time on helping members manage their angry feelings about the organisation, or on developing trust within the group. If this is not done, the trainer with their carefully planned programme may become frustrated or insensitive when the group is unable to engage straight away. Anticipating how learners may present is particularly important when using external trainers, who need to be briefed about such issues so that they can respond appropriately. The quality of such briefing can unfortunately be highly variable, sometimes placing the external trainer in a difficult and unforeseen situation.

Set training goals and objectives

The expectations of the commissioners, together with the needs and context of the learners, provide the information upon which specific training goals and objectives can be identified. Jarvis (1995) states that learning outcomes must be specified in terms that are:

- explicit
- relevant
- agreed
- understood
- realistic
- timely
- measurable.

Earlier, the distinction between aims as broad directions for teaching, and objectives as describing what the learner should be able to do and know by the end of the training event, was drawn (Jaques 1992: 64). In competency-based training these objectives are extended to specify, in measurable terms, how the learner is expected to be able to apply learning in their work. Thus Jaques's design of group learning programmes describes two levels of planning:

1   *Strategic*: overall aims, structure, content and teaching method (the focus of this and the next chapter);
2   *Tactical*: handling the group process as it unfolds, channelling it towards the overall aims of the programme (as discussed in Chapters 6 and 7).

(Jaques 1992: 115)

The complexity of setting learning outcomes was also discussed earlier, and it was recognised that learning is not a purely rational and linear activity, as feelings, unconcious processes and the unexpected play a major role. Nevertheless, specifying aims and objectives do provide 'an intentional framework in which both intuitive and spontaneous changes can be made' (Jaques 1992) and within which trainers and learners can negotiate both means and ends. Without such a framework there is a danger of hidden agendas and motivations arising, leading to anti-learning group behaviour, manipulation and poor or even negative outcomes.

In the light of these factors, the setting of training goals and objectives requires the trainer to:

- identify overall goals for the event that are relevant, realistic and timely;
- identify specific and measurable objectives as to what learners should be able to know or do by the end of the course;
- identify specific outcomes enabling the application in practice of the knowledge and skills learnt on the course;
- place these learning objectives in a logical sequence so that the learner can see a progression of learning tasks and challenges;
- identify at whom the training is aimed and for whom it is appropriate;
- specify any prerequisites; e.g. previous training required, level of experience required or current job roles;
- specify any pre-course preparation;
- clarify whether any elements of the course are to be assessed;
- clarify whether the course attracts credits for NVQ or other award-body purposes;
- identify trainers' and learners' responsibilities in achieving the objectives of the training programme.

EXAMPLE

Title: Effective supervision of staff working in the mental health field

Aims

The overall aim of this training programme is to equip the Eastshire Social Services Dept team managers in mental health services with the knowledge and skills to supervise staff in accordance with the Service's Supervision Policy and standards.

Course structure: 3 days + 2 days

This training will consist of a total of five days' training split into a three-day module followed by a two-day module six weeks later. All course members will be expected to undertake preparatory work before both modules, including for module 2, bringing a video tape of a supervision session conducted by the participant. This will be analysed in *small group* settings only.

Module 1 The aim of this module will be to provide a theoretical underpinning and to identify the key skills required for effective supervision of staff in the area of mental health services. It will combine knowledge and skill development, including critical reflection, skill rehearsal and the analysis of supervision issues. The course content will be based on 'Supervision in Social Care', supplemented by additional material.

The learning objectives for this module will be:

- to understand and be able to explain the principles and pur-poses of supervision to supervisees;
- to understand and be able to use adult learning theory to analyse their own supervisory practice;
- to understand the components of a viable supervision contract and the processes required to negotiate one;
- to understand the role of anxiety and be able to describe how the supervisor can utilise anxiety in a constructive way in supervision;
- to understand the concept of reflective practice and be able to describe how this is facilitated through supervision, particularly in exploring values and promoting anti-discriminatory practice in supervision.

The learning outcomes from this module will be to:

- bring written evidence by the second module of negotiating a supervision contract with at least two supervisees;
- provide a video tape of supervision, with a written analysis of the process in terms of adult learning theory.

Prerequisites

All participants must be in managerial positions in which they have direct responsibility for the supervision of staff undertaking mental health work. All participants are expected to complete both modules and the course assignments.

Credit rating

The evidence generated by course participants of their learning during and after this course can be retained for submission in portfolios for the Advanced Award.

State objectives for each session

If the learning experience is to be coherent so that one session leads logically to the next, it is important to state the objectives for each session within a programme, and to be able to indicate how the methods relate to the learning objectives. Otherwise the selection of methods can become random, reflecting more the trainer's preferences than the learner's needs. For instance, doing one role play after another without pause for reflection is both unlikely to meet the learning objectives and likely to leave members unable to move on to the next session. In addition, where specific objectives for a particular session are unclear, it is more likely that direction will be lost if, for instance, the trainer is challenged or the group generates powerful emotional processes. This can be a particular problem in the final session of training events, which can lose direction and purpose if not properly thought out. It is often said that it is easier to loosen a tight structure than to tighten a loose structure. Thus at the start of any particular session, it should be possible to explain to learners the objectives and purposes of methods used. Using the example of the supervision training outlined above, the trainer should therefore be able to explain:

- how each session fits with one of the five over-arching learning objectives – e.g. 'This session is on understanding the elements of, and how to negotiate a viable supervision contract.' Note: this will be easier if these objectives have themselves been placed in a logical sequence;

- how what we are doing now fits with what went before, in terms of subject coherence – e.g. it would be important to address definitions and purposes of supervision before tackling supervision contracts;
- what parts of the learning cycle this session is aimed at – e.g. experiencing, reflecting, analysing, planning or rehearsing;
- what values, knowledge, experience, skill or dynamic are being explored;
- how this session builds a bridge to the next session, explores experience or attitudes, contributes to understanding a theory, or rehearses a particular skill.

Maintaining the engagement of the learners is a continuing process. It can ebb and flow like a tide throughout a training event. Explaining the purpose of a session and the areas of learning that are anticipated acts both to reassure and motivate, especially when risks are being taken – for instance, in experiential learning. Thus when the course is entering more challenging aspects, it can be useful to signpost this so as to prepare learners and assure them as to how they will not only be led into a powerful experience but also out of it. The programme planner described in the next section enables the trainer to plan each session in a training event, around the key issues outlined above, with the result that the trainer has a detailed and explicit understanding and rationale for every part of the programme.

Select training methods, place in learning sequence, set time-scales

This is the heart of the matter: the selection of methods to match learning needs and conditions. As methods and how they relate to experiential learning theory are addressed in the next chapter, they will not be discussed in detail here. At this stage the initial tasks are the following:

- to begin with known elements: start and finish, meals, free time;
- to block out the time schedule on a large sheet of paper and start filling it in, locating, in a logical sequence, each of the main objectives to a particular session;
- to design the programme from start to finish, starting with the overall aims and objectives for each session – in other words, do

not start by putting a favourite exercise in the middle of day two and trying to fit everything else around this;

- to write down the aims of each session even if at this stage the methods have yet to be formulated.

At this point, a more specific programme planning tool can be useful to ensure that the detailed planning integrates aims, methods and outcomes, identifies which parts of the learning cycle are being targeted, and considers how the learning group may respond in terms of its stage of development and needs. To illustrate such a framework, an example of planning for a session of the supervision training course outlined earlier is given.

Programme session planner

Course: Supervision of staff (16 participants)

Objective 3: To understand the components of a viable supervision contract and the processes required to negotiate it

Time: Day 2: Session 1: 9.30–11.00

Aims

Knowledge To be able to understand the elements of a supervisory contract; and the different stages and potential processes involved in negotiating a viable contract both administratively and psychologically; to identify the components of existing supervisory agreements and the processes required to be able to evaluate their quality.

Values Exploring why a contract is important in terms of addressing power issues, transparency, choice and negotiability, and in modelling a partnership approach to staff–manager relations.

Skills No focus during this session – to be covered in following session.

Note: the aims could be written as specific competencies where this is applicable.

Identify link with previous session

End of day 1, work undertaken on supervision histories will illustrate the problems created by lack of clarity between supervisor and supervisee.

Method

9.30   Key messages from day 1: reflection in pairs, then shared with group
9.35   Explain purpose of this session
9.45   'Quick-think' in two groups, placing ideas up on a flip chart:
       a   what should be covered in a supervision contract?
       b   what values can be modelled by using a written supervision contract?
9.50   Feedback onto flip charts from the two quick-think task groups
10.00 Presentation, covering:
       a   importance of written contracts in addressing power and authority issues openly, and in modelling partnership practice through the negotiation, choice and clarification of mutual rights and responsibilities;
       b   elements of a contract;
       c   stages of contract formation: mandate, engagement, ambivalence and formal contract; importance of the process of negotiation;
       d   recording and reviewing of supervision contracts.
10.30 Questions arising from the group
10.40–11.15   Reflection in pairs:
       ●   review the nature and detail of existing supervisory agreements;
       ●   what are my supervisees and I clear about?
       ●   in how many cases is there a written contract?
       ●   what areas of supervisory expectations or authority have not been raised?
       ●   what areas are disputed or confused?
       ●   what steps will I take to address gaps or confusions?

Elements of experimental learning in the session

Conceptualisation: quick-think exercise anmd presentation.
Reflection: examining quality of existing agreements.
Experimentation: action to be taken to improve existing contracts.

(note: the next session will need to focus on extending the active experimentation by involving the group in a role-play exercise in which they rehearse the process of negotiating a contract. This will move the group into experiencing.)

Potential group responses

This session may generate some storming, as it is challenging; for instance, there may be:

- resistance to formalising supervision, which could be displayed in the group as flight ('I haven't got time to do this') or fight ('This isn't necessary');
- anxiety about the prospect of raising uncomfortable issues in existing supervisory relationships, which could generate denial ('I've discussed all these things already') or a degree of help-lessness ('How do I raise this?');
- concern and struggle about power issues in terms of what is negotiable or not, especially over confidentiality.

Programme balance

In designing any session the trainer needs to establish an effective balance between teacher-centred and learner-centred methods – for example, presentation of theory, knowledge or case examples, with reflection on experience, action exercises or skill rehearsals. Much will depend on the trainer's knowledge of the group's needs, their professional maturity and work context. For instance, a learning group which has not worked together before that is expected to deal with an emotive and unfamiliar subject area, such as HIV/Aids training, will need the presentation of information before it can be moved into more participatory modes of learning. Groups sometimes complain about training courses being nothing but a succession of instructions to 'break into small groups and discuss', and are signalling a wish for solid input and action-learning work. It is also worth remembering that generally people are more alert in the mornings, which are therefore better for theoretical work, leaving afternoons for action-exercises.

Size

Another key dimension is the size of the learning group. Larger groups (between eighteen and twenty-four) function very differently from smaller groups. Individuals are less confident to speak, feedback from small group work takes longer, and for the trainer it is much harder to read what is going on. However, very small groups, eight or fewer, present a different problem. Here each individual participant has much greater responsibility for the group process, and individuals will feel more exposed. Also, in very small groups the level of personal disclosure can become an issue and the boundary between training and therapy or personal supervision needs to be maintained. In small groups too there may be a more limited range of experience, diversity and skills to draw upon. Thus very small groups can be as demanding as large groups for the trainer. For the single trainer working on skill development, a group of between twelve and sixteen is optimal. This also splits down into three or four small groups for more detailed work. At this point careful thought needs to be given as to who should work with whom in small groups. Ensuring gender and racial balance is usually preferable unless there are reasons, for instance, for single gender/race groups. On multi-disciplinary courses, there are times when single discipline groups are necessary. If there are different grades of staff in the room, so that some learners are there with their managers, there is a need to think about whether such pairings should work together.

Group size is also important when considering whole group participatory sessions. Twelve members is probably the largest size if everyone is to feel reasonably comfortable to speak, as opposed to listening to a presentation. That does not mean that whole group sessions cannot be useful with larger groups, but it becomes a different group interaction. Whole group sessions are important in checking in with all participants as to how they are experiencing the course in order to check how all members are finding the course, not just the more vocal and confident ones. This simple discipline can be very revealing, either in confirming that all is going according to plan, or the converse. It is often an opportunity for learners to raise other issues that have not been vocalised at the start – for instance, about what is going on in their work places, or about a response to an earlier exercise, or to other group members. This 'taking the temperature' exercise should be done at least once per day, in order to help the trainer pace the course and consider any modifications to the programme. It is also important to try and record everyone's response, otherwise it can be all too easy to focus only on one or two of the strongest responses.

Finally, trainers normally have too much material (out of their anxiety about having too little!) and need to be prepared not to use all of it.

On occasions, however good the planning, the programme may require modification. The ability to be flexible is a strength, not a weakness, and demonstrates sensitivity to group needs. Alternatively, the trainer may make a judgement that the group needs to focus on the objectives in the programme and that it would be unhelpful to make changes.

Allocate elements within training team, preparation for co-training

Much depends on whether there is more than one trainer. If so, it is necessary to think carefully about who does what and why, and what signal this sends out to the group in terms of power and modelling. This applies both to the planning and delivery stages. As Chapter 7 discusses co-training in depth, this aspect is not explored further here. However, it is worth stating that two heads are not always better than one, especially if there are tensions and rivalries between the trainers, which can impact disastrously upon the group, which then becomes contaminated with the unresolved co-trainer dynamics. One participant on a course related that their experience of this had been so bad that it had made them frightened of attending any further training. The message is that co-training requires proper preparation if its undoubted benefits are to be fulfilled.

Assess and plan for the logistical tasks

Practical matters are not peripheral aspects to the learning experience. Recalling the discussion in Chapter 5 about the importance of the physical environment and needs in creating a secure and supportive learning climate, it is crucial that attention is paid at the planning stage to these elements. If these are not resolved beforehand, difficulties with venue are often very difficult to resolve once the event has started. One of us arrived to give a workshop on the impact of child protection work, to discover that the venue was a night club, whose carpets were sticky with spilt drink, which reeked of the smell of alcohol, whose lighting consisted of low-voltage spot lights, and where the chairs were designed to ensure that one did not sit down! Some of the participants even recalled that their parents had frequented the venue as a dance hall a generation earlier. What message was being given about staff care? Practical arrangements contribute powerfully to the state of both the learners and the trainer. So:

- ensure that course advertisements, application forms, selection process and joining instructions, maps and course registration are clear;
- check out venues for space, large rooms and syndicate rooms;
- check out what is likely to be happening in adjacent rooms, especially in terms of noise – replenishing the bar stock is a serious distraction to learning!
- check out the comfort of chairs, check out wheelchair access and whether there is a loop system, check out heating and ventilation;
- check out lighting – good natural lighting makes a huge difference;
- check out refreshments, including special dietary needs, and ensuring a vegetarian option; check timings with venue;
- agree how messages for participants will be kept, check what telephone provision exists;
- ensure that course handouts are presented in an accessible format;
- ensure that there is a supply of felt pens, sticky tape/Blue-tack, flip-chart paper, OHP, screen and video if required – check whether there is a photocopier for use in emergency;
- if the training is residential, clarify sleeping facilities, catering, bar provision, leisure facilities, recreational options.

Plan learning transfer tasks and post-training learning support

As this is the subject of Chapter 10, the comments here will be brief. Trainers sometimes, and managers often, underestimate quite seriously the complexity involved in transferring learning acquired in the context of a training course back into the work place. The result is that trainers may assume naïvely that participants will somehow just be able to transfer their learning unprompted and unaided. Trainers may thereby fail to understand that course design does not finish when the learners depart, but involves establishing a plan from the outset for learning transfer. This is more than asking learners to form an action plan during the last half hour of the course. Learning transfer starts by engaging with relevant managers at the commissioning and planning process, for it is managers who are critical to the success of the transfer process. Agreeing with managers how participants can discuss, rehearse and apply the course material on return must occur before the course ever starts, rather than being left to the participants as they walk out of the door.

Plan an evaluative component

Again, this aspect is covered in detail in Chapter 11, so there will only be brief comments here. Evaluation of training is becoming increasingly important, and required at a level 'beyond the happy sheets' that participants complete as they leave the course. In broad terms, the best evaluations are obtained over time through multiple sources of observation. These are best when conducted over time, involving both staff who have attended the course and their managers, and focusing not just on behavioural/practice changes, but also on levels of knowledge and changes in thinking or attitudes. For instance, as a simple exercise it is very instructive to ask participants returning to a second module on the supervision course described earlier, to explain what theory and knowledge had been retained from part one, and how they have made use of it. A simple quiz can be a very revealing device, as well as being fun. Sometimes, until learners are asked, they are unaware of what they have learnt or how they have used it. Hence evaluation not only measures, but also assists, the integration of learning.

SUMMARY

- Careful design and planning is crucial, to ensure effective learning, and that the power invested in the trainer is used constructively to achieve the agreed objectives.
- There is a distinction between overall aims as broad directions for teaching, and specific objectives as describing what a learner should be able to do and know by the end of a training event.
- Outcomes occur at both intentional and unplanned levels, and over a wide time-scale, so that planning cannot predict all outcomes from training.
- Careful planning should not block unplanned opportunities for learning.
- Planning starts at the point of commissioning a training event, and managers need to be engaged at some level in the planning process. Decisions need to be taken as to what involvement learners or service users may have in the planning process.

- Each component or session of a training event should have specific objectives which must relate to the overall aims, what came immediately before, the experiential learning cycle, and an analysis of the learning group's needs and processes. A programme planning format has been presented to assist with this process.

- A trainer's checklist was presented, which can be used to assess the learning opportunities afforded by plans for any particular event.

- Programme design is crucial to effective learning, and might be best conceptualised as a tight–loose approach. In other words, detailed clarity about the aims, objectives and management of the training event should be matched with a flexibility to modify, and very occasionally jettison, these plans, if the needs and mood of the learning group so require.

Chapter 9

Methods to facilitate learning

Purposes, pitfalls, preparation and process

> This chapter explores:
>
> - factors to consider in the selection of training methods;
> - description of principal training methods;
> - how different methods produce different types of learning;
> - potential pitfalls and process issues to consider.

This chapter is closely linked to Chapter 8, which considered how to plan a training event. It was stressed that the design of a training event should not be built around the trainer's favourite exercises, but on an analysis of learning needs and objectives. A 'Programme session planner' format was presented in Chapter 8, which provided a framework for the design of training sessions. That framework needs to be understood in reading this chapter, as it underpins the selection of the specific training methods described here. The reader should therefore be acquainted with the contents of the previous chapter before reading this chapter.

The aim of this chapter is to describe the principal training methods relevant and appropriate to the context of social care training, and to relate the use of these methods to the learning theory presented in Chapter 2. It is not therefore a 'cookbook' from which readers may select new or unusual ingredients to spice up their courses, nor can the discussion cover all the practical points related to using these methods. Rather, the emphasis here is on exploring in general terms the potential learning purposes, pitfalls, preparation required and processes to manage these methods in order to maximise their benefits. Trainers are sometimes confronted by the uncomfortable experience of a well-tried method suddenly failing them when used in a different group. Seemingly straightforward methods, frequently used on training courses, can produce very different outcomes, depending on the trainer's understanding of their purpose and ability to manage them with different groups of participants. In other words, there are no foolproof methods. The aim of this chapter is to deepen our understanding of the nature and impact of the principal methods available to the social care trainer. Its underlying premise is that the efficacy of any training method lies as much in the manner, flexibility and context of its use as in the specifics of the method itself. Before describing the range of training methods, the chapter starts therefore by examining ten key factors that should be considered in the selection of any particular method.

Selection of training method: ten factors to consider

Aims and objectives and intended outcomes

The starting point must be to select methods that will achieve the learning objectives. This requires a detailed planning format so that each session within an event, however short, is related to the principal learning objectives, as demonstrated in Chapter 8 with the 'Programme session planner' format. However, within each session, as shown in the example given in Chapter 8, there may be more than one learning component; for example, several micro-objectives covering knowledge, values and skills, each of which needs a different method. Conversely, one method, such as a case study can yield multiple learning benefits. The method should relate to a specific learning outcome or outcomes, which in turn should relate to key programme objectives. If it is unclear how a method can be related to the course objectives, it should not be used until this is clarified. Often the problem lies less with the selection of methods, however, and more with learning objectives or planning processes that are not specific enough. Good methods will not work properly if they are laid on top of bad planning. In addition to being clear in their own head, the trainer must also explain the purpose, process and intended outcomes of all methods to learners.

Clear and specific programme planning should ensure that methods relate not only to the achievement of learning objectives in terms of knowledge, values and skills, but are based on an understanding of how adults learn. This was described in Chapter 2 (p. 50) with reference to Kolb's Experiential Learning Cycle. Kolb's Cycle suggests that the kinds of problem-solving which lead to changes in behaviour and thinking, requires engagement with all four elements of the Cycle. Thus trainers need to plan a programme in which structure, psychological environment and methods enable learners, at different points, to experience, reflect, conceptualise and actively experiment. Methods need to be selected from the perspective of what areas of learning they are intended to generate.

The selection of appropriate and effective methods occurs when learning objectives are matched with relevant parts of the Experiential Learning Cycle through a method which enables specific learning objectives to be achieved. It is possible to distinguish between four broad types of learning, which relate to the Learning Cycle:

1   Cognitive/intellectual/verbal/theoretical/knowledge-based learning – e.g. understanding a theory or a piece of research.
2   Experiential/emotional/affective/personal-awareness learning – e.g. exploring the feelings generated in working with a certain user group.
3   Reflective/creative/generating ideas/making connections – e.g. enabling learners to make connections between values, knowledge and skills in one area of practice with those in another.
4   Behavioural/skills/practice/experimenting/action learning – e.g. rehearsing interviewing skills.

A programme using only one group of methods, and thus focusing only on certain parts of the Cycle, will generate limited learning outcomes. For instance, a day filled with theoretical presentations, focused largely at the conceptualisation stage, will fail to address the need for sharing and reflecting on experiences and reactions to the presentations, and active experimentation in terms of the action implications of the material.

However, the starting point (as Chapters 5, 6 and 7 have demonstrated) is for the trainer to create and maintain a secure group learning environment. Without this prerequisite, learners and groups will be unwilling to engage or share their experience, at the very first stage of the Cycle. Thus in terms of methods, the first task is to select methods that enable learners to feel secure, to engage and to share experience.

Learning group's process and stage

Chapter 6 explored the significance of group dynamics in mediating the potential responses of learners to training. In selecting methods careful attention must therefore be paid to both the stage and state of the learning group's processes. In particular, the trainer must assess the degree of cohesiveness, trust, openness and commitment of course members. Even apparently non-threatening exercises may be met with resistance in groups that lack basic trust. Moreover, the fact that some members might be keen on challenging exercises does not mean that everyone is ready, or can voice their discomfort if they disagree. Recalling the discussion in Chapter 7 on the balance of challenge and support in groups, a role play with a high-challenge–low-support group would be a much riskier endeavour than in a high-challenge–high-support group. Equally, an unfacilitated discussion, perhaps around a case study, in a low-challenge–high-support group might have little impact on participants critically appraising their work. The group's need to stay cosy would prevent difference being explored.

Prior experience of learners

In Chapter 5 the significance of learners' prior experiences was considered. It was recognised that an individual's openness, trust and engagement in learning were influenced by a wide range of factors stemming from personal, professional and social experiences. While it is difficult for the trainer to know in a group setting how this affects individuals and how they are disposed towards particular training methods, information about this may come from the pre-course recruitment process, personal knowledge of participants, responses to previous training, briefings from managers and information from learners given during a training event. A participant may have indicated beforehand to the trainer that they have recently had a very negative experience of role play.

In addition to information about individual attitudes and confidence as learners, the trainer needs to take into account any information about how a particular group has responded to different training techniques. For instance, a group may be undertaking an extended piece of training such as a post-qualifying course and will have developed responses to different methods. Course tutors often remark how open or, conversely, difficult or unconfident a group is, which can provide some guidance on which methods are likely to be more appropriate. One of us discovered that the group had only the previous day been through an extremely demanding and emotional training session with another trainer, based on extensive use of videos with adult survivors of sexual abuse talking. Any experiential method used before the group had debriefed the previous training experience would be likely to overload the group. It is important therefore to establish what experiences a learning group has been through just prior to the current event. Finally, there is also a need for the trainer to consider the experiences of the group within their wider organisational or inter-agency context. The group may be one that has been neglected by the agency, has received little training, or is currently facing the uncertainty of another restructuring within their agency.

Follow-up opportunities

A related factor is the question of whether the group will have follow-up opportunities. This links to the point made earlier about whether the group has only come together for this particular training course, and will disperse after the training, or is an ongoing one. Where there are follow-up opportunities, and the group is a cohesive one, more challenging material can be sustained over a longer period during the training, and it is possible to agree that less time be spent on addressing organisational issues arising, as these can be picked up later by the group. In other words, slightly less attention needs to be focused on beginnings and endings than with a stranger group.

Learning styles

The recognition that learners have different learning style preferences is another factor influencing selection of method. In Chapter 2, four main learning styles were noted: activist, reflector, theorist and pragmatist. Here again there are limits as to how far the trainer can know individuals' styles. Nevertheless, it is reasonable to suggest that in most learning groups there will be a range of learning style preferences, which may be influenced not just by personal history but also by occupational role. Thus manual workers, or those undertaking basic care tasks, are likely to prefer more concrete demonstrations and action methods to abstract debate. These preferences also reflect professional cultures, so that doctors, and to a lesser extent police, for instance, are generally more comfortable with didactic presentations and a 'chalk and talk' than are social workers and nurses. To summarise: activists will prefer action-orientated methods; reflectors like to observe and investigate feelings and values; theorists like formal presentations of research; while the pragmatists enjoy problem-solving exercises. What is important is that the methods are varied to accommodate different learning style preferences, and not just the trainer's preferences.

Trainer: competence, confidence, relationship and boredom

The trainer's competence, experience and confidence in using any method is a further factor to consider. This does not mean that the trainer should not use a new method – after all, there must always be a first time. One of the great strengths of co-training is that new methods can be tried out, with the extra support of a co-trainer. However, in using any method the trainer must know why it is appropriate, and how to employ it. Simply imitating, as opposed to applying, a method used by another trainer in a different context carries dangers. The trainer's confidence in their method, in the specific context, is also important, especially where more challenging and exposing methods are used. For instance, in requesting participants to bring video-taped recordings of their practice for analysis in small groups on training events, the trainer's public confidence, based on previous experience of the method, in the value of the learners taking this risk, has considerable impact on an apprehensive group. An analogy might be drawn with the way in which the dentist tells us to lie back as it won't hurt. The trainer's confidence with even a tried and tested method can vary according to the learning group. Thus running a quiz with managers might induce much more anxiety for the trainer than with practitioners.

However, a related factor in terms of trust and confidence is how well the trainer is known by the group. More challenging methods are likely to be acceptable, and therefore effective, where the trainer's approach and competence are well understood by the learners, and the trainer understands the strengths and vulnerabilities of the learning group. Trainers can also become bored by their methods, and assume that learners too will be bored. The result can be that the trainer introduces new methods too quickly or loses sight of the fact that the learners may not have encountered those methods. A group may still need to undertake familiar introductory exercises, for instance, because it has to go through its 'forming' stage. In changing methods, trainers must beware of ignoring the stages of group development.

Timing

The effectiveness of a method depends on the timing. If the timing is wrong, the method will not be fully effective at best, or counter-productive at worst. The facilitation of group learning requires a beginning, a middle and an end, and therefore the length and structuring of a training course has significant implications as to which methods are best at what stage. In general terms, because learning is based on exploring and utilising experience, methods that assist reflection on experience are preferable at the start or the end of a course as opposed to starting or ending with a powerful experiential exercise. The shorter the course, the less time there is to prepare the group for more challenging action and experiential methods or to debrief them afterwards. This can have implications for methods used on modular courses where learners come together, for instance for three hours once per month. This can mean that group cohesion has to be re-established each time, thus limiting the time available for learning. Timing is also connected to sequence, as discussed in Chapter 8. A continuous stream of theoretical presentations, or reflective exercises, however good, would be unbalanced, creating either indigestion or frustration. A manager on one course gave feedback that, although he had enjoyed it and learnt a good deal, he found the diet of presentation followed by small group discussion, followed by feedback on flip charts repetitive. He wanted some action exercises to generate some experience of what practice might feel like.

Size of group

The size and composition of a group are two of the most powerful determinants of group behaviour. Large groups behave differently from small groups (four to eight participants). Methods that work in a group of one size may not work in that of another size, as discussed in Chapter 8. This does not rule out the use of methods other than presentational ones in larger groups (twenty-four plus). Participatory and experiential exercises are possible even in very large groups (forty plus), as long as there are enough facilitators to work in sub-groups, and to observe the whole process. Indeed, there can be a tendency to rule out these methods with very large groups, when they can be very effective, if the objectives are very clear, and methods are carefully chosen and managed. An example might be where the aim is to enable a large network such as a multi-agency group of senior managers, middle managers and practitioners to come together to explore their functioning as a whole system. By training in small, often single-tier groups, it can be hard to appreciate the impact on staff and service users of the agency or professional network as a total system.

Very small groups, on the other hand, pose other challenges, in terms of the potential exposure and demands on each member, including the trainer. There are few hiding places in small groups. Some exercises simply cannot be done unless there are sufficient numbers; for instance, where role plays or action exercises are designed to explore a range of perspectives.

Composition

Composition refers to the make-up of a group, including the trainer(s), and covers features such as:

● role (professional, volunteer, carer, user, politician);
● agency or discipline;
● grade (manager, practitioner);
● gender, ethnicity, age, disability;
● external relationship (stranger group, occasional group, established group).

The more diverse the composition and the less established the group, the more time it will take for the group to form and generate the cohesion required to attempt more challenging methods. Such groups are likely to need methods which focus on sharing and engaging in each other's experience of work. There may be limited understanding of mutual roles, which need clarifying before they can move on to more reflective, analytic and action-orientated methods.

The composition also has implications for power relations within the group, as well as between the trainer and the group, which in turn have implications for choice of training methods. For instance, there may be a blind person in a group, and the trainer, unaware of the fact, has planned an exercise based on visualisation and art work. Another example is where there is a single black worker in a group and the trainer plans a role play in which the client is to be a black person. Here there is a real danger that the black worker may feel obliged to take the client role, thus replicating the oppressive process of how black service users lack choice or culturally appropriate services.

Physical environment

If the trainer has not checked out the venue, nasty surprises can await them. They may have planned a number of small group exercises that require participants to move between groups, only to find on arrival that the venue is a steeply tiered lecture theatre. Other venues such as hotels or work places can be very exposed. For instance, in hotels, bar and reception areas are sometimes offered as syndicate group spaces. These appear uninterrupted at the start of the day, but by lunchtime members of the public are around, and small group discussion for instance, or video analysis of practice, becomes impossible. Where large conference rooms in work places are used, interruptions, the arrival of refreshments, paging systems, or other workers and service users passing by outside the room, can make it extremely difficult to run some action exercises where again learners may be very exposed. In selecting methods, the trainer needs to know the physical layout of the venue, and consider the impact of other factors over which they may have little or no control.

Awareness of these ten factors means that the trainer needs to be armed not only with a clear plan before the course begins, about methods to be used, but also ideally to have knowledge of other methods which can be brought in if some of the unpredictable factors described above arise. The ability to modify methods on the spot is also extremely important, not least because some of the best methods are created spontaneously when the trainer is able to pick up on unplanned learning opportunities, or respond to methods suggested by groups. The more familiar the trainer becomes with a method, the more learning they are able to achieve through it, and the more responsive they can be to facilitate unanticipated opportunities for learning. On a practical note, it is helpful for the trainer to keep a learning diary to record how different methods work, and ways of improving them. Such aides-mémoire come in very handy when the trainer feels short of ideas, or feels that every course must have new methods.

We turn now to examine specific training methods.

TRAINING METHODS

Traditionally, training methods are divided into two main groups:

1   Trainer-centred methods (sometimes referred to as teacher-centred).

2   Learner/group-centred methods (sometimes referred to as student-centred).

Methods can also be distinguished in broad terms along four other dimensions:

1   High personal involvement vs. low personal involvement.
2   High challenge/exposure vs. lower challenge/low exposure.
3   Emphasis on co-operative methods vs. competition.
4   On the job vs. off the job (training courses).

In this book generally the focus is on methods to be used with 'off-site' learning.

It may be noticed that methods cannot be easily divided up as to which aspect of Kolb's Learning Cycle a method targets. The reason is that almost any training method, including lecture formats, can target more than one, and sometimes all four stages in the Cycle, according to how they are applied. For instance, depending on the content of a formal presentation lecture – such as the sharing of a traumatic experience by a survivor – it may engage listeners in their own experience, as they identify with the speaker, more than in analysis and conceptualisation. For this reason, the methods described below are not organised around the Kolb Cycle but under four main method groups:

1   Presentation-based methods
2   Group discussion methods
3   Experiential learning methods
4   Reflective methods.

Under each heading, a variety of methods are presented, explaining how they can be used to access different parts of the Learning Cycle, and issues and potential pitfalls to consider in using them. Tables 9.1, 9.2, 9.3 and 9.5 cover each of the four method groups. In considering the use of any of these methods, however, it cannot be emphasised too strongly that the choice must relate to the context and condition of the learning group, and the competence of the trainer. Every method requires preparation, explanation and skilled delivery, followed by a structured reflective framework so that the learning from a particular presentation or exercise can be elicited.

Presentation-based methods

This includes the trainer-based group of methods mentioned above. However, because these methods do not just involve presentation by the trainer, it seems more helpful to widen the description to presentation-based methods. The distinction between presentation-centred and learner-centred methods is in the role of the trainer. Learner-centred does not imply, in the context of group training programmes, self-directed learning, but that the learning is being elicited *from*, as opposed to knowledge being transmitted *to*, the learner. Many learner-centred methods require a very active role from both learner and trainer. However, the majority of presentation-centred methods cast the learner in a much more passive role.

Lecture

Although this is the most obvious case of a presentation-centred method, it should not be neglected. Indeed, the strong 'experiential learning' traditions of social care training in recent years have sometimes resulted in a lack of theoretical and research presentation. Participants complain that they have not been given sufficient knowledge and theory to respond to. The issue therefore is as much to do with preparation, relevance, timing and delivery of a formal presentation, and how it is followed up in terms of reflection, critical analysis and action areas for practice. Sloppy, short, unfocused 'inputs', with poor visual aids and uncritical transmission of theory, practice or research have devalued the place of the lecture within training programmes. It is also erroneously thought that a lecture cannot be integrated within experiential learning. This is a misunderstanding of the term 'experiential', as if it restricted learning only to 'having experiences'. Within Kolb's Cycle, lectures can have a valuable role not only in the transmission of knowledge and theory but also in stimulating reflection, and provoking an emotional engagement in a subject – as, for instance, where service users talk about their experiences.

Audio-visual presentation

This refers mainly to the use of commercially produced training material, or sometimes material recorded from television programmes, or recording of a lecture/speech given elsewhere. Commercially produced audio-visual material can be put to many uses in training, depending on its content, and can be very powerful in its effect on a group, especially where the material brings users 'into the room'. Careful preparation and clarity as to what learning is being sought is essential, and the trainer needs to be familiar with the material. It can be interwoven with reflective work, by pausing and exploring observers' reactions, or acting as trigger material in terms of asking, 'What would you do at this point?'. Debriefing such experiences carefully is essential. When audio-visual material is used in this way, the distinction between presentation-based and participatory learning is removed. The role of the learner is as a very active, responding participant. Trainers will also need to consider copyright requirements when using such material.

Theatre/creative presentation

The use of dramatic presentations with professional acting companies has become increasingly popular both in direct practice work as well as in training. Its value lies in the ability to use dramatic metaphors to address complex, conflictual or emotive issues, and involve audiences in this at the same time. Its learning benefit is thus less at the conceptual level than at the experiential level, providing a very good platform for subsequent reflection. Careful briefing of the actors is critical so that they address the professional issues appropriately.

Depending on the content and type of delivery of any of these presentation formats, they can generate heavily charged emotional material, hence the need to consider the ten factors described above. The trainer must be alert to signs of emotional distress and this may indicate the need for co-training.

Demonstration

In a demonstration, either the trainer or someone else with a particular expertise demonstrates a skill, either in role play or in a real scenario. Demonstration might also be done using video presentation, which is of course much safer for the trainer! Modelling is an essential part of skill development, especially in relation to inter-personal skills. In social care training, the skill being modelled might typically be interviewing, or managing some kind of group process. However, in our experience, modelling of skills is under-utilised in training programmes. This can stem from a view that expertise should not be demonstrated, as it is elitist, or that expert demonstration will leave learners despairing that they can never achieve such a standard. On the other hand, learners certainly notice if the trainer can only discuss an area of practice theoretically, and is unable to demonstrate its application in practice.

Demonstrating complex interactional skills is not the same as demonstrating moving and handling skills, in that there may be different views as to what is happening, and therefore what a 'skilled response' might be. It should be stressed that the demonstration focuses on only one way to perform the skill, but it does represent one experienced worker's application of their knowledge, values and skills to practice. Demonstrations can result in considerable and productive debate about the nature and appropriateness of the skill being shown, and reflection on individuals' skills. Because of this the trainer cannot easily fulfil the role of both demonstrator and facilitator of the group's observations. Two trainers are needed.

Finally, attention should also be paid to who the 'expert' is. Indeed, this applies to much of the preceding discussion about presentations. The role of the 'expert' is a very powerful one. If presenters are predominantly white, male, heterosexual and able-bodied, this will convey oppressive messages about status, patriarchal and Eurocentric control of knowledge, and the marginalisation of similar or greater expertise held by women, ethnic minorities, gay/lesbian or disabled groups. Similarly, if the 'expert' is always from one discipline – for instance, a psychologist – at inter-agency training events, it will also

Table 9.1 Presentation-based methods

Benefits	Considerations
Provides clear exposition of complex material	Must be linked to reflection on the material to be recalled and relevant
Gives an overview to stimulate debate	Must be well prepared and delivered by someone with expertise
Can access expertise not held by trainer	If using outside speakers, must be sensitive to group context
Good for transmitting information, but can also stimulate emotional responses	Choice of presenter re. gender, race, discipline crucial
Targets cognitive/intellectual but also experiential learning	Timing crucial
	Needs good handouts and visual aids
	Less likely to suit all learners, can demotivate or marginalise
	Can facilitate powerful emotional content: debriefing essential

inhibit learners from identifying with, or making use of the expertise because they feel alienated from their own expertise.

Group discussion methods

Small group discussion (four to eight learners) is probably the most frequently used, and sometimes over-used, of all training methods. It can further a wide variety of learning aims, such as encouraging participation, building group cohesion, generating energy, sharing of experience and knowledge, exploration of values and perceptions, analysis of differences and commonalities, generating ideas and facilitating risk taking. Its attraction is that it can be used very flexibly during a training event, with the focus selected either by the learners or by the trainer. Small groups can be structured or unstructured in terms of task, facilitated or self-directed.

The apparent simplicity and flexibility of small groups, however, can mask their unpredictability and complexity. It is tempting to feel that having set a small group exercise the trainer can relax, even prepare for their next course, when they should be observing group interaction and intervening if necessary. Small groups, whatever the task, often generate responses other than those requested, which can have a powerful effect on the larger group and on the course as a whole. For instance, a small group discussion may provide an opportunity for learners to share their experiences about the course, including any dissatisfactions, or a small group may become dominated by the concerns of one member who chooses to use that forum to share a personal issue. The wrong combination in a small group can result in anti-learning groups forming who simply reinforce negative attitudes towards the training, or an attitude that 'nothing can change'. In an inter-agency event lack of thought as to composition of small groups may result in staff from the same agency sitting together, or the creation of a group in which there is only one member from that agency, who feels very isolated. Unstructured composition of small groups can create gender and racial imbalances which marginalise those in a minority, causing them to begin to disengage or lose confidence to contribute.

All these examples illustrate that the make-up, tasks, objectives, monitoring and feeding back of small group work requires preparation and thought if it is to contribute effectively to learning. Bergevin *et al.* (1963: 95) claim that a good group exists when

● it is of interest to all group members;
● all members have sufficient information to participate;

- it is clearly instructed;
- different perspectives can be offered.

Having made some general observations about the use of small groups, we move now to identify different types and tasks for small groups.

Buzz groups, snowball groups, cafeteria-style groups

All of these groups are good for energising learners, moving them around, making links between people, and getting interaction, ideas and feedback going between the group and with the trainer. While the first two types are better at generating reflection or strategies quickly, the cafeteria-style group can be useful for more considered responses involving some analysis.

Buzz groups

The term 'buzz group' is used when two members share their reaction to a presentation of some sort. Trigger questions might include: 'Which bits did you react most strongly to?' or 'What surprised you most?', 'What made/did not make sense?'.

Snowball groups

This is an extension of buzz groups, except that the initial pairs then join forces with another pair, discuss for ten minutes, then join up with another foursome, discuss, then feed back.

Cafeteria groups

In a large audience, participants are seated in groups of six or eight at round tables, so that they can respond to formal inputs as a discussion group. This is a useful method for integrating presentations and work-ing in a participatory way with large audiences. Convenors for each group can be appointed and flip-chart paper and pens are provided so that they can feed back. The advantage of this arrangement is that participants can be arranged in a variety of ways: by team, agency, discipline, interest groups, manager/practitioner groups and so on. This allows them a base group within a very large audience or during a conference event. However, getting feedback from a large number of small groups in a very large room can be laborious. A useful short-cut is to get the convenors from each group to meet over lunch, compare all the feedback and synthesise it into one or two summary sheets.

Quick-think

This method has commonly been referred to as a 'brainstorm', but it is now recognised that this is an insensitive use of language in terms of those who suffer from epilepsy. The method involves the group generating as many responses as they can to a chosen trigger theme or word – for instance, 'partnership' – which are then written on a flip chart. These can be feelings, ideas, associations, myths or assumptions in response to the trigger word or theme. This is probably one of the simplest, most common and effective ways of freeing up thinking, energising and valuing a group's ideas. It can be undertaken with large or small groups, works on the basis that quantity breeds quality, and relies on the deferment of judgement – by not pausing to analyse each idea. This encourages the less experienced and newer members to contribute, because all comments, as long as they are not offensive or oppressive, are permitted. It is important to generate as wide a group of responses as possible, and to note both participants who are not contributing and those who dominate. The trainer needs to record all responses and to beware of beginning to sift, slow up or 'rationalise' the process by trying to re-state a response in the trainer's own words, or pausing to emphasise what the trainer regards as key highlights.

Panels, debates, interviews, fishbowls, quizzes

These methods are based on the Socratic idea of using structured questioning to externalise the learner's thinking by eliciting:

- what the learner knows;
- what the learner knows but is unaware they know;
- what the learner does not know;
- what the learner does not know and is unaware they do not know.

All of these methods can be useful as learner-centred methods of presenting or drawing out knowledge, theory, values and practice approaches.

Panels and debates

These enable groups to work together on presenting and articulating a professional issue. They test critical reasoning and can be useful in getting learners to look at an issue from a perspective that they would not normally adopt. However, because they can be dominated by a few members who are particularly vocal, and may be an exercise that quieter members find daunting, they are more effective in small groups or panel teams. Like the other methods described in this section – interview, fishbowl and quiz – the motivation for learners behind them lies partly in the adrenalin created by introducing a degree of intra-group competition. These methods also focus learners not only on the clarity of their own thinking but also on their observations and analysis of others' thinking.

Interview

The group may be asked to elect an interview team and prepare areas for the interviewers to cover. The interviewee can also be asked to comment on areas that were not explored. The interview can be particularly useful in working more interactively with a visiting 'expert' in probing their knowledge from the learner's perspective, and allowing the learners to retain control of their learning. In this way the 'expert' is reframed as a resource to the group.

Fishbowl

Three members are seated in an inner circle and asked to start discussing a proposition, such as 'Confidentiality and multi-disciplinary working are incompatible'. The rest of the group sit in the outer circle. Once the discussion is under way, any member of the outer circle can replace someone in the inner ring to make a point, as long as the person in the inner ring is not speaking at that point. The aim of the fishbowl is to get as many people in the group involved in giving their views on a subject. It is therefore best with groups of no more than twenty.

Quiz

The last method in this section is the quiz. Although at face value it might appear patronising, in fact small group rather than individually based quizzes appeal directly to the aspect of play which has a significant role in the learning process. Senior managers as well as practitioners relish the challenge of being 'right', and the method can provoke useful debates, in addition to its primary value in eliciting and exchanging knowledge or evaluating levels of knowledge within the group. For instance, on a development day for an Area Child Protection Committee, a quiz was designed to test members on their knowledge of committee structures, tasks and management data. The lack of knowledge among a significant proportion of the group provoked a very healthy debate. Different kinds of quiz can also act as effective methods of revising earlier knowledge or theoretical models. One way of doing this is to put up on flip charts visual symbols or diagrams representing key models. An example comes from a course for trainers. The Kolb Cycle was put up on a flip chart, but without any words, and small groups were asked to fill in the missing words and explain the model to the rest of the group. Such exercises often reveal interesting information about exactly how a model was understood or not, and can open the way for the trainer to correct any misunderstandings. They also demonstrate that repetition has an important role in cognitive learning.

Feeding back and concluding from discussion groups

The value in all structured discussion groups lies not just in the discussion, but in the quality of the small group's conclusions and feedback, and in the way this is utilised by the trainer. Feedback without any further analysis or encouragement of cross-group debate other than a word of thanks from the trainer, is a meaningless exercise. Sometimes it is better to specify that feedback to the whole group is not sought. However, in the majority of cases it is an essential part of the task to hear the conclusions drawn from these structured discussions and debates. This can give the trainer an opportunity to probe thinking by asking how a certain conclusion was reached and to get the group to explore different perceptions and conclusions. Taking feedback from structured discussions is a complex business but is as important to the learning as the work undertaken during the structured discussions.

A very simple feedback structure based on the Kolb Cycle would contain these five questions:

1   What did you observe during the presentation or exercise?
2   What feelings were generated during the exercise or presentation?

Table 9.2 Group discussion methods

Advantages	Considerations
Flexibility for range of learning tasks	Room layout needs to be suitable
Good for sharing, reflecting, analysing experience and generating strategies	Avoid over-use of small group discussion
Engages learners with each other	Selection of small group vital: gender, race, discipline, grade, degree of experience, etc.
Generates energy	
Makes positive use of competition without putting individuals on the spot	Tasks, and nature of feedback required need to be clear: put in writing
Stimulates ideas, creative thinking	Process needs managing as it can provoke wider, unplanned or unwanted discussion
Validates and explores groups' knowledge, values, perceptions, feelings	Trainer needs to check in with small groups on progress (not switch off), and ensure they remain focused
Can provide immediate feedback	
Checks learners' grasp of subject	Can be frustrating if discussion too quick for some learners
Explores consensus/difference	
Small group enables risk taking	Skilled management of feedback by trainer crucial
Assists quieter learners to contribute	
By giving different tasks to small groups, a wide range of work can be covered	In large groups, trainer must decide on aim and extent of feedback, otherwise process can become laborious and group lose focus
Rehearses the confidence to explain one's practice	Avoid reinterpreting feedback
Encourages group's responsibility for own learning	Encourage group to interpret its own feedback

3   What links did you make with other areas of your professional knowledge, experience or beliefs?
4   What have you learnt from the presentation or exercise?
5   What can you apply to your practice?

Experiential learning methods

A wide variety of activities go under this heading, with the potential to create powerful and deep-level learning experiences. Here, therefore, even more than with other groups of methods, the need to assess and prepare a learning group for using these methods is essential. Negative experiences of badly managed role plays or other experiential learning methods can put both learners and trainers off using such methods at all, despite the fact that they are an integral component of effective practice learning. Given the range of potential learning from these methods, and their emotional potency, the trainer's clarity of purpose and care in making use of such methods is vital.

While all of these methods involve some enactment of experience, they can be used for a variety of purposes to target different parts of the Learning Cycle. For instance, a role play may help learners to appreciate the experience of being a service user (experiencing), or it may be used to rehearse a specific skill (active experimentation). However, the safety and success of these methods also depends on the underlying cohesiveness of the group, as these methods are more exposing and emotionally demanding than the other methods described so far. It is important that in using such techniques the focus is clearly educational rather than therapeutic. While individuals may find an exercise therapeutic for them, this is a secondary and personal bonus.

Role plays, games and simulations

Role plays

These enable the learner to experience something about which they are intellectually aware. This increases their emotional understanding of a role, and is particularly good for exploring processes and skills associated with addressing interactional problems and relationships. However, not everyone finds this medium easy, not least because sometimes they have been subject to a badly managed role play in the past. Hence careful preparation and explanation to the group of the learning objectives and process of the role play are necessary. Information before the course should also have made clear whether role plays and other experiential methods are to be employed.

Role plays should normally be done in small groups, as exposure to a whole group can be very daunting, unless the trainers play the more demanding roles such as the workers. Even in small groups, role plays usually require facilitation until the group becomes more confident about itself, and clear about the framework both for running and debriefing the role play. However well planned, the results of a role play cannot be wholly predicted. Learners are frequently surprised by how far and fast they can get into role, even if the role play lasts only a few minutes. This stems from our natural tendency to project one's own experiences, feelings or thoughts onto the roles and experiences of others, usually without realising it. Indeed, many aspects of experiential learning rely on the idea of projection, and it is important that trainers are familiar with this when using experiential techniques.

Projection, however, means that the boundary between role playing and the acting out of the individual's own issues, feelings or attitudes in the role can be crossed extremely quickly. While this can be a potentially rich source of unexpected learning, it depends on the trainer's good debriefing of the experience. Trainers need to be alert to angry or distressed individuals volunteering to take the role of a vulnerable or angry person in a role play. Observers too can be very affected by role play, either through identifying with those in it, or simply by the emotion generated. Trainers should not neglect, therefore, the audience's needs to debrief after watching a powerful role play.

Another issue is ensuring that the audience do not become passive spectators. They can therefore be asked to observe different aspects of the process, different actors, or observe from different perspectives – for example, 'Pretend that you are the child in this family observing this interaction, what feelings, concerns and needs does it raise?' They can then feed back 'experiential' rather than intellectual observations. The concept of projection also means that comments made by observers may well say as much about the attitudes of the observer as the behaviour of the observed.

Doubling

Different observers are asked to track different players during the role play to speculate on what that person might be feeling or thinking at any point. The trainer can stop the role play and invite doubling. An observer touches the role player on the shoulder, stating, for instance: 'I am the patient and I am feeling patronised but unsure what to say to the doctor.' This is an approach which can extend the benefits of role play through active participation from the observers.

Simulation

These are an extended form of role play in which a whole process, rather than just one small section, is enacted. Examples might include a residents' meeting, a case conference or a management meeting. Simulations require careful preparation to ensure that they are realistic, but their advantage is that they extend role playing to tackle more complex processes. The emphasis is much more on problem solving, and looking at group decision-making processes. Simulations thus require a substantial time allocation, perhaps as much as three to four hours to allow for adequate preparation and debriefing. A major difference between simulations and the other methods is that the simulation involves more or sometimes all course members, which means that they are all likely to get heavily into role. Debriefing is thus even more imperative and will take longer.

Hypothetical

The narrator prepares a series of short cameos involving a number of roles; for instance, family members and professionals, taking a situation through a number of stages. It could, for example, be focused on bereavement counselling involving the following sequence: informing the relatives; the relatives back in their own home; the relatives telling others (friends and so on); the family one year on. As each cameo is narrated, with the role players for that cameo seated in front of the audience, the audience is invited to speculate in turn on what each of the players might in role be feeling, or needing. After this, the players respond simply to their own experience of listening to the narration and to comments from the audience about their character. A series of five cameos, including audience comments and character feedback, should take no more than forty-five minutes. This method, which is different from a role play, can be used to obtain the participation of larger audiences, where the aim is to explore complex processes and how they unfold over time.

The hypothetical has the advantage of not requiring players to act, or invent lines for their character. Instead, each character simply draws on their own feelings and thoughts evoked by the unfolding narration and the feelings and thoughts directed from the audience onto their character. The hypothetical works on the basis of the audience's projections, which can reveal much about the nature of the audience's own understandings and attitudes, in this case to a bereavement situation. As with the role play, much depends on careful preparation, and debriefing of both audience and characters. Frequently the most powerful learning comes from the latter, who often come to appreciate experimentally how one dynamic in the helping process compounds another over a period of time.

Other creative methods for experiential learning

Creativity and play make a very significant contribution towards learning. After all, it is through play that young children learn and communicate. It is easy to neglect this dimension when dealing with adult learners, especially if they are managers in suits. Unfortunately, some approaches to games in learning settings have been counter-productive, in terms of being inappropriate, aggressively competitive or patronising.

It is perhaps more useful therefore to distinguish between play as a medium for learning and playing games. An example of the latter would be an ice-breaker exercise at the start of a training event, where the trainer gets participants to chuck a bean bag around the group as a fun way of facilitating introductions and energising a group. In relation to specific games for use in training, many practical texts have been written, references to which can be found in the bibliography. The focus here is different.

The existence of 'right' and 'left' brain preferences is now well known. Thus, while 'left' brain learners prefer logical, analytical and linear approaches, 'right' brain learners prefer more imaginative and intuitive approaches involving patterns, art, colour and music. Using play, rather than playing games, is about accessing creative, intuitive knowledge held at an emotional, unconscious or experiential level. Depending on the exercise used, play may be used to bring learners together or for more reflective and analytic purposes. An example one of us used,* was in development work with a very large inter-agency group comprising an Area Child Protection Committee and three large sub-committees. Each of the four groups was asked to make a physical representation of how it related to the other three groups, using materials provided such as paper, glue, straw, paper-clips, scissors, colour magazines and so on. The models were then presented and this provided the framework for an analysis of inter-group relations.

Neuro-linguistic programming (NLP) has also discovered that people think and learn with a preference for a particular combination of senses (Lawlor and Handley 1996). Thus some will find visualisations helpful, others will find auditory prompts and associations helpful, while others will find physical activity helpful. Trainers could then think about how subject matter could be reinforced and linked by methods such as mind maps, music or exercise.

---

*   This exercise was developed from an original idea by Gerrilyn Smith.

Space does not permit more than a brief mention, in this section, of a wide range of approaches to enhance creativity and tap into unconscious processes. These can enable rapid access to experiences, perceptions, feelings, memories and areas of personal, group or organisational awareness that are held at a subconscious level. For that reason these are also potentially very powerful techniques, because it is impossible to anticipate what will be produced, or how it will impact on a learning group. The timing must therefore be considered carefully, in terms of allowing sufficient space for reflection. The group's capacity to respond to such material is highly dependent on their confidence in the trainer. The trainer also needs to be aware that some participants, notably those who are 'intellectualisers', may dismiss such approaches and seek to opt out in a way which can undermine the group's confidence in their use.

Sculpting

The basic method involves getting group members to portray a particular relationship by creating a physical representation, using other group members in a silent physical portrait as statues. This method makes use of body and visual imagery. They can be positioned so as to depict features such as closeness or coldness, dominance or submission, dependence or autonomy. Each group member is chosen to represent either an individual (a user), a group (carers' network) or an institution (agency). Normally an individual or small group directs the sculpt to demonstrate their perceptions and experiences. Once the sculpt is set up, the trainer can go round and ask each person to describe what their pose feels like, and whom they can or cannot see. A sculpt can be used to depict relationships, dynamics or processes at strategic, operational, inter-agency or inter-personal levels. Sculpts can also be set in the past, present or future. The sculpt can then be done from different perspectives; for instance, from the perspective of a service user or a disabled person. A further development can be to rearrange the postures into some desired improvement of working relationships. This takes the learning process on from experience, through reflection to active experimentation, whereby new relationship frameworks are 'played with'. The physical experience of being different, albeit only for a brief moment, can be a strong motivator for change.

Sculpting can highlight power relationships between individuals or groups, not only through the physical postures, but also via the feedback from those in the different positions within the sculpt. Sculpting can provide a strong medium for those who may not normally be heard, or who are less articulate, to have a different type of voice. It can throw into sharp relief oppressive processes such as isolation, marginalisation, lack of access and alienation from sources of power and decision making. Again the physical experience of confronting such power imbalances and structures can be a powerful force for change, as long as the group is prepared for, led through and debriefed with considerable care afterwards. Although sculpting is possibly one of the most risky and physically intimate methods that a trainer can use, its potential benefits can be great. One modification is to state that individuals within a sculpt do not have to have a point of physical contact with other people in the sculpt.

Art work

This too can be focused either on relationships or on the more internal worlds of individuals, to depict in visual form areas such as team processes, feelings or self-perceptions. Once again it is a medium which can generate strong images, because, like sculpting, it is based on subconscious material. Neither the trainer nor the learner can fully anticipate what will emerge. Like sculpting, art can give a different voice to quieter or less powerful members, a parallel with the therapeutic use of art with children or those with communication difficulties. A care assistant can describe the dynamics of a residential home more powerfully in one drawing than all the verbal analysis of the manager. One danger to avoid is too much interpretation of a drawing by others. Instead, others can be invited to react to different drawings as if they were in a gallery, but interpretation should be left to the 'artist'.

Guided fantasy

This involves the trainer asking the group to close their eyes, while the trainer takes them through a guided fantasy using a story-telling approach. While this type of technique is often used on a stress management and relaxation course, it can also facilitate emotional understanding. For instance, in exploring the effects of attachment disruption, a guided fantasy in which participants imagine themselves at home as a child, and being suddenly removed from their parents, can be very powerful. The trainer must, however, be clear where the fantasy is to end, and how the material generated within individuals is to be shared. Once again this method can release strong emotional responses, and

Table 9.3 Experiential learning methods

Advantages	Considerations
Engages at experiential and feelings levels	Pre-course information needs to be clear that such methods are to be used
Chance for unexpected to arise as learning opportunity	Demands more trust, greater exposure
Enables complex dynamics, patterns and processes to be explored	Cannot be done if group not safe
Increases levels of openness	Ensure there is enough time
Can bring subconscious and unresolved issues to surface	Clarity of purpose, preparation and space for debriefing are critical
Can be used to rehearse skills	Unpredictable outcomes
Provide behavioural evidence of theory and knowledge	Some learners have had bad experiences of such methods
Increases group cohesion and emotional energy	'Intellectualisers' may resist or undermine
Creative mediums can give quieter learners a powerful 'voice'	Some learners may need support if unconscious material surfaces
Can highlight power and discrimination issues	Clear boundary with therapy
Promotes strong engagement and recall of learning because of emotional link	Confidentiality rules must be clear
	Trainer must have confidence in method and ability to process issues arising
	May require co-trainers
	Role plays may focus on only a few members
	Observers' tasks need to be clear

learners needs to be clear how the exercise fits with the programme's objectives, in order that training does not become therapy. It is important to assure participants that they are in charge of what they wish to share. This method, as with art work, can, result in disclosure of highly personal material. The trainer must therefore be clear at the outset what the purpose of the exercise is, and what sort of feedback is to be sought, as well as how any personal disclosures will be responded to.

Reflective methods

Although these methods are integral to making use of role play and other experiential approaches, they require separate discussion in this section. Giving learners an experience, however powerful, will not be of benefit unless they are successfully able to reflect upon it. If not, at best the experience may be forgotten, or at worst may be left unravelled, confused and undebriefed.

Reflection is at the heart of making use of experience and is necessary at all four stages of the Learning Cycle. Unfortunately we sometimes do not always approach reflection in a structured way. In part this is a consequence of the fact that there has been insufficient attention to helping professionals learn what it is to be a reflective professional. The result, on training courses and in the work setting, is that observation, reaction, analysis, strategising and rehearsing become merged in ways that do not support effective learning. For instance, notice how easily participants watching a role play leap in with comments such as, 'I've had that happen to me, and what I did was . . .' or 'Why didn't you think of asking her . . .?'

As a result, not only is any structured reflection lost, but those involved in the role play have been prevented from reflecting on their work. Instead, they are forced to consider why they did not do what has been suggested, even if they do not regard the idea as helpful. This in turn distracts them from critical self-reflection and analysis. They may end up feeling misunderstood, and in receipt of considerable and unsought 'advice' about their practice that does not connect meaningfully with their experience or their needs.

A clear reflective framework for analysing role plays, discussion of cases or video recordings of interviews can prevent this happening. This should separate observation, reflection, analysis and preparation for future action. There should be an emphasis on asking open questions which provoke reflection and which reduce the danger of the discussion being contaminated by the questioners' own assumptions and biases. Providing a set of reflective questions based on the Learning Cycle – for instance, in analysing a role play – can be very helpful, as demonstrated in Table 9.4.

Although a debriefing exercise may not cover all these questions, this framework helps learners, both as observers and observed, to direct their reflection. It also has the advantage of reassuring participants that they are not going to be on the wrong end of a free-for-all session of criticism. It should also ensure that all four stages of the Learning Cycle are attended to, so that reasoned conclusions and specific action steps are elicited.

Table 9.4 A structured framework for reflection

1 *Preparing for experience*
  ● What were you planning to do in this interview?
  ● What was your role?
2 *Observing experience*
  ● What did you say/do?
  ● What did the patient/client/supervisee do/say?
  ● What surprised you?
3 *Reflecting on experience*
  ● What feelings did you experience during the interview?
  ● What did this experience remind you of/was similar to?
  ● What parallels with real life did the simulation offer?
4 *Analysing/conceptualising experience*
  ● What assumptions have been challenged/affirmed?
  ● How would you explain/understand what was happening in that session?
  ● How would it have been different if you had been male, white, etc.?
5 *Preparing for the next piece of work?*
  ● What might you do differently as a result of what you learnt?
  ● What are the pros and cons of different options?
  ● How can you prepare for the next stage?
  ● What would be a successful outcome for you from the next stage?

Case study

This has been included in this section as it allows learners, working on either real or fictitious case material, to reflect on and study a problem in a complex form (Jaques 1992: 94). Case studies offer a wide range of potential learning opportunities:

● application of research and theoretical knowledge;
● exploration of emotional responses;
● exploration of value judgements;
● to challenge denial;
● exploration of different roles; e.g. a multi-disciplinary group can be asked to examine a case study looking at how different disciplines would understand and approach the issues;
● examination of role conflicts;
● generation and evaluation of practice standards.

The important points to note are that the material needs to be relevant to the learners' context, contain problems in which there may be a range of options and have a point of identification for all members. Thus, in a

Table 9.5 Reflective methods

Benefits	Considerations
Integrates new experience with prior experience, knowledge, skills	Requires clear structure
Disciplined method for reflection to ensure benefit from experience	Learners may need to be taught how to reflect, especially how/what to observe
Assists recording of experience	Reflection occurs over time
Prepares for further learning	Avoid the rush for judgement/ solutions/actions
Identifies training needs	Lack of reflective opportunities at work can leave an accumulation of unreflected experience that can flood the learner
Enables different perceptions of an experience to be offered in groups	
Individual reflection sustains learning	Boundaries with reflection on personal issues need to be clear
Enables bridge to be built between training and work setting	
Promotes transfer of learning to work	
Reflective diaries/logs can provide portfolio evidence	

group that contains several disciplines it would be essential that the case study material has all the disciplines represented in it. It is also necessary to ensure that the case studies are socially representative in terms of features such as gender, race and class. Once again the instructions for how the case is to be examined need to be specific.

One powerful approach to case study for inter-agency training can be to use material from published inquiries into practice – for instance, in the mental health or child protection fields – in a disguised form. The impact on participants, regardless of whether they have accurately analysed risk and provided an effective intervention plan, of hearing the outcome of the real case can serve to deepen their theoretical understanding by attaching some emotional significance to it.

Individual reflection

So far we have looked at reflection from a group learning perspective. However, individual reflection also needs to occur, both within training courses and, more importantly, alongside and beyond the training course. There are a number of simple devices which can assist.

Learning diaries/incident logs

These can be maintained on a regular or occasional basis, and they can be structured to suit a variety of reflective needs. They can be used to record successes, critical incidents, feelings/moods, insights, questions and so on. They can highlight future training needs. For instance, on a leadership course for residential managers, members were asked to maintain a leadership log between modules to record significant leadership incidents. They were asked to record three incidents when they had performed well and badly, and to analyse in which contexts they performed better or worse. The incident log was also used as a basis for seeking feedback from colleagues about their perceptions of the same incidents. The log enabled them to establish a baseline leadership profile and to identify specific leadership skills for further work. Logs and diaries also assist in integrating on- and off-site learning, and for maintaining links with the training process. Finally, they can provide evidence for portfolio purposes.

Self-evaluation checklists

This is a useful tool for helping learners establish a baseline before starting a piece of learning, and marking their progress. It also helps to identify specific development needs. A variant on this is to get course members to design their own self-evaluation framework, if there is the time to do this. It is important with any external self-evaluation tool to give the respondents a chance to contextualise it, either by adding items that are relevant to their job and which are not included, or by getting them to delete areas that are not relevant. The more ownership and credibility the checklist has, the more valued are its results.

Mind maps

Finally, as was noted at the outset, people have very different preferences for how they best remember and integrate complex learning. For those who find visualisation helpful, mind mapping is a good technique. And in order to illustrate rather than describe this, a mind map of this chapter is presented (see Figure 9.1).

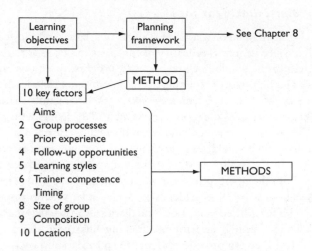

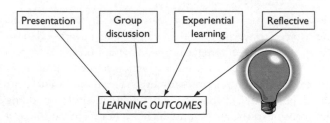

Figure 9.1 A mind map summary of key messages from Chapter 9

Chapter 10

Transferring learning into practice

Issues and frameworks in learning transfer

This chapter explores:

● what is learning transfer, and why it is so important;
● models and research about learning transfer;
● strategies for maximising the transfer of learning from training to job performance.

Six months after an extensive period of training on partnership practice and change targeted at all first-line child care managers in a social services department, follow-up evaluation indicated that the managers had found the training very useful and wanted some refresher training. This was arranged, and the refresher training began with participants being asked to recall what theoretical material had been useful and what practical steps they had taken to apply this.

What emerged was a picture that for many trainers is increasingly familiar and disheartening. This included poor recall of the theory, diffidence about whether they had fully understood it and thus anxiety about trying to share it, few people having read the literature provided and little shared action within or across teams to implement learning on a joint basis. As this somewhat gloomy picture emerged, the group was asked to explore the contrast between their original enthusiasm as depicted by the post-course evaluations, and the low rate of their learning transfer – i.e. putting their original learning into practice in their jobs. In response to this question they described a number of barriers to the transfer of their learning:

- an agency culture where 'doing' not thinking, reading, exploring or feeling were valued;
- where 'models' were perceived as being for students;
- a lack of time to apply the learning;
- a lack of support, coaching or feedback from their managers to apply the course material;
- the sheer volume of other change going on which they had to learn about in order to survive organisationally;
- the absence of local opportunities to continue learning together;
- becoming an isolated learner once the formal course structure ended.

The participants expressed a clear need for some repetition of the theoretical models, which they continued to regard as relevant and valuable. Thus the refresher day focused on

- consolidating their grasp of theory;
- exploring what they had learnt/applied which they did not recognise until they had an opportunity for reflective discussion;
- understanding the complex journey from theory to practice;
- exploring the barriers to learning transfer, particularly isolation;
- identifying local action learning groups based on people who worked together;
- reviewing personal motivation to take their learning forward;
- identifying current local and agency-wide initiatives or issues of shared concern to which the models could be applied.

Although the participants were initially somewhat depressed by their lack of progress, the mood quickly lifted as they discovered that they had learnt more than they had thought, were given permission to appreciate the complexity of learning transfer, and addressed the isolation which had undermined their confidence. Too often the expectation by agencies, learners and, worst of all, trainers is that transfer of learning back into job performance will start automatically when the training ends. When this philosophy of 'train and hope' does not prove successful, trainers, managers and learners can each end up blaming the others for the lack of training outcome.

This chapter sets out to unravel the complexities of learning transfer and to offer a framework and strategies to maximise the positive impact of training on performance. It is clear from the example above that the process by which what is learnt in training transfers into better performance on the job is a complex one, influenced by a range of factors.

However, this vital subject is short on both research and attention. Despite the assertions made in leading management books that 'training is highly related to organisational excellence' (Peters and Waterman 1982: 142), the research basis for such optimism about the power of training to raise performance is lamentably low (Analoui 1993: 6). Eraut, writing about in-service training for teachers, puts it in a nutshell when he observes:

> The common practice of providing input without follow up is almost bound to fail because it underestimates by an order of magnitude the amount of support that is needed, and because it fundamentally misconstrues the nature of professional learning in the classroom . . . .The learning of practical knowledge is little discussed and little studied.
>
> (1994: 37)

These observations could apply equally to training in social care.

Despite these limitations, the issue of transfer is a fundamental one for everyone involved in training. As Bell (1993) has stated, the first goal of training is to meet users' and carers' needs. Second, training exists to promote the achievement of organisational goals. If training cannot demonstrate how or whether it contributes towards these two goals through the transfer of training into performance, then it matters very little whether it achieves its third goal, which is to meet the professional development needs of individual staff. Finally, the ability of workers to transfer and adapt their learning into a variety of different contexts is becoming increasingly important because of the continuously changing contexts of their work. Indeed, CCETSW's definition of professional competence includes the ability of social workers to apply skills, knowledge and values to new situations, and to distinguish these from skills or knowledge that have a unique application (CCETSW 1991). It is hoped that this chapter will help to enlarge the reader's understanding of the issues involved in the successful transfer of learning into performance, as well as offering some practical strategies at both the planning and delivery stages of the training cycle.

WHAT IS TRANSFER?

Annett and Sparrow (1985: 116) describe the transfer of training to be 'the benefit obtained from having had previous training experience or experience in acquiring a new skill or adapting an old skill to a new situation'. This focus on skills alone, however, leaves out the importance of values and knowledge in the transfer process, and says nothing about the value of the transferred learning to users. Dickson and Bamford (1995) state: 'Positive transfer is the degree to which trainees effectively apply knowledge, skills and attitudes gained in a training context to the job.' Curry *et al.* describe transfer of learning as the application of learning acquired in training to the job, by ensuring that workers 'receive the right training with the right support at the right time to facilitate transfer and client impact' (Curry *et al.* 1991: 112). This definition makes explicit that transfer is effective if it results in positive effects on the services to users, echoing Bell's (1993) assertion that the first goal of training is to meet users' and carers' needs. Three key points emerge from these descriptions of transfer:

1   Transfer of learning involves acquiring knowledge, values and skills and applying these to the job.
2   Transfer requires organisational support.
3   The ultimate test of effective transfer is whether it benefits service users.

FOUR TYPES OF TRANSFER

Transfer can be considered in four main ways, each of which results in different outcomes: (1) specific/vertical; (2) general/lateral; (3) negative, and (4) zero effect (Analoui 1993: 14; Annett and Sparrow 1985: 120; Curry *et al.* 1991).

First, specific, near or vertical transfer refers to knowledge, skills and values learnt which are similar or exactly the same as those found in the work place. This type of transfer relies on the idea of 'identical elements', so that the more similar what is being transferred is to the job task, the more successful the transfer. An example would be learning moving and handling skills. But this model requires the learner to recognise the similarity of the task to newly acquired knowledge or skills. Equally, they must be able to recognise the relevance of prior knowledge and skills to a new task, otherwise transfer will not occur. The more specific or specialist the knowledge or skills involved, the more difficult it can be to recognise the application in another context. For instance, probation officers having to supervise sex offenders often fail to appreciate the relevance of their previous experience in supervising other violent clients.

Second, general or lateral transfer refers to knowledge, skills and values that can be applied across a wide range of new situations, or to situations of a similar complexity. This process of generalisation is based on the idea of pattern recognition, lateral thinking and making connections between past and current situations. However, for generalisations to work, there is also a need to be able to discriminate as to what is appropriate or relevant to transfer across situations, otherwise overgeneralisation may occur. For instance, student social workers may apply task-centred theory to every case, thereby failing to use other theories which may be equally relevant.

General transfer also relies on 'formal discipline' theory, whereby skills are seen to derive from a number of core abilities such as information processing, memorising and reasoning, which can be adapted to a wide range of contexts. In terms of professional competence, these would include Eraut's 'process knowledge' skills, described in Chapter 2. These cover skills that are essential to good professional practice, which, it is often erroneously assumed, professionals possess or acquire without requiring any specific training. Eraut (1994: 107–16) lists five key process skills:

1   *Acquiring information*: interviewing and observation skills, and interpretation of information.
2   *Skilled behaviours*: a complex sequence of actions that becomes so internalised that it is performed almost automatically, so that workers can cope with high volume demand and rapid decision making.
3   *Deliberative processes*: planning, problem solving, analysing and decision making, which require a combination of theoretical, situational and practical knowledge and judgement, and where reliance on procedures is inadequate.
4   *Giving information*: the ability to give information clearly and in ways that can be heard and understood by service users, and to provide the information that is likely to be most relevant to the service user.
5   *Metaprocesses or reflection*: self-knowledge and self-management to direct one's own behaviour to engage effectively in the processes described above. It requires the reflective capacity to self-evaluate critically what one is doing, thinking and feeling – to stand outside oneself, and be prepared to examine assumptions and actions.

Third, negative or inappropriate transfer refers to learning that makes it more, rather than less, difficult to learn a new skill. This can occur through the intrusion or application of previous work practices, values or theories which are unhelpful or inappropriate to a new situation. An example might be workers from a residential setting on a training course who claim that there is no need to review their recording practices because 'We've always done it this way'. However, it is important to distinguish between the uncritical repetition of entrenched bad habits, and the process of undergoing temporary de-skilling and loss of performance that often accompanies the initial application of new skills and knowledge. We rarely do the right thing the first time following training, especially when what is to be transferred are complex problem-solving skills, knowledge and values.

Fourth, zero transfer is when there is no impact from training on performance. However, it is important to note that zero transfer impact is not necessarily the same as saying that nothing was learnt. Some learning is unconscious, or is only transferred into the work place under supportive conditions, as the example at the beginning of this chapter showed. Thus managers may report zero training transfer, when in fact the learning is suppressed within a work place culture in which the unwritten message is 'Don't rock the boat, leave things as they are round here'.

Let us now try to summarise the above. Bridges (1994) makes a useful distinction between transferable skills – for instance, specific computer skills – or presentation skills and the transfer of learning, which requires a much deeper grasp of underlying principles and general performance skills. The idea of transferable skills might apply to 'near transfer' situations, whereas the concept of transfer of learning is closer to generalisation, where both the context and the application of knowledge and skills and values will be more complex. For instance, the application of an assessment framework from a training context to the management of cases would require more than a transfer of skills, because judgements must be made about when to apply or modify assessments in different cases. This requires more than the transfer of skills and knowledge; it requires a transfer of learning.

Cree and Macauley (1997) suggest that traditional ways of conceptualising knowledge and skills as separate entities have been misleading. In order to facilitate a transfer of learning, knowledge and skills need to be developed simultaneously. In order for transfer to occur – for instance, using a newly taught assessment framework – 'knowing that' (knowledge) and 'knowing how' (skills) need to be assimilated alongside the strategic understanding of knowing what to do when. This reiterates discussion in Chapter 2 about the distinction between individual competences (specific capabilities) and competence as a deep-level, integrated understanding and ability to co-ordinate appropriate internal, cognitive, affective and other resources necessary for successful adaptation, application and transfer of learning (Wood and Powers, in Eraut 1994: 181).

INADEQUATE ANALYSIS OF TRANSFER ISSUES IN THE PLANNING AND DELIVERY OF TRAINING

Training transfer is affected by a range of factors beyond the design and delivery of the training event. These factors include organisational cultures and support, the nature of what is to be learnt and transferred, and the capacity of the learner. Unfortunately, naïve assumptions about transfer in the minds of managers, commissioners of training, trainers and learners have contributed to an inadequate analysis of transfer issues. These faulty assumptions include the following:

- transfer of learning automatically follows a training event;
- all learning during training will result in behavioural changes on the job;
- the learner is the principal or sole agent of transfer;
- the teacher/training method is the principal or sole agent of transfer;
- what is taught is what is learnt;
- effective transfer is demonstrated by the worker becoming immediately more competent and confident on return from training;
- transfer relies on the depth of 'technical' learning – e.g. the learner's grasp of the specific knowledge, skills or values taught in training;
- that work-place conditions do not have to be modified in any way to enable transfer to occur.

In one of the few books specifically about transfer, Analoui (1993) observes that the major deficit in most approaches to transfer is the failure to appreciate the impact on transfer of organisational culture and work-place conditions and dynamics. In describing the organisation as a dynamic learning environment, she refers to the rules, culture, norms, power structures, values both overt and covert which socialise all members of the workforce. She states:

The main reason training is not transferred is not because ineffective learning has taken place, but because the transfer of learning
has been prohibited by colleagues, bosses, clients, either formally or
informally, preventing the learner from displaying the knowledge or
skills acquired. . . . These changes to attitudes or behaviour have to
be informally approved by peers, and supervisors.

(Analoui 1993: 52)

A powerful example of this process can be found in the implementation of some anti-discrimination training, whereby individuals returning
to challenge practices and attitudes may be ostracised. Analoui goes on
to state that effective transfer requires organisational support, particularly from the immediate supervisor, but also for the learner to possess
the ability and social skills to cope with the 'social assault course' of the
transition between training and its transfer into the social system of the
work place (1993: 124). The learner's personal confidence, professional
acceptance and ownership of the learning will have considerable influence on the individual's approach to negotiating these transitions.

CREATING AN ENABLING CLIMATE FOR THE TRANSFER OF LEARNING: TRANSFER AS A SOCIAL AND TECHNICAL PROCESS

Transfer depends on the organisational context in which learning
occurs. Positive, developmentally orientated team and agency contexts
will enable transfer to take place in a way that rigid, rule-driven contexts
will prohibit. Too many stories exist of professionals who have been
sponsored by their agency to undergo extensive pieces of professional
development in order to examine an agency problem, which they are
then blocked from applying on return to the agency. Often the individual leaves in frustration to join another agency where their learning will
be utilised.

Analoui's analysis suggests that a 'socio-technical' model is needed to
understand transfer fully. This is in line with Eraut (1994: 33), who
stresses that a 'significant proportion of learning associated with any
change in practice takes place in the context of use, and that there is
little immediate transfer of learning from one context of use, e.g. a
training event, to another, e.g. workplace'. This means that we must
plan for transfer from the outset of any training venture. Effective
transfer therefore combines three phases:

1   Planning for transfer from the outset.
2   Acquisition of technical learning related to the specific knowledge, skills and values required to perform the job.
3   Social learning and skills, including understanding the social structure of the work place, how to maintain group membership, how to understand others' expectations, how to engage others in changes that enable the individual to transfer their learning into practice (1994: 105).

An exclusive emphasis on technical learning, however good, will fail to address the fact that for individuals to improve their performance, others – especially those in their immediate team and close professional network – will need to be involved and on-side. Therefore training for transfer must address technical and process-knowledge needs, in order to equip learners to be not just technically proficient, but also an effective member of their organisation. This indicates that often the most effective transfer occurs when those who work together learn and train together (McFarlane and Morrison 1994).

PREDICTING TRANSFER

A further implication of this thinking is that predicting the extent and nature of training transfer is very difficult. This is so for several reasons.

*   *The difficulty of analysing social care practice.* Specifying competences and analysing job components, skills and attitudes can only go so far in describing practice. Style, intuition, situational factors, and the creativity involved in tackling complex and unpredictable human problems mean that no performance can be reduced to applying a set of distinct skills, values and knowledge. The ability to know how to act when it is not clear what should be done is as necessary as being able to specify what should be done in prescribed circumstances.
*   *Learning and the development of practice are cumulative processes.* Individuals transfer their learning into practice over time, and in different stages. Our intellectual, emotional and behavioural understandings of an area of practice may all be at different stages at the same time, continually being refined and reappraised. Thus an intellectual appreciation of discrimination may precede an emotional realisation of what it means, which in turn may precede changes

in behaviour and practice. All of these are stages along the transfer route.

- *Transfer does not occur only at a conscious level.* A supervisor returned to the second part of supervision training course, reporting little success in making use of part one. However, when asked about the behaviour of her supervisees, she revealed that they seemed to be more open about feelings. Although initially perplexed by this, when it was explored she began to see that she had changed her approach to supervision without realising it, and that this had given staff permission to discuss the emotional content of the work. Without that reflective opportunity, it is possible that the supervisor would not have recognised and owned the very real transfer that had gone on. Transfer may need to be elicited from the learner, particularly where the learning is in less tangible areas such as values or emotional understanding.

  The critical role of the supervisor cannot be underestimated in this process. Regrettably, for middle managers and above, the availability of more senior managers to act in a reflective capacity is a serious gap for many middle managers.

- *Learning may become compartmentalised.* Although we should expect training in one skill to benefit another skill if there are common elements of task or psychological process, this requires the individual and the agency to recognise the common elements. However, while job analysis can play a very useful part in identifying common elements of skills and knowledge between different jobs, it too has limitations. As Annett and Sparrow comment: 'There is no handy off the shelf source of information on how much transfer can be expected between pairs of skills' (Annett and Sparrow 1985). Moreover, the breakdown of core competences within the NVQ system into discrete elements of knowledge, values and skills has contributed to the compartmentalisation of learning.

- *Anxiety prevents or distorts transfer.* The impact of anxiety on learning was discussed (Chapter 1). The concern with managing risk, in mental health, child protection and criminal justice settings has been a powerful driver in gaining additional funding for training, and in galvanising agency commitment to training. However, the hidden message can be the covert expectation that training will 'prevent' disasters occurring, and that following training staff should be able to 'get it right'. This anxiety may be made worse for individuals who have been trained, now appreciating what should be done and what procedures should be followed, but knowing that the necessary resources or systems are not in place to enable them to apply their new learning. In this context transfer may be displaced into procedural conformity and rigid practice, with little room for experimentation, or staff may become immobilised from putting their learning into action for fear of failing.

- *Prior experience influences transfer.* Learners do not come as blank slates. Their previous learning experiences, motivation and self-confidence all play a powerful role in determining their response to new learning, as do their current perceptions of the nature of the professional task, their managers and their organisation. Trainers regularly encounter individuals within an agency group sharing the same difficult working environment, who make far more practical and positive use of the training than other participants.

Because of these difficulties in predicting the extent and nature of training transfer, there is 'no easy way to say with certainty just how much any given achievement or skill will transfer to another, or how far general problem-solving and inter-personal skills can be transferred into totally new situations, and what training methods facilitate this' (Annett and Sparrow 1985: 124).

It is not surprising, given the paucity of research, that trainers can make overly optimistic assumptions about transfer. However, despite the fact that the precise mechanisms of transfer remain unclear, trainers are not completely in the dark. Research undertaken on the effectiveness of in-service training in teaching, health and social work provides some firm clues as to what facilitates positive transfer, and how trainers can positively influence this.

WHAT DOES RESEARCH TELL US ABOUT THE PROCESS OF TRANSFER?

Parker and Lewis (1980), drawing on models of change, developed a specific model called the transition curve (Figure 10.1). This describes the process of change, with particular reference to organisational or imposed changes, which offers further insights to the transfer process.

The first stage of shock in response to change, especially where this is imposed, is quickly followed by denial at the reality or extent of change or the need to adjust to the change. The feelings of threat, imminent loss, powerlessness and anger can result in denial, as indicated at stage 3.

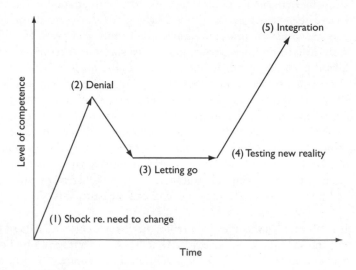

Figure 10.1 Transition curve
Source: Parker and Lewis (1980)

As an example, only a fortnight before the implementation of the Children Act 1989, a group of workers with whom one of us was working were denying that the Act would change anything. Others claimed that they were already doing everything that the Act required so there was no need to change.

The third stage is depression and letting go, when denial gives way, often reluctantly, to an acceptance that change is happening. This stage may be accompanied by feelings of dependency, temporary helplessness, passivity, anger and, most critically, reduced competence and confidence. At its worst, a lack of support at this stage, this may result in disengagement and giving up. However, with support, the individual is able to start to let go of the previous reality, and ways of doing things, in order to make the changes necessary to engage constructively in the new context. This marks the beginning of recovery. However, this can only happen effectively if previous knowledge, skills and values that are relevant to the new context are affirmed. Otherwise the outcome may be compliance rather then integration, assimilation and real change.

Stage 4 marks the point where the new reality is tested out, in terms of discovering which previous skills, values and knowledge, and relationships can be relied upon to address the demands of the new context. Although there will still be some fears and a reduced level of performance, the road to change and integration has begun. The identification of future training needs can begin. However, full integration takes time, and can be disrupted if further change occurs before confidence has fully returned. For example, in responses to changes in community care legislation, many social services departments also set about major organisational changes. In other words, further change occurs while understanding of, and the ability to work in, the new context is still tentative. Frequent organisational changes in recent years have depressed some workers' expectations about the possibility of positive outcomes from such changes, and have generated a feeling of 'here we go again'.

Factors affecting the ability to transfer learning

Analoui argues that all learning and change is a process of initiation, negotiation and integration, which may be more or less smooth or bumpy (Analoui 1993: 92). This is attested to by a number of research findings on transfer, mainly looking at in-service development work with teachers. These studies identify a range of factors affecting training transfer.

Factors affecting transfer

- The motivation and expectations of the learners – 'Is it worth it?' (Marsh 1989).
- The level of self-confidence, self-efficacy and self-esteem of the learner (Gist *et al.* 1991).
- The opportunity for learners to develop their own ideas (Doubler 1991), and be involved in joint problem solving which is away from the job (Townsend 1996).
- The importance of social and supportive interaction between learners (Doubler 1991).
- The flexibility, analytic skills, competence and empathy of the trainer (Husein 1988).
- Starting where the course members are, negotiating agendas and being encouraged to use one's own experience (Husein 1988).
- Recognition that choice of method is less important than the extent to which learning is negotiated and structured, and feedback is given (Allen 1985).
- The cultural fitness of the programme (Husein 1988).

- The organisation's commitment, response and sustained support after the training.
- Tailoring post-training support to the needs of individual staff each of whose transfer process is different (Doubler 1991; Eraut 1994).
- The provision of developmental supervision (Townsend 1996).
- Coaching and mentored classroom support to observe and feed back on practice (Doubler 1991).
- Observing the practice of different experts and hearing their thinking aloud (Eraut 1994).

Doubler's (1991) study of teachers changing their teaching of science provides rare detail on the transfer process in action. He concluded that there was no automatic transfer of changes in teachers' thinking into classroom practice, that there are tensions for the teacher between old and new strategies, and that the transfer process is very individualistic for each teacher. Instead, transfer was observed to be an incremental and gradual process, often very fragile at first, which occurred when teachers

- became more reflective;
- focused more on children's ideas;
- moved away from right/wrong thinking;
- became less directive;
- changed the types of questions they asked;
- received ongoing and practical support, including being observed, being allowed to test out ideas, and having time to reflect and build on practice.

Although Doubler's study was on the transfer of learning from training into classroom practice, there are many obvious parallels with the transfer of learning into practice in social care settings.

In summary, research points to four key factors which influence the transfer of learning:

1   Learners – their motivation, capacities, expectations, needs and knowledge.
2   What is to be transferred – its complexity, specificity, immediacy, newness and relevance.
3   Training – negotiability, values, design, methods, location, timing.
4   Organisation – culture, values, support, stability, supervision.

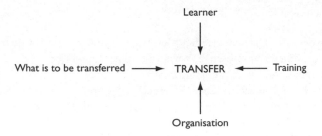

Figure 10.2 Four transfer factors

STRATEGIES FOR PROMOTING TRAINING TRANSFER

The remaining part of the chapter will focus on how each of these factors can be addressed in order to maximise the potential for learning to be transferred into practice. Underpinning all these strategies, however, must be a partnership for learning between managers, trainers, learners and service users, for it is upon the quality of this partnership that transfer depends (see Figure 10.3).

Transfer factor 1: The learner's contribution to transfer

Individuals' capacities to learn are not fixed, but can be enhanced and extended if the learner is motivated. However good the training programme, individuals will not learn if they do not wish to. Moreover, as we have seen in Chapter 5, each individual's approach and motivation

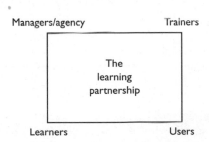

Figure 10.3 The learning partnership

to learning are influenced by a range of historical, situational, physical and cultural factors. These include:

- life experiences, values, needs, tolerances, ambitions, power dependencies, frames of reference, ways of seeing the world;
- prior experience of learning situations;
- levels of self-confidence and self-efficacy;
- current and historical family, social and work roles;
- intellectual, social and emotional skills;
- ways of memorising and perceiving;
- prior professional knowledge, skills and values;
- preparation, motivation and expectations towards new learning;
- nature and awareness of their own learning styles, ability to self-evaluate.

In terms of strategies available to individual learners to enhance their capacity to learn, one of the most useful approaches lies in the understanding and expanding of one's learning style. In Chapter 2 Honey and Mumford's (1982) four principal learning styles were presented. These were activist, reflector, theorist, and pragmatist.

All individuals, including trainers, therefore have natural preferences, strengths and weaknesses in their learning style. For example:

- activists, who like to leap in and try things out, may be poorer at observing, reflecting and analysing before acting;
- reflectors, who like to observe and stand back, may be anxious about making mistakes, taking decisions, acting before all the facts are known or giving something a go;
- theorists, whose strength lies in approaching things in a systematic and logical manner, may be weaker when it comes to taking pragmatic decisions, having to 'fly by the seat of their pants' or dealing with strong feelings;
- pragmatists, who are strong on problem solving and trying out new ideas to solve practical problems, may be weaker in dealing with feelings or waiting until a full analysis of the situation has been completed.

Dickson and Bamford (1997) draw a distinction between two main approaches to learning. The 'holists' approach material in a more inclusive way, looking for broad relationships within it and identifying underlying principles and generalities. In contrast, the 'serialists' tend to become caught up in the narrow detail of specific aspects and applications, as a result of which they can find generalisation of key principles, knowledge and skills to other areas of work more difficult. Taking into account the idea of learning styles, the individual can work on enhancing their transfer capabilities through extending their learning styles and addressing those areas in which they are weaker. The starting point is for the learner to identify their own learning styles, which can be done through Honey and Mumford's Learning Style Questionnaire (1982). In a subsequent publication, Honey and Mumford (1986) have suggested a number of practical ways in which learning styles can be expanded, to which the reader is referred for some useful checklists of possible strategies. However, the following examples of strategies for strengthening each learning style will give some ideas about their approach. Thus to improve

- activist style: do something new, such as co-working with a colleague;
- reflector style: develop a structured decision-making or review record;
- theorist style: develop a reading programme – e.g. one hour per week to read a journal;
- pragmatist style: examine the pros and cons of different approaches to a problem.

Enhancing the individual's responsibility for learning

Enhancing the role of the learner in the transfer process cannot be achieved unless the individual is clear about their responsibility for learning. Although this is often discussed in the ground rules at the start of training events, defining an individual's responsibilities for their learning is not straightforward. It is also affected by the discipline from which the worker comes. Health trained professionals tend to have a clearer sense about their individual responsibility for learning than social work staff, because of different traditions and arrangements for the delivery of training, and the requirement of health professionals to re-register periodically with professional bodies. Confusions exist as to where the boundary lies regarding the agency's responsibility for the individual's learning, and the degree to which individual profesionals are responsible. Moreover, the common misconception that learning means 'attending a course' further confuses the discussion.

Individual workers have responsibilities at three stages of a learning process:

1   Identifying a learning need and preparing to meet it.
2   During a training event or other learning process.
3   After a learning event, to facilitate transfer into their practice.

At each stage – before, during and after training – the individual's responsibilities can be identified at the four points of Kolb's Experiential Cycle; that is, to identify their needs or experience, reflect on them, analyse them, and decide on further action. Examples are given of this in the matrix in Table 10.1, which is designed as a practical means for identifying the learner's role in their learning and thus enhancing successful transfer. It might also be used in conjunction with the learner's supervisor. Clearly, these are illustrative questions only, as there are many other questions with which learners need to engage.

Table 10.1 Learner reflection matrix

	Before training	*During training*	*After training*
Experience: Identify my learning needs/ experience	I wish I could do my job better; I was unable to manage that situation.	Is this what I need? Do I feel safe to contribute?	What happened when I returned to work?
Reflect: Explore my learning needs/ experience	Where/when do I feel I could do things better?	What am I feeling? What connections am I making?	Who asked what I had learnt? Did I manage situations differently?
Conceptualise: Understand and put in context	What existing skills have I got? Is this a training need?	How am I understanding the learning? What values underpin this?	What does my learning mean for my work, and my service users?
Active experiment: Decide on action	Decide what to do about my learning needs: seek training or other learning opportunity.	Do I have a clear picture of what this new skill is, or how to apply it in my job?	How can I rehearse my new skills? Who will observe me?

Transfer factor 2: What is being transferred where

The second key transfer factor concerns the nature of the learning to be transferred. Four different types of transfer can be identified:

1 Simple vs. complex learning.
2 Specific vs. general learning.
3 Immediate vs. long-term learning.
4 New learning vs. re-learning.

The more exact and specific the learning to be transferred – for instance, computer skills – the easier the transfer. This may account for the fact that much of the research on transfer has focused on verbal and motor skills learning, because this is much easier to measure than learning involving values, feelings and more complex applications. The more complex, the greater the situational variables; the more discretion and judgement involved in whether to use a particular skill or theory, the harder the transfer process.

Another variable is how urgent or immediate the transfer process will be. Thus, if the learning has no immediate relevance – for instance, if training on new legislation is introduced a long time before the new arrangements come into force – transfer will be adversely affected. Finally, as the example at the start of the chapter showed, re-learning will promote easier transfer than new learning.

Location

Another factor influencing transfer is the location of training. Analoui argues that location has a significant impact on transfer, in that, broadly speaking, the further away the training is from the work place, the more difficult the transfer process: 'the proximity of the learning situation and trainee to the actual work environment provides opportunity for social as well as technical learning and thus the potential for effective transfer is increased' (Analoui 1993: 61). For example, an evaluation of training on managing challenging behaviour demonstrated that transfer took place more readily when the training occurred in the residential unit rather than externally. In other words, on-site learning reduces the degree of social learning and transitions that learners must do both in negotiating membership of a training course, and in bringing such learning back to the work place. However, Analoui also states that, for complex learning requiring a high degree of technical input, such as problem-solving and dealing with difficult and emotionally laden areas, off-site training is preferred. Therefore, as Analoui (1993: 123) shows in Table 10.2, the complexity of the transfer process alters according to how many transitions must be negotiated.

At (1) the learner attending a training course at a point where they are negotiating a new job and a new work place has not only to integrate the technical knowledge and skills to do the task, but also face considerable social learning to understand and begin to operate effectively in their new work environment. In contrast, for a learner attending a course from a familiar work place and a familiar job (4), the amount of social learning is far less, as the 'rules' are known, leaving them freer to focus on the 'technical' skills and knowledge being acquired.

While transfer is generally accelerated when those who work together also train together, assessment is required as to whether this is the most advantageous approach. For instance, teams often need to get away from the work place to move into 'learning' mode, or individuals in a very 'stuck' work-place environment might well need to join a different group on an off-site training course. Thus the degree of social learning or transition required to put new knowledge and skills into action is not simply a function of the location of the training, but has as much to do with the culture and functioning of the work place.

Summarising this section, the implications for trainers in promoting transfer are as follows:

● they must understand the learner's current work context;
● they must assess the degree of transition that groups and individuals will need to negotiate in order to transfer learning – e.g. it is important to know how long learners have been in post, or whether they are about to change roles;
● training content and outcomes must be carefully matched to the nature of the learners' work roles and the competences required in the roles;

Table 10.2 The learning transfer continuum

(1)	*(2)*	*(3)*	*(4)*
New job New work place →	Familiar work New work place →	New job Familiar work place →	Familiar job Familiar work place

Source: Analoui (1993: 124)

- entry criteria need to be clear to ensure that learners have the necessary prior experience, knowledge, skills and roles to be able to make use of the learning;
- it is vital to provide work-based opportunities for learners to try out their learning in real situations, to observe themselves in action, receive feedback and analyse their practice;
- where general skills, knowledge or processes are being taught, learners should be assisted in identifying a practical context to which the learning can be applied as soon as possible.

Transfer factor 3: The training process

The key to transfer is that it must be embedded in the thinking and planning of managers, trainers and learners from the outset. If it is bolted on as an appendix at the end of a training event, the potential for effective transfer has already been significantly reduced. Learners are pondering what awaits them at their desk, and the course mood has already begun to move into endings and withdrawal. Managers look forward to staff returning to pick up their work, and hoping that something from the course will have rubbed off, while the trainer's attention has already begun to move to their next training event. It is a scene familiar to every trainer, who departs with the vague hope that at least some of the members will use some of the material. After all, as a trainer remarked, 'A 50 per-cent hit-rate is pretty good round here'. How different the atmosphere can be, when instead participants are leaving to undertake assignments, video themselves at work and are returning to share their discoveries, so that transfer is built into the programme from the very start.

The TOTAL model (Transfer of Training and Adult Learning) (Curry *et al.* 1991) provides a framework as to how transfer can be integrated into each stage of the training cycle: needs assessment, setting objectives, programme design, methods, delivery and evaluation. In this way training transfer becomes the over-arching goal of the programme, embedded in every element, not just in the final module. In this discussion we shall provide an overview as to what this means at each stage of the training cycle, referring as necessary to more detailed discussion in other chapters.

Curry *et al.* emphasise the need to assess at each stage of the training cycle potential barriers and facilitators affecting transfer, at three levels: managers/agency, training, learners. These can then be collated into an overall assessment of the transfer environment (Table 10.3), in which

Table 10.3 Transfer assessment grid

Facilitating factors	Before	During	After
Training needs assessment			
Training objectives			
Programme design			
Delivery methods			
Evaluation			
Agency level			
Training level			
Learner level			
Barriers	Before	During	After
Training needs assessment			
Training objectives			
Programme design			
Delivery methods			
Evaluation			
Agency level			
Training level			
Learner level			

Source: Adapted from Curry et al. (1991)

facilitating factors and possible blocks are identified. Armed with this information, strategies for overcoming or circumnavigating blocks can be generated, thus raising transfer prospects.

First, training needs assessment must be linked closely to the management of performance, through the identification of the competences required for the particular task. Regular training needs analyses using a variety of methods are necessary in order to maintain an accurate picture of workforce needs, in relation to agency goals, user needs and professional standards. Further discussion about training needs assessment can be found in Chapter 3.

Key considerations include the following:

- How comprehensive and reliable is the training needs assessment, at organisational, professional and individual levels?
- Who owns the training needs assessment?
- Are all the needs expressed training needs?
- How closely does it relate to agency plans and goals?
- Are there clear performance standards and competences against which training needs can be tested and training outcomes can be measured?

Second, regarding the development of training objectives, in general terms the more specific and performance-orientated the learning objectives, the more likely transfer is to occur. In contrast, non-specific objectives will almost certainly weaken the transfer potential. For example: 'This course will look at aspects of grief and loss, and will therefore help participants to improve their counselling skills.' A specific objective might state: 'The objective of this course will be to apply the grief counselling model in three cases within the first two months.'

Chapter 8 is referred to for more detailed discussion about setting training objectives. Dickson and Bamford (1997) also emphasise the need for relevance in terms of setting training objectives. In order for objectives to motivate learners and have meaning for them, the aims and content of training programmes must have utility, desirability, practicality, appropriateness, and adaptability.

Key considerations include the following:

- Are training goals and objectives clear and specific?
- With whom have these objectives been negotiated?
- Are they consistent with agency and service goals?
- Are learners aware of the link between training and agency goals?
- Do the objectives specify the performance expected as a result of the training?
- Is the expected behaviour and contribution of the learner explicit?
- Is the role of the supervisor in supporting this training explicit?

Third, with reference to programme design and delivery methods, as these are closely linked, they are discussed jointly here in relation to transfer. In Chapter 8 programme planning and design were explored, and in Chapter 9 training methods were discussed.

The quality of the trainer plays a crucial part in the learning process. Brotherton states:

> Research indicates that the instructor cannot rely on the student's own ability to discover what is useful through experience, nor can much occur through self development. Positive assistance is required so as to structure the experience in the direction of new understanding, development and personal expansion.
>
> (Brotherton 1991)

Without in any way denigrating the value of self-directed learning, our experience is that in a climate of insecurity and continuous change, the role of the trainer and the supervisor in facilitating and motivating learners is vital.

In relation to the impact of methods on training outcomes, Allen's research led to this conclusion:

> It is not the methodology but the extent to which methods make use of interaction, negotiation, structured activities, and feedback. The assumption that adult learners are self directed is not supported, they wanted direct guidance, and needed to be taught how to be self directed learners.
>
> (Allen 1985)

Having established that the role and conduct of the trainer is a vital ingredient, other research based on interpersonal skills training proposes a number of factors in the design and delivery of programmes which will promote the likelihood of successful transfer (Dickson and Bamford 1997):

● *Train loosely.* Programmes should not be too rigid, regimented or predictable, otherwise learners may become too cosy in their learning, and cease to think about application or generalisation issues. Variety and challenge can be maintained by offering a range of training methods, exploring a variety of case examples and strategies and viewing differing demonstrations of skilled, and poor practice, behaviours.
● *Promote mediation.* Transfer is promoted when learners can make appropriate connections between knowledge, values and skills used or taught in one context, and other practice or work contexts. Identifying the underlying principles and general skills required for good practice assists this process of applying learning in one context with application in another. Learners should therefore be provided with opportunities to explore the application of learning to their specific work contexts.
● *Fluency learning.* In Chapter 2 the skill acquisition model by Haring *et al.* was presented, which emphasised the need to go beyond the basic acquisition of a skill, during training, to proficiency and generalisation, in order to integrate and maintain the new skill in practice. Another way of describing this, in terms of promoting transfer, is that training programmes need to provide opportunities for moving from basic acquisition to increased fluency in the use of specific skills and models of practice. This is

facilitated when skills and models are taught in a logical sequence in which levels of complexity are gradually increased. Enhancing fluency may also be done by requiring workers to audio or video record themselves using new skills in their actual work, or to be observed, and then to return for further analysis and consolidation of their learning.

- *Goal setting.* Finally attention should be given to learners anticipating situations in which their new knowledge or skills may be compromised, and developing relapse prevention strategies, such as realistic and specific goal setting, and identifying a colleague who can act as a learning transfer partner. The partner might, for example, agree to observe practice or undertake some co-work.

Key considerations:

- How culturally 'fit' are the methods?
- How does the composition of the group (continuing vs. one-off group) and location of the training (on site vs. off site) help or hinder transfer?
- How far do the methods provide for skill rehearsal, feedback, coaching?
- How does the programme specifically prepare learners for the transition back to work?
- How far are the managers of the participants involved in the training process?
- How might timing of the training affect the potential for transfer; e.g. what else will be happening in the work place that might help/hinder transfer?

Fourth, evaluation: Chapter 11 addresses evaluation issues. It emphasises that training must be evaluated against performance and practice outcomes, in addition to the learner's immediate post-course reactions and their cognitive learning. Establishing a clear evaluative process is a powerful catalyst for transfer, because it builds on the fact that what gets done tends to be that which is measured. Evaluation strengthens expectations that transfer should be visible in actual practice, establishes practice-based transfer targets, provides direct feedback to the learner, and helps to identify factors which hinder the transfer process.

One very practical technique is to ask trainers to provide learners at the end of a course with a 'transfer postcard', addressed to the trainer, which the learner is asked to return after three months (Curry *et al.* 1991). To offer confidentiality, it may be preferable to issue a stamped addressed envelope in which the transfer postcard can be sent. The postcard is filled in with the learner's transfer action plan at the end of the training course, and then evaluated by the learner at the end of a set review period and returned to the trainer. This places some personal responsibility on the learner to evaluate what has been transferred. The postcards returned to the trainer can then act to build a transfer database in the organisation. Where two identical training courses have been run, this method provides a useful comparison between two groups as to the extent of training transfer.

Key considerations:

- What is being measured: immediate reaction, memory, changes in job behaviour, enhancement of practice?
- Do the evaluation criteria match the training objectives?
- Do they involve observation of transfer by others – supervisor, users, colleagues.

ORGANISATIONAL STRATEGIES

Although this is the final factor to be discussed, it may well be the most significant, as the research cited earlier in this chapter stressed the critical role played in the transfer process by the learner's immediate manager. Organisational strategies for transfer also bring into focus the agency's overall attitude to staff development and performance management. For training is one element of a much broader human relations framework of recruitment and selection, induction, supervision, appraisal and discipline which, if not functioning well, will inevitably blunt the impact of even the best training. In order for the organisation to play its part in the transfer process, the strategic role and mandate of the training function must be understood and owned throughout the organisation, and managers in particular must know how their role as staff developers should complement the training function.

Transfer will be assisted where managers are involved in annual performance reviews and appraisals so that individual and team training needs and performance targets can be identified. However, the manager's biggest contribution to the transfer process rests in their supervisory role:

- helping the worker to analyse their learning style and blocks to learning, both personal and organisational;
- assessing the training/development needs of the worker/team, and how these can be met through a variety of development work, including both on- and off-site learning opportunities like training, projects, co-working, assignments, secondments, observations, mentors, action learning;
- providing practical and emotional support to workers before, during and after undertaking training;
- assessing service delivery and user needs;
- regular and constructive coaching and feedback to the worker, including observation of practice;
- assisting the worker in planning transfer of learning into their work via individual and team opportunities to utilise new knowledge and skills;
- regular meetings to check on progress of transfer plans.

However, if managers are to carry out these developmental functions, they will require both the permission and supervisory skills to invest time and energy into this aspect of their role. No transfer strategy can work effectively if managers are not given the time, training and support to play their vital developmental role alongside trainers and their own staff.

Once again, practical frameworks can assist. Based on the Transfer Grid of Curry *et al.* (1991), transfer strategies can be plotted, taking into account the contributions of different stakeholders: learners, trainers, managers/supervisors. In the illustration given in Table 10.4, the grid has been illustrated with reference to team strategies.

At an organisational level, effective training transfer needs to be underpinned by strategies at both the macro (policy, performance management systems) and the micro (supervisory/team/worker) levels.

Key considerations:

- How, at a policy level, can trainers, managers and learners agree their respective roles and responsibilities in the transfer process?
- How can a competence framework be used to assist the transfer process?
- How can the trainer involve relevant managers from the outset?
- How does the agency equip its managers to act as developmental allies?
- How can teams be equipped to act as active learning groups?
- How can successful transfer methods and outcomes be disseminated?

Table 10.4 Team transfer strategies grid

Before	During	After
1 Team involved in training needs assessment, and relating these to team goals	Team provide cover for colleagues on training courses	Individuals discuss training, and review potential uses for team. Contribute to team transfer log
2 Team identify how training could assist with cases/areas of work	Team organise co-work to try out models of work taught on training	Team assess impact on cases. Contribute to transfer log
3 Team identify future team development needs	Team brief facilitator jointly and set goals	Team establish annual review day, and start team development diary

Source: Adapted from Curry *et al.* (1991)

SUMMARY

- Training transfer can be defined as the extent to which knowledge, values and skills gained in training are applied appropriately in the job.
- The precise mechanisms of training transfer remain under-researched, and it is still assumed too often that transfer will automatically follow training.
- Four types of transfer were identified: specific or near transfer, general or lateral transfer, negative transfer and zero transfer. A distinction was made between transferable skills and the transfer of learning.
- Transfer was understood as having two stages: first, acquisition of 'technical' knowledge and skills during training; second, the transfer of these into different working contexts after training. Successful transfer not only requires good technical learning, but also an understanding of work-place norms and dynamics, and the ability to negotiate and transfer learning back into the working environment.
- Four major influences on transfer were identified: the learner, the nature of the learning to be transferred, the training and the organisational context. A number of practical strategies for enhancing transfer were identified in relation to each of these four influences.

- In order to promote more effective training transfer, attention needs to be paid at each stage of the training process to transfer implications. Practical and emotional support from the learner's supervisor and team colleagues were identified as extremely important.

Chapter 11

Beyond the happy sheet

This chapter explores:

- the purpose of training evaluation;
- what needs to be evaluated;
- a goal-based model for training evaluation;
- factors that influence the effectiveness of evaluation;
- specific issues related to evaluating inter-agency training.

It is a tradition with training courses for the trainer to ask participants to complete an evaluation sheet at the end of the training. This form is often referred to as the 'happy sheet'. A study completed in 1989 found that 90 per cent of organisations, responsible for training 80 per cent of the workforce in the UK, utilised this method of evaluation alone (Training Agency 1989). The Social Services Inspectorate (SSI) in their report on targets and achievements of the Training Support programme (SSI 1997) noted that despite moneys being available for evaluation activities, many local authorities focus on gaining immediate feedback from course participants and in some cases their managers. Few had a framework for longer-term, systematic evaluation to measure the contribution of training to the quality of service provision. This means that trainers and the organisation, in the main, receive some feedback on the feel-good factor but not enough information to analyse exactly what course participants have learnt, how much they will retain and how the training will impact on practice.

It is surprising that in an area of practice where accountability is such a major concern that evaluation of training to social care staff has received such little attention (Jones *et al.* 1995). Given that accuracy is such a central issue in social care, it is surprising that this focus on

immediate end of course evaluation often results from an implicit belief that training is generally useful and therefore evaluation is not necessary. Others consider that any evaluation that goes beyond the training room is just too complex and time consuming and that managers are not interested anyway (Sheal 1997). However, the introduction of market economics to public services, the restructuring of training units and competitive tendering have all begun to raise questions regarding the cost and effectiveness of training. In addition, managers at all levels in organisations continue to question whether training can contribute to the quality of services provided and to the outcomes for service users and their carers (SSI 1997). These questions require those engaged in training activity to consider ways of identifying how the resources expended on training impact on the quality of service provision and the competence of staffs if training should remain a priority area for funding.

The whole concept of evaluation can be overwhelming as trainers and managers struggle in a maze not knowing how and where to start or where to go (McMahon and Carter 1990). In this chapter we attempt to find a way through the maze by considering the following questions:

- What is evaluation?
- Why should it be done?
- What is involved?
- How do you do it?
- How far can you go?

There is no definitive path through the maze, and indeed more than one centre, depending on where the trainer wants to go. Each trainer needs to find their own path to the agreed centre, depending on the map and resources provided by the commissioner of the evaluation. The aim of this chapter is to ensure that all those entering the maze have some idea as to where they should be going, what should be included on the map and what are the appropriate resources to complete the journey.

TRAINING EVALUATION IN SOCIAL CARE SETTINGS: WHAT IS IT AND WHY SHOULD IT BE DONE?

What is it?

Definitions of evaluation of training are broad ranging but include some key features. First, the focus is on assessing the value of training

(Manpower Services Commission 1981; Bell and Beard 1996; Hamblin 1974). Second, evaluation is about the measurement of the effectiveness of training (Hamblin 1974; Goldstein 1993). These definitions beg the question of value and effectiveness to whom and of what. For example, should the focus be on financial or professional value and effectiveness? Within profit-making organisations this can be clearly identified: the purpose of training would be to increase profitability for the shareholders, yet this is not so clear within social care organisations. Third, how do we measure training effectiveness? In manufacturing this can be done in terms of level of productivity, but are the same measures relevant in social care settings? Would we want to measure the effectiveness of an Approved Social Workers' course for mental health workers, in terms of an increase or decrease in the number of people sectioned under the Mental Health Act 1983?

In order to clarify what is meant by evaluation in social care settings it may be of more use to consider the purpose of evaluation in these settings.

Why do it? The purpose of evaluation

As described at the beginning of the chapter, evaluation in social care training units has tended to concentrate on internal validation, within the training room. The evaluation has focused on participants' perceptions as to whether they learnt anything and how they experienced the training. However, as training has become a more structured, accountable activity in social care settings the focus has shifted (Robson 1995). Trainers, others in the organisation and service users are asking questions that require external validation. This means an evaluation that takes place beyond the training room exploring the ability of the learner to apply training to practise within their work setting.

There are a number of groups which have a vested interest in staff training. These are shown in Figure 11.1.

These groups will, to a greater or lesser extent, be interested in evaluating quality and standards in the following areas:

- *Training*: in terms of equipping the workforce with the required knowledge, values and skills to contribute to the achievement of organisational goals.
- *The trainer*: their ability to facilitate group learning to agreed aims and objectives.
- *Professional practice and staff development*: the impact of learning

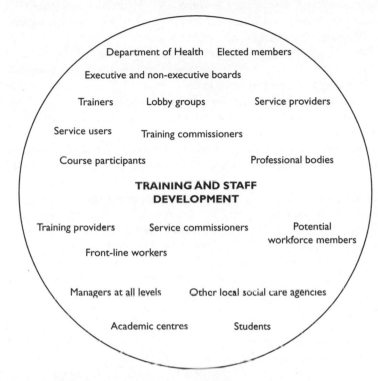

Figure 11.1 Social care training stakeholders
Source: Promoting Inter-Agency Training (PIAT)

from training programmes on learners' work practice and their professional development.

- *Achievement of organisational goals*: ways in which training impacts on achieving and promoting organisational objectives.
- *Interface with external influences*: promoting, through training, effective inter-agency collaboration in its dealings with other organisations, both at a local and national level.
- *Working in partnership with service users*: promoting user empowerment and anti-oppressive practice.

Clearly, different aspects of evaluation will be emphasised by different stakeholders depending on their specific interests. For example, the manager of a training unit, commissioning training from an external trainer, may be interested in the quality of the trainer and the way in which they facilitated group learning. A service user may want to evaluate the way in which the trainer consulted with users in designing and delivering the course.

Formally subjecting a course or a training strategy to a structured evaluation process can convey the message that this training is important, and thus money is being invested in the evaluation. This raises the profile of the training and it becomes an event not to be missed.

In addition to the formal approaches to evaluation, course participants will informally evaluate courses through discussion with each other and with colleagues. This results in situations where certain courses are perceived as well worth attending while others are perceived as a waste of time. Trainers, both internally and externally, are also subject to this informal evaluation. For example, an internal trainer may get a reputation for being humorous and their courses are seen as enjoyable and worth attending, with little consideration of long-term learning. Other trainers may be perceived as challenging and confrontational and to be avoided, even though they may have more impact on changing practice. Likewise, a training manager may commission an external trainer, if feedback is satisfactory, on the grounds that course participants said they enjoyed the course, and they may recommend the trainer to another training manager. Thus an informal grapevine system of evaluation exists which may sometimes be more influential than formal evaluation and yet be based on little more than personal likes and dislikes.

As can be seen, training evaluation in a social care setting serves a number of purposes and needs, addressing a variety of levels – input, output and outcomes. However, they all have some common themes inasmuch as those with an investment in training are interested in determining the value and effectiveness of training. It may be that they are interested in this in terms of achieving organisational goals, or it could be for others that their interest is in their own personal development. Whatever the purpose, the trainer and the organisation need to identify what is involved in assessing the value and effectiveness of training.

WHO DOES IT?

One of the issues to consider when undertaking a training evaluation centres on who should be undertaking the evaluation. Neutrality can only be achieved by using an external assessor. This is often a costly process, and it may only be considered appropriate if the training to be evaluated involves a significant investment in terms of training and staff resources. An example might be a training strategy that offers three levels of training for all staff working with older people regarding recognition, assessment and intervention in cases of adult abuse. Alternatively, an external evaluation can be important if training is a response to a critical incident; for example, an SSI inspection or a child death. In cases where external accreditation is involved evaluation may combine both an internal and external examination.

If, as we will argue, evaluation is an integral part of the training process, it is likely that the responsibility for evaluation will fall on the training unit. This can be difficult for a number of reasons. First, trainers will inevitably have a vested interest in demonstrating that they are effective. Second, the level at which they will be able to undertake an evaluation will depend on the position of the training unit and the perception of training within the organisation. If the training unit is marginalised and training seen as irrelevant to achieving organisational goals, it is unlikely that the organisation will invest time and resources in training evaluation. On the contrary, if the training unit has a high profile and training is assumed to be beneficial in terms of influencing practice and service delivery, the organisation may be reluctant to invest in an evaluation that is only likely to confirm what they already believe. Finally, evaluating training is no mean feat and requires skills in terms of understanding and applying research methods. Trainers may not necessarily have the relevant skills for this task or there may be no recognition of the time and training required to undertake effective evaluations.

Evaluation can, however, be undertaken effectively by trainers if they are provided with a clear framework which emphasises that training is integral to achieving organisational goals and that there is a commitment and responsibility for learning and evaluation at all levels within the organisation. The following elements, as identified by Bell and Beard (1996), provide the key components of this framework:

- staff training and development are a resource that is integral to the achievement of organisational goals;
- senior managers identify goals for the training section within the context of organisational goals;
- line managers recognise and assume responsibility for staff development;
- the specific outcomes for a training course are clearly specified before the event;
- the level and methods of evaluation are agreed at the start of the training process;

- evaluation is considered in terms of measuring actual outcomes at whatever level, against the initially agreed criteria;
- evaluating data are used from a wide range of different sources;
- outcomes are reported back to senior managers and other stakeholders, including the workforce;
- evaluation is introduced gradually and built up to become comprehensive and part of the culture of the organisation.

(Bell and Beard 1996)

WHAT IS INVOLVED?

Factors to take into account

Any training evaluation needs to take the following factors into account:

- learning is an ongoing process;
- evaluation is part of the training cycle;
- any evaluation is likely to contain a degree of subjectivity.

Each of these will be considered in more detail below.

Learning as an ongoing process

Learning is an ongoing process. However, we need time to process the learning by reflecting, observing and making use of the experience, analysing and creating meaning from the experience. Once we have done this then we prepare and actually apply the learning to practice. It is only at this stage that there is likely to be a learning outcome in terms of a change in practice.

However, Gray and Gardiner (1989) emphasise that learners may go through the process of learning at different levels, as indicated in Table 11.1.

They argue that different learners will respond to learning on a training course in different ways. For example, a course on practice guidelines for working with adults from ethnic minority groups with mental health problems may be interpreted in a very narrow way by some learners. They may react to the guidance at a superficial level (level one) and will then apply the guidance to work with service users in a tokenistic manner, adhering to the guidance but not actually addressing the individual user's needs. Another learner may consider

Table 11.1 Levels in the processing of learning

Reaction to learning end of course	Processing learning post course	Outcomes (3–6 months)
Level one narrow and focused	reproductive and superficial	focuses on facts and information
Level two recognition of diversity and complexity	constructive and deep	understanding of meaning and able to interpret
Level three demonstration of versatility	ability to generalise and changes perception	generalises and applies

Source: Gray and Gardiner (1989)

the underlying issues that have resulted in the guidance (level three). They may begin to think about the way in which mental health services do not only offer a poor service to users from ethnic minority groups but also that the needs of other minority groups are not addressed, and consequently apply the learning from the course to improve practice with these service users.

The more significant the learning that takes place on a training course, the more likely it is to impact at a significant level on practice. However, Gray and Gardiner indicate that different factors can influence this process. For example, a learner may leave a training event with a narrow and focused understanding of the learning. If the supervisor spends time with the learner after the course, reflecting on the learning and facilitating the way the learning is processed, it could result in the learner gaining a better understanding and consequently applying the learning and interpreting it in a diverse and deeper rather than a narrow, focused way.

A training evaluation needs to take these factors into account at each stage of the learning process. This is discussed in detail later in the chapter.

Evaluation as part of the training process

Evaluation that occurs at the end of the training cycle can often have the feeling of an add-on, almost as an afterthought. This is demonstrated in

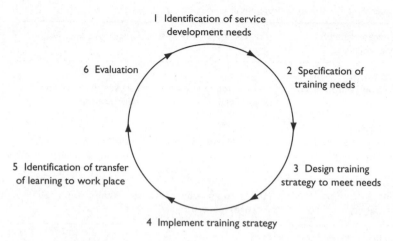

Figure 11.2 The training cycle

many training sections by the use of standardised end-of-course evaluation sheets, often linked to quantifying information through the use of a
computer package. The use of these forms highlights two of the features
that underpin a reactive approach to evaluation. First, that evaluation is
a retrospective activity, obtaining standardised feedback once the course
has been completed, with no evaluation regarding the process that led
to that particular training course being commissioned and delivered.
Second, a standardised format assumes that there are key features of any
training event that need evaluating, with little recognition of the unique
features of each individual training course.

While reactive evaluation serves a purpose, as will be described later in
the chapter, what is clear from the evaluation needs of interest groups is
that a more proactive approach has to be taken to link evaluation into
the training cycle (see Figure 11.2).

Throughout the training cycle commissioners and providers should
be evaluating both task and process, to ensure that evaluation is
contextualised. As Rae states: 'evaluation starts at the birth of the
programme' (Rae 1991: 11).

Table 11.2 highlights the different elements of the training cycle and
the way in which evaluation can inform effective decision making
regarding training and learning at each stage of the process. The
components of the evaluation process itself are considered in greater
detail later in the chapter.

Table 11.2 The links between the training cycle and the evaluation process

Training cycle	Evaluation process
Identification of service development needs which have training implications. This leads to a specification of training needs.	Has the organisation been realistic in its expectations of training? What other factors are likely to influence meeting service development needs?
Design strategy: Make explicit the training intent in terms of designing a training strategy to meet service development needs. Prioritise and plan training activities to meet the needs. Define these in terms of learning objectives and performance specification. Identify trainers.	Does the training strategy satisfy the specifications outlined by the commissioner? Are the right members of the workforce targeted for training? Is the planned training likely to meet the desired learning outcomes and performance standards required by the commissioner? Have trainers got the appropriate knowledge, skills and values?
Implement: Delivery of the training programme and the way in which learning objectives are achieved.	How effective is the delivery process in terms of achieving the learning objectives?
Transfer of learning: This is the way in which learning is transferred to practice	How effective has the training programme been in terms of acquiring competence? What has facilitated or blocked the transfer of learning to practice? What impact has learning had on practice?
Evaluation: How effective has training been in promoting staff development, improving service delivery and meeting organisational goals?	Has the whole training process had an impact on service developments? How could the process be improved? What are the areas for future development?

Evaluation as a subjective process

In our opinion one of the reasons that there has been so little evaluation of training in social care settings is that there has been little acknowledgement of the limits of an evaluation in terms of objectivity. Commissioners of evaluation have been searching for models that will provide objective responses, and when these have not been found have tended to give up or focus on the collection of quantitative data.

At the outset of a training evaluation it should be recognised that the evaluation will contain significant areas of subjectivity, for the following reasons. First, evaluation has a political dimension to it. The type and style of evaluation selected and the criteria chosen are likely to reflect the interests, values and goals of the commissioners of the evaluation (Robson 1995). For example, if the evaluation has been commissioned by the senior management team who have been asked by the SSI to improve training in the area of drug misuse, they will have a vested interest in demonstrating that this has been effectively achieved. Second, any evaluation of training effectiveness, in social care settings, centres largely on collecting qualitative data. It is inevitable that subjectivity will exist, as the evaluation will rarely allow for an objective, non-participatory observation of events (Bramley and Pahl 1996). As Bramley (p. 13) states: 'Evaluation is never absolute truth.' The aim is to provide valid evidence which can be utilised by the client to inform decision-making while recognising that training evaluation is unlikely to be totally objective. It is on this basis that methods of evaluation will now be considered.

HOW DO YOU DO IT?

Models for evaluation

In the section above consideration has been given to the purposes of evaluation in social care settings and some of the issues that need to be taken into account when planning an evaluation. We now turn to models of evaluation in order to identify ways in which the needs of those commissioning evaluations of training can best be met. The most commonly utilised models of evaluation are those based on the work of Kirkpatrick (1967) and Hamblin (1974). These models are goal-based, with the focus of the evaluation centring on the extent to which the goals have been achieved.

Kirkpatrick offers a four-dimensional model that considers evaluation from the micro to the macro in terms of four goals:

- *Dimension 1 – reaction.* The immediate reaction during and after a training event from the participant. The goal here is to establish the learner's immediate learning and satisfaction with the training event.
- *Dimension 2 – learning.* The extent to which the participant has acquired new knowledge, values and skills. The goal is to identify

the learning that remained with the learner after the training programme is completed.

- *Dimension 3 – behaviour.* The impact of the training on the ability of participants to improve their job performance. The goal here is to evaluate the way in which the learner has applied their learning to practice.
- *Dimension 4 – ultimate goals.* The consequences of the training for the organisation in terms of goal achievement. The goal at this level is to establish the extent to which training has impacted on the quality of service to users and the attainment of organisational goals.

Bell and Beard suggest that there are two further dimensions to level 4: first, outcomes for others who are in contact with the organisation – for example, other agencies; and second, national outcomes in terms of advancing professional credibility (1996).

Hamblin has taken this model and adapted it. He believes that each dimension cannot be considered in isolation. Rather, the dimensions are interconnected in the following way:

TRAINING
leads to
   REACTIONS
which lead to
   LEARNING
which leads to
   CHANGES IN BEHAVIOUR
which lead to
   CHANGES IN ORGANISATION
which lead to
   CHANGES IN THE ACHIEVEMENT OF ULTIMATE GOALS.

Both models mirror the three functions of training in terms of meeting individual, professional and organisational needs. Training is intended to influence the individual, their professional practice and the achievement of organisational aims. Hamblin's model provides a framework enabling trainers to consider the impact of training on the individual by considering their reactions to the training; for example, did they enjoy the course? What do they feel they learnt? By considering changes of behaviour one can consider not only the individual response but also the impact on professional practice. For instance, as a result of the learning from the training event, have participants developed their skills to complete a certain task?

Exploring changes in the organisation focuses on the organisational objectives. For example, as a result of the training, are participants able to work more effectively with the identified user group? The evaluation of the attainment of ultimate goals examines the way that achieving organisational objectives impacts on the community at large. For example, training for staff working with older people to keep them in the community can raise the standard and profile of the service and reassure the broader community that their needs are likely to be met effectively in old age.

The model emphasises that learning is an ongoing process and that the impact of training, as described throughout this book, begins at the training event and continues when the learner leaves the room. Hamblin also emphasises that the consequences of training can impact beyond the organisation. Thus the goal-based approach provides a framework for evaluating the immediate, short-term and long-term effectiveness of training.

The key issues in using Hamblin's model, according to McMahon and Carter (1990), centre on:

- purpose
- control
- cost
- benefit.

Each of these will be considered in detail.

Purpose

This describes what it is that the trainer can realistically aim to evaluate at each stage. Unless the trainer is clear about the limitations of evaluation at each level, the evaluation itself is meaningless. For example, a reaction evaluation may give some indication of the way the learner intends to use the learning in practice. It cannot evaluate what has been learnt and how this will be applied in practice. In our experience this has often led to confusion, trainers assuming that, because a learner says they will do something at the end of the course, it is taken for granted that they are equipped to do this, ignoring all the other factors that can influence the transfer of learning into practice.

Control of variables

One of the crucial factors to bear in mind, when undertaking a training evaluation, is the influence of variables on the evaluation process. These include the quality of supervision, organisational change and staff turn-over, which are often beyond the control of the trainer in terms of evaluation. Each level of evaluation includes not only the factors that influence the previous level of evaluation but additional factors of its own. The further away from the immediate reaction to the training course, the more complex and wide-ranging are the variables affecting the evaluation of training impact. This can be a major issue in attempt-ing evaluations at higher levels.

Costs

The greater the level of sophistication of the training evaluation, the greater is the cost. It is a complex task costing a training evaluation. Although one can identify the costs in terms of salaries and overheads, consideration also needs to be given to opportunity costs (Rae 1991) These are the hidden costs incurred while trainers, learners and managers are completing the evaluation and not contributing to 'out-put'. Often the amount that an organisation is prepared to spend on evaluation will be determined by its perception of the actual cost of the training itself. However, in the same way in which so many factors influence the costing of evaluation, it is impossible to place an objective cost on the price of training. For example, the fact that an employee received training on moving and handling may have influenced their practice so that they avoided a back injury which might have cost the employer in terms of compensation.

Benefits

Benefit outcomes are very much linked to the level of evaluation under-taken. For example, it is more useful to managers to know that the training has had an impact on improving quality of service provision than that course participants enjoyed the training programme. This in turn may not be as significant as the extent to which the overall conduct of training contributes to improving organisation performance (McMahon and Carter 1990). These different parties are concerned to discover whether different benefits follow training, which in turn affects their approach to evaluation.

In order to facilitate an effective evaluation, consideration needs to be given to the purpose for the evaluation in terms of these components. As can be seen in Figure 11.3 the broader the scope of the evaluation the more costly and less control there is over other variables. However,

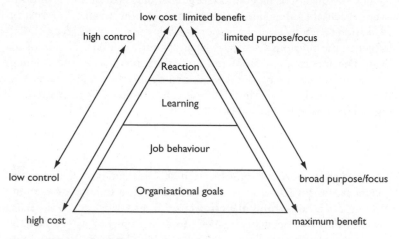

Figure 11.3 The strengths and weaknesses of different levels of training
evaluation
Source: Based on McMahon and Carter (1990)

these are often the most beneficial levels of evaluation as they have the broader focus. Deciding on the level of evaluation requires an assessment of the strengths and weaknesses of the evaluation model for the commissioner's purpose.

It may be that one component will be the determining factor in its own right. For example, if the commissioner is very clear about the budget available, this can be used to determine the level of evaluation. Alternatively, the commissioner may want to ensure that the evaluation is one that is controlled with results that are unlikely to be influenced by other factors. In this situation it would only be possible to undertake an evaluation at the reaction or possibly the learning level.

Establishing a baseline

Before one can begin to undertake an evaluation of training it is necessary to establish the current knowledge, values and skills of the potential learners. The Hamblin model of evaluation is enhanced if a baseline is established. This enables any change to be measured against a yardstick. However, this requires careful consideration in terms of methodology. Baselines can be achieved in two ways: either by assessing the knowledge, values and skills of the learners before they start on a training course; or by utilising a control group to compare and contrast the learning of those who received training against those who did not. Both approaches present problems.

Potential learners' assessment

If participants make a self-assessment, it enables them to identify their own learning needs. However, it is difficult for participants to remain objective, particularly when they are asked to assess their attitudes and feelings rather than skills (Rae 1991).

A problem can arise regarding the time of the self-assessment. As outlined in Chapter 5 learners approach training with their own fears and anxieties. If learners are sent questionnaires before the training, they may feel anxious that their responses indicate that they know less than others who may be attending the training, and this may deter or demotivate them from the course itself. An evaluation at the start of the course, that feels like an examination or test, is likely to inhibit course participants or raise anxiety levels, which in turn may distort the responses. Less formal approaches – for example, a group quiz – may provide a general indication of the group's level of knowledge but will give little information regarding individual learners.

The line manager may provide an assessment of their perception of the course participant's knowledge, values and skills in the particular area to be covered by the course. The advantage of this is that the line manager should have some measure of the participant's ability and be able to compare this with that of other members of the team. However, it can be problematic if the line manager is unfamiliar with the particular area of practice and may not be in a position to make a judgement. Consideration also needs to be given to the manager's bias towards the participant, which may positively or negatively influence their assessment and the learner's response. Issues can also arise regarding what information should be communicated to the trainer.

The dilemma for the trainer is whether to use methods of evaluation which establish a baseline for individual learners that may impact on the actual learning process, or attempt to establish a more generalised group baseline that may not provide accurate information about individuals. Hence the importance of a training needs analysis of the workforce which identifies the baseline and is linked to the evaluation process. Notwithstanding these limitations, self-evaluation with management and user feedback can indicate learner gain.

Use of a control group

Learning takes place without training. It is for this reason that any evaluation that attempts to measure the impact of training on learning should consider using a control group. This involves using two groups of staff who are matched in terms of work setting, level of experience and job competence. One group participates in the training and the control group does not. The level of knowledge, attitudes, skills and job performance of both groups are assessed before and at periods after the training. If both groups provide similar results in the evaluation process it is unlikely that the training has had an impact on learning. However, if the control group shows significantly less change than the trained group, one can begin to consider that the training has influenced learning and job behaviour. This method of evaluation is useful inasmuch as it provides a benchmark against which to measure the effectiveness of training, but it requires a great deal of negotiation and may raise issues of equity for the control group (Bell and Beard 1996).

However, the use of a control group does not necessarily guarantee objectivity. Creating a well-matched control group is difficult because of the significant number of variables which can exist and which can be difficult to quantify – for example, the impact of past and present personal, professional and organisational experiences on attitudes to learning, training and the job and the quality of management supervision and support. All of which reinforces the fact that evaluation cannot be objective.

WHAT DO YOU DO?

Methods for evaluation following the Hamblin model

Having identified a model for evaluation, reflected on the purpose of each level of evaluation within the model and discussed factors to consider before commencing the evaluation, we turn to methods of evaluation using the Hamblin model. This will be done by exploring the focus at each level of evaluation in terms of questions that the evaluator is likely to want answered, and the tools available to gain answers to these questions. The issues that the trainer are likely to encounter at each stage of the evaluation process are identified and discussed.

Stage 1 – reactions during the training event

Focus

- Does the content facilitate meeting the task?
- Does the trainer's style facilitate effective learning?
- Are blocks to learning being managed by the trainer?

Tools to evaluate learning task and process

- Informal feedback during coffee or lunch breaks.
- Feedback sessions incorporated throughout the programme.
- Learning journals enable the learner to record on a daily or sessional basis their reactions to the training and to evaluate what they have learnt; however, they may not share all their views with the trainer.
- Written trainer review (Buckley and Caple 1995), whereby the trainer details their perception of reactions to the course in terms of meeting learners' needs and learners' responses to methods. The evaluation also includes an analysis of the trainer's reactions in terms of management of task and process issues. Learner reaction to recruitment, selection, administration and physical setting can also be included.

Tools to evaluate trainer effectiveness

- *Self-evaluation*. This requires the trainer to evaluate their own performance in terms of agreed criteria. This can be very difficult to achieve as the trainer is an integral part of the learning process and it is impossible to 'stand back' objectively and observe group interactions while remaining part of the process. However, it is important that the trainer learns to reflect like this.
- *Direct observation or audio/video recording of trainer practice.* This involves an observer providing feedback to the trainer on the way in which they performed their role.
- *Evaluation from participants.* This requires learners to give feedback to the trainer on the way they are managing the learning process. It can be done as an integral part of the programme, for example, the trainer can ask participants at the end of each day for feedback regarding the pace of training, the methods used. Alternatively, learners can complete a written form at the end of each day.

- *Evaluation from co-trainer.* While still containing a subjective element, this is also likely to be subjective, but can provide useful information regarding immediate reactions to managing the co-training relationship and the sharing of responses to the reactions to process and task.

Who is involved?

- Course participants and trainer.

Considerations

Ongoing evaluation during a training event enables the trainer to reflect and alter the programme so as to ensure that the needs of the learners are being met, in line with the aims and objectives of the course. This is important so that trainers remain sensitive to the group process. The problem can be that both participants and learners are engaged in the actual learning process and will be evaluating parts of the course in isolation rather than in the context of the whole event. Evaluating throughout the training course is also time consuming. A range of methods are required that engage participants, so that they do not feel as if they are being burdened by an irksome task or that the evaluation distracts learners or trainers from their main task.

Immediate post-training reactions

- Focus.

This can be divided into three areas – organisational, trainer's performance and course content:

1 Organisational

- Were recruitment and selection clear, enabling participants to make decisions regarding the appropriateness of the course?
- Were equal opportunities policies applied in order to access training opportunities?
- Was pre-course information relevant and did it arrive well before the course?
- Was the venue comfortable, accessible and conducive to learning?
- Were refreshments varied and of high quality?
- Were special needs acknowledged and catered for?

2 Trainer's performance

- Was the training delivered within an anti-oppressive framework?
- Did the trainer have a sufficient knowledge base? For example, were they aware of practice issues as encountered within the agency?
- Did the presentation styles promote learning?
- Were a variety of training methods used that reflected the different learning styles of participants?
- Was the trainer supportive and did they create a safe environment for learning?
- Was the training set at the right level to meet the needs of the group in terms of prior knowledge and skill level?
- How did the trainer manage group process – for example, encouraging participation, managing conflict?
- How was feedback managed?

3 Course content

- Was the material up-to-date and relevant?
- Did it incorporate agency policy?
- Did the material reflect difference in terms of race, gender disability, etc.?
- Was the material presented in a variety of ways?
- Was there sufficient time to allow for reflection?
- Did the material promote the development of knowledge, values and skills?

Tools

- *Pre and post questionnaires.* The form is likely to consist of a series of questions focusing on the areas described above. Variety can be introduced by using a range of questioning techniques, including open-ended questions, multiple choice, tick boxes and levels of satisfaction scales.
- *Instant reaction sheets.* Formal/informal verbal feedback, structured group review with learners.
- *Blank sheet review.* Participants are given a free rein to comment on anything they feel is relevant. Attention is given here to seeking feedback and measuring change with no preconceived perceptions of ways in which training will influence the learner. This is achieved by focusing on opinions. Participants are asked to identify the

achievements of the training programme. These can be broad ranging, and one of the criticisms of this approach is that it is difficult to gain a consensus by which opinions can be judged. For example, how does one rate success if responses include comments like 'I think I'll do things differently', 'I can't remember much about it?' However, this approach can be useful in terms of identifying some of the wider-ranging costs and benefits of training that may be lost by more focused approaches. It is very participant-centred and may provide information on unanticipated outcomes.

Who is involved in the evaluation process?

● The learner and trainer.

Considerations

An instant reaction sheet, distributed at the end of a training course, as described in the introduction to the chapter, is the most common form of reaction evaluation and is also a relatively cheap and easy method of evaluation. However, although it is useful for measuring immediate responses to the training, it brings with it a number of problems resulting from its familiarity and over-use. Most learners will have had previous experience of using these forms and may have completed them in a very routinised way, not appreciating their purpose. One course participant stated that he felt that completing the 'happy sheet' was rather like saying 'thank you' to a host at the end of a party. No matter how dreadful the party, most people tell the host they enjoyed it. Likewise no matter how poor the quality of the training, most learners do not want to hurt the trainer's feelings. These sheets are also completed at a stage when learners are feeling tired and wanting to get home. As this is the case, it is not surprising that course participants who complete the evaluation sheet are more likely to focus on tangible factors like poor seating or dreadful lunches rather than on the quality of the learning experience, which requires them to think back to an experience from which they have just 'switched off'. Alternatively, learners who have found the course an enjoyable experience may be in a state of euphoria. This may be reflected in a course evaluation form that eulogises the content and trainer, focusing on the here-and-now without considering the relevance of training to practice.

Despite these limitations, reaction evaluation is important. It recognises that training is more than learning: it is about enjoyment and gaining some satisfaction from the course and that learners are also more likely to put their learning into practice if they feel positive about the learning experience. It also provides an opportunity for learners to comment on training from a user perspective. If this level of evaluation is to be taken seriously then it should be incorporated into the training programme with an appropriate time allocation and not considered as an add-on with the final comment from the trainer: 'By the way, can you complete the evaluation sheets before you leave?'.

Second, learners are more likely to complete the form if they are made aware of the way in which the information will be utilised by the trainer and the organisation and will be of benefit to themselves and other learners. Third, trainers tend to assume automatically that reaction evaluation is an individual, often anonymous activity. Some of the most effective reaction evaluations that we have done have been completed as a group activity, enabling learners to discuss and debate comments made by others and providing more precise and specific information for evaluation. For example, the trainer heads up sheets of flip-chart paper with words like 'venue', 'food and drink', 'administrative arrangements', 'course content', 'methods', 'trainer style' and so on. Each learner is given a felt-tip pen and asked to put comments on each sheet. Once this is completed, the trainer and learners read the sheets and the trainer initiates a discussion, getting learners to compare, contrast and elaborate on the comments.

Stage 2 – learning evaluation

Focus

- What has the participant gained in terms of cognitive knowledge – e.g. theory and research findings?
- What skills has the learner acquired or developed as a result of the training?
- In what ways have the learner's thinking changed?
- How have the learner's attitudes and values changed following the training course?
- Are there other factors that could account for changes in the learner's knowledge, skills and attitudes?

Tools

- Tests, quizzes.
- Learning logs.

- Simulations could be undertaken on a training course to establish that the learner has acquired the relevant knowledge, values and skills and are common on Memorandum of Good Practice training courses, when the learner demonstrates their ability to video interview a child to be a witness in court, often using actors in the role of the child.
- Competency matrices assess learning by focusing on identified requirements and measuring the learner's knowledge, values and skills against these standards.
- Practical tests.
- Post-course interviews.
- Call-back days.
- Evaluation of personal video.
- End-of-course assessment.
- NVQ and PQ competencies.
- Written assignments to test knowledge.
- Supervisor assessment.
- Semantic differential scales, which assess the strength of a particular attitude using a rating scale, and can be used at the beginning of training, after which the learner is reassessed at the end of the course or a number of months after the course is completed.

Who is involved in the evaluation?

- Learner, service users, line manager, trainer, mentors and assessors.

Considerations

There are a number of issues regarding the way that learning is measured. First, the term 'knowledge' can be interpreted in a number of ways. In social care training it is important that learning takes place at both cognitive and experiential levels. Much of what we learn has a high emotional component and it is easy to respond to learning at this level without fully comprehending at a cognitive level. For example, we use the Vince and Martin Learning Cycles on training courses for supervisors and trainers. Learners immediately respond to these cycles, identifying and relating at an emotional level. What becomes apparent is that, unless time is spent ensuring that they are understood at a cognitive level, the learners can go away having misunderstood the learning – a classic example of a little knowledge being a dangerous thing.

Skill measurement requires criteria that are not easily standardised.

For example, Davies (1996) found that central to nursing practice was the ability to be autonomous and independent, but these are skills that are difficult to put into operation, observe and measure because they are abstract ideas – hence the importance of standards and competencies. Another danger can centre on the assumption that knowledge and comprehension automatically translate into skill. As skill evaluation is not testing for intelligence it is necessary that a flexible, open-ended process is utilised that considers variations of the problem and the range of responses (Jones *et al.* 1995).

'Attitude' change is also difficult to measure and is often confused with skills in terms of evaluation. Jones *et al.* note that attitudes can be defined in a number of ways:

- as a perception that the individual holds about themselves or others;
- as a perspective which provides a frame of reference for living;
- as an expectation which centres on a notion of what can be done or expected of others;
- as opinion or personal judgement of what is right.

Frequently we talk about evaluating changes in attitudes without clarifying exactly what we mean. In addition, it is difficult to measure attitudinal change because there is a lack of understanding as to the way in which attitudes are linked to knowledge. For example, to what extent does information influence attitude change? Likewise the relationship between skill acquisition and attitudinal change is also unclear (Jones *et al.* 1995).

However, attitude and value change are still very important – for example, in terms of anti-oppressive practice – and need to be tested at both intellectual and practice levels; for instance, via case studies or observed practice.

Stage 3 – changes in job behaviour

Focus

- How effectively have the knowledge, skills and attitudes acquired from the training been transferred to the job?
- What opportunities has the learner had to consolidate their learning into practice?
- What have been the barriers that have influenced the transfer of learning to the work place?

- Have all the training needs required to do the job been met?
- What factors promoted or prevented the transfer of learning?
- Were the methods of training delivery appropriate and relevant for the job?
- Could the training outcomes have been achieved as effectively through alternative methods?
- What other factors contribute to change in job performance?
- How have the team/supervisor supported the transfer of learning to job behaviour (Buckley and Caple 1995)?

Tools

- Direct observation of practice.
- Assessment of action plan, learning journal.
- Portfolio.
- Work-place assessment.
- Interviews with service users.
- Critical incident reports, which involve collecting information regarding behaviours that are 'critical' to undertaking a task effectively; these are then collated, standards established and performance is measured against these standards.
- Performance appraisal and staff appraisal.

Who is involved in the evaluation?

- Learner, service user, line manager, trainer.

Considerations

High-quality job performance is one of the main reasons for providing training in social care settings. Yet, the all important transfer of learning and training to the work situation is the 'Cinderella' of evaluation. If the value or true worth of investment in training and development is to be identified, it needs to be the 'belle of the ball'. (Bell and Beard 1996)

Evaluation of the impact of training on job performance can be complex, as other factors – such as work setting, support of managers and colleagues and workload pressures – will impact on the learner's ability to apply their learning to practice. In these situations the environmental resistance plus the individual's own anxieties can act as powerful barriers to changing job behaviours (Sheal 1997). Any evaluation of changes of job behaviour needs to be undertaken in conjunction with an assessment of the obstacles, or indeed the alliances, within the work setting that impact on the learner's ability to improve job performance (as described in Chapter 10).

Evaluation of training at this level has a number of benefits. It involves learners and managers and can also involve service users in the training process, giving a message that not only is training important but also that they are important (Sheal 1997). It also provides an opportunity to ensure that the link between training and practice is made apparent to both learners and managers, and enables future training needs relevant to job performance to be identified.

Stage 4 – achieving organisational goals

Focus

- To what extent has the training improved services for users?
- To what extent has the training resulted in the attainment or furthering of organisational goals?
- How has the training improved the well-being of the organisation in terms of morale, levels of staff turnover, absenteeism, disciplinary action?
- How has training affected the profile of the organisation within the community and nationally?

Tools

- *Organisational climate surveys.* These measure the influence of training as one component that contributes to the effectiveness of the organisation.
- *Bench marking surveys.* These are surveys that compare performance against an agreed standard; e.g. it could be previous performance or best practice.
- *Feedback* – from user groups, internal and external inspections, or other agencies and organisations.
- *The quasi-legal approach.* A panel is established, and evidence is presented from all interested parties regarding the training programme and its perceived impact on attaining organisational goals; for example, learners, managers, trainers and service users. This raises issues regarding the weight given to different sources of

evidence and the bias that may be introduced with the different agendas of the different interest groups.

Who is involved in the evaluation?

● Learner, service user, line manager, senior management, training unit, other relevant organisations.

Considerations

This level of evaluation links training outcomes with organisational effectiveness and recognises the impact that training can have at all levels within the organisation. However, continual organisational change within social care settings can make goal evaluation at this level both difficult to achieve and meaningless.

This can be illustrated by an example. A training strategy focusing on managing challenging behaviour was devised to meet the needs of foster carers. At the initial training needs analysis consideration was given to the evaluation process. It was decided by senior managers, fostering support workers and foster carers themselves, that the training should impact on organisational goals by reducing placement breakdowns, the thinking being that staff would be better prepared for managing difficult behaviour. The training was delivered and the evaluation process began. However, within twelve months the situation within the organisation had changed to such an extent that it was impossible to separate out the impact of training. For example, budgets had been cut and residential establishments closed so that foster carers were keeping young people who might well have been placed elsewhere if alternative placements had been available. The result of this was that on paper there was a reduction in placement breakdowns but it was impossible to link this to training alone because of the other changes that influenced the process.

INTER-AGENCY TRAINING: HOW FAR CAN YOU GO?

So far in this chapter we have recognised and considered the complexities of evaluating training in a single agency setting. The evaluation process becomes even more complex within the inter-agency arena. This is because the framework for inter-agency training is often far less well defined than for single agency training. As outlined in Chapter 4, the management and support structures for inter-agency practice are still embryonic, and there is often an organisational lack of clarity regarding the purpose of inter-agency working, let alone a clear understanding of the training remit. A development group run by PIAT (Promoting Inter-Agency Training) considered these dilemmas and the implications for evaluation in terms of inter-agency child protection training. The conclusion was that irrespective of written policies and agreed working structures a clear aim does emerge in terms of inter-agency practice, and that is to develop effective working relationships across professional and organisational boundaries in order to meet the needs of service users. Thus the aim of the training within this arena is to provide structured opportunities for personal, professional and organisational development for groups of multi-agency professionals in order to gain greater understanding of roles and constraints and to promote and develop effective working relationships. The purpose of the evaluation should consequently be to measure the impact of the training on inter-agency working practice and service delivery for users.

We shall now consider the focus for evaluating inter-agency training at each level of the Hamblin model.

Reaction during the training event

This is a particularly important area of evaluation for inter-agency trainers, as they are training a diverse group of participants who will have different philosophies, expectations and priorities in terms of working together. The focus of the evaluation should be on the ways in which these differences are being managed on the training course in terms of task and process. The purpose of the evaluation is to identify issues enabling the trainer to address them to promote a climate for effective learning.

Immediate post-training reactions

The purpose of evaluation at this level, as with single agency training, is to identify learners' immediate response to the training. The focus should be on ways in which the training experience has affected the learner's immediate understanding of different professionals roles and responsibilities and the learner's attitudes, knowledge and skills towards inter-agency working.

Learning evaluation

Learning from inter-agency training should bring about mutual understanding of professionals' different roles and a greater ability to combine skills to meet the needs of service users (DoH 1991a). It is therefore important that the focus is not just on knowledge but also on measuring changes in values and attitudes.

Changes in collaborative practice

The focus here should be on the ability of the learner to apply their learning to their inter-agency practice. Schmidt (1997) sees inter-agency working practice or collaboration as a shared responsibility to solve problems and make decisions regarding meeting the needs of service users. It should be changes in approach to these areas of practice that are the areas for evaluation at this level.

Inter-agency goals

The focus should be on ways in which the training impacts on meeting the needs of service users through inter-agency practice as reflected in organisational goals regarding inter-agency practice and in line with local and governmental guidance on joint working.

The issues

Although within the Hamblin framework one can identify the focus of the inter-agency training evaluation at each level, there are certain issues which need to be considered that are likely to influence the actual ability to evaluate the training at each level. These are summarised here and discussed in more detail in Chapter 4.

Professional differences

There are differences between professionals that will influence their approach to training. While some of these can be identified and addressed through reaction to training evaluation – for example, different roles and responsibilities – there are others which are not as easy to identify and address yet they may have a major impact on the training event and learning (for instance, problems relating to culture and philosophy).

Lack of commitment from managers to evaluation

As described above, any evaluation beyond the immediate post-training reaction requires a commitment from managers and supervisors within the organisation. What is striking in the literature is the lack of management commitment to inter-agency training and subsequent evaluation (Shaw 1994; Weinstein 1994).

Training and other variables

Training does not take place in a vacuum. Ling *et al.* in Weinstein (1994) highlight such variables as resources, departmental policies, staffing and individual personalities influencing inter-agency practice over and above the influence of training. We have discussed above how the trainer often has little control over these variables in a single agency setting. This is likely to be exacerbated in an inter-agency arena, and will influence the level to which the trainer can realistically evaluate the impact of training.

In preparing this chapter it was apparent that there are very few large-scale studies of the effectiveness of inter-agency practice (Schmidt 1997), let alone of the effectiveness of training in this area (Weinstein 1994). Yet government documents such as *Training for Community Care: A Joint Approach* (DoH and SSI 1991) and *Working Together under the Children Act 1989* (DoH 1991a) indicate that inter-agency training is essential if different professionals within social care are to work effectively together. What appears to have emerged is an implicit understanding that inter-agency training is an effective vehicle for promoting inter-agency practice. However, as budgetary cuts continue to affect social care agencies, causing them to turn inwards (Armstrong 1996), questions will inevitably be asked regarding the costs and benefits of inter-agency training. Evaluation is essential to prepare ourselves for the attack.

SUMMARY

At the start of the chapter we emphasised that undertaking a training evaluation can feel like entering a maze. In conclusion, what is evident is that there is no one correct path through the maze. The path for each trainer will be determined by the directions and resources provided by the commissioner of the evaluation. With this in mind, the PIAT evaluation group devised the following principles for undertaking effective training evaluation:

- *State the purpose of the evaluation.* This should take into account the specific interests of the stakeholders who are commissioning the evaluation.
- *Accept that there is no perfect model for evaluation.* There is no objective model for evaluating training in a social care setting. However, the organisation, trainers and service users can benefit from training evaluations within the limits of the available models.
- *Be clear about the level at which evaluation can be realistically undertaken.* The Hamblin model of evaluation identifies four levels of evaluation – reaction to training, learning, impact on job behaviour and meeting organisational goals. It may not be possible to evaluate at all levels. The level of evaluation that can be effectively achieved is likely to be influenced by cost, purpose, benefits and areas of control.
- *Set evaluation in context, considering the personal, professional, organisational and political factors.* The subjectivity of the evaluation can be reduced if there is an acknowledgement of the factors that influence the process.
- *Specify benchmarks for measurement.* Training evaluation needs to take into account the level of knowledge, values and skills of the potential learners, before the training commences. Consideration also needs to be paid to the fact that learning is an ongoing process that continues once the learner leaves the training room and that learning does not necessarily always impact on job behaviour or the achievement of organisational goals. In addition, evaluation is part of the training cycle; any benchmarks for measurement should take into account all aspects of this cycle.
- *Engage participants, managers and service users in the evaluation process.* An effective evaluation requires the views of all those who are likely to be affected by the impact of a training course.

Bibliography

Aiken, M., Dewar, R., Di Tomaso, N., Hage, J. and Zeitz, G. (1975) *Coordinating Human Services*, San Francisco: Jossey-Bass.

Aitken, M. (1992) in C. Hallett and E. Birchall (eds) *Co-ordination and Child Protection: a Review of the Literature*, Edinburgh: HMSO.

Allen, B. (1985) *Teaching methods for the training of educators for the professions*, PhD thesis, Surrey University, pp. 39–45.

Analoui, F. (1993) *Training and Transfer of Learning*, Aldershot: Avebury.

Annett, J. and Sparrow, J. (1985) 'Transfer of training: a review of research and practical implications', *Psychological Issues*, PLET, 22, 2: 116–24, Warwick University.

Appleton, J.V. (1996) 'Working with vulnerable families: a health visiting perspective', *Journal of Advanced Nursing*, 23: 912–18.

Argyris, C. and Schon, D. (1974) *Theory in Practice: Increasing Professional Effectiveness*, San Francisco: Jossey-Bass.

Armstrong, H. (1996) *Annual Reports of Area Child Protection Committees*, No. 2, DoH ACPC series.

Ashworth, P. and Saxton, J. (1990) 'On "competence"', *Journal of Further and Higher Education* (1992) 14, 2: 8–25.

Audit Commission (1992) *Community Care: Managing the Cascade of Change*, London: HMSO.

Baldwin, D. (1996) 'Some historical notes on inter-disciplinary and interprofessional education and practice in health care in the USA', *Journal of Interprofessional Care*, 10, 2: 173–88.

Baldwin, J. and Williams, H. (1988) *Active Learning: a Trainer's Guide*, Oxford: Blackwell.

Baldwin, T. and Ford, K. (1988) 'Transfer of training – a review and directions for future research', *Personnel Psychology*, 41, 1: 63–105 (Spring).

Balloch, S. (1996) 'Experience of training in the statutory social services', in N. Connelly (ed.) *Training Social Services Staff: Evidence from New Research*, London: National Institute for Social Work.

Bamford, T. (1990) *The Future of Social Work*, in S. Banks *Ethics and Values in Social Work*, London: Macmillan, p. 106.

Bandura, A. (1977) 'Self-efficacy – towards a unifying theory of behavioural change', *Psychological Review*, 84, 2: 191–215.

Banks, S. (1995) *Ethics and Values in Social Work*, 1st edn, Basingstoke: Macmillan.

Barr, H. and Waterton, S. (1996) 'Summary of a CAIPE survey: interprofessional education in health and social care in the UK', *Journal of Interprofessional Care*, 10, 3: 297–303.

Bell, L. (1993) 'Tossing the coin', *Discussion Paper in the Future of Social Services Department Staff Development and Training Units*, Joint Initiative for Community Care, Milton Keynes: LGMB/ADSS.

Bell, L. and Beard, A. (1996) *Get Going: a Guide to the Evaluation of Training*, Milton Keynes: Joint Initiative for Community Care.

Benne, K.D. and Sheats, P. (1948) 'Functional roles of group members', *Journal of Social Issues*, 4: 41–9.

Bergevin, P., Morris, D. and Smith, R. (1963) *Adult Education Procedures*, New York: Seabury Press.

Biggs, S. (1992) 'Purchasing and providing training for community care: the place of care management', *Special Edition of Social Work Issues. Care Management Implications for Training*.

Bion, W. (1961) *Experience in Groups*, London: Tavistock.

Boydell, T.H. (n.d.) *A Guide to the Identification of Training Needs*, London: British Association for Commercial and Industrial Education.

Bramley, P. (1976) *Evaluation of Training: a Practical Guide*, London: British Association for Commercial and Industrial Education.

Bramley, P. and Pahl, J. (1996) *The Evaluation of Training in the Social Services*, London: National Institute for Social Work.

Braye, S. and Preston-Shoot, M. (1995) *Empowering Practice in Social Care*, Buckingham: Open University Press.

Bridges, D. (1994) 'Transferable skills: a philosophical perspective', in D. Bridges, *Transferrable Skills in Higher Education*, Norwich: University of East Anglia, pp. 7–16.

Brookfield, S.D. (1986) *Becoming a Critically Reflective Teacher*, San Francisco: Jossey-Bass.

—— (1996) *Understanding and Facilitating Adult Learning*, Milton Keynes: Open University Press.

Brotherton, C. (1991) *New Developments in Research on Adult Cognitions*, Nottingham: University of Nottingham, Psychology Dept.

Broudy, H. (1980) 'Personal Communication', in M. Eraut, *Developing Professional Knowledge and Competence*, London: Falmer Press.

Brown, A. (1994) *Groupwork*, 3rd edn, Aldershot: Arena.

Brown, A. and Bourne, I. (1996) *The Social Work Supervisor*, 1st edn, Buckingham and Philadelphia: Open University Press.

Brown, R. (1996) *Group Processes: Dynamics Within and Between Groups*, Oxford: Blackwell.

Brummer, N. and Simmonds, J. (1992) 'Race and culture: the management of 'difference' in the learning group', *Social Work Education*, 11, 1: 54–64.

Buckley, R. and Caple, J. (1995) *The Theory and Practice of Training*, 3rd edn, London: Kogan Page.

Burgess, H. (1992) *Problem-led Learning for Social Work: The Enquiry and Action Approach*, 1st edn, Whiting and Birch Ltd.

Burgess, H. and Taylor, I. (1995) 'Facilitating enquiry and action learning groups for social work education', *Groupwork*, 8, 2: 117–33.

Burton, K. (1996) 'Child protection issues in general practice: an action research project to improve inter-professional practice', Essex: Area Child Protection Committee (unpublished).

Campenelli, P., Thomas, R., Channell, J., McAuley, L. and Renouf, A. (1994) *Training: an Exploration of the Word and the Concept, with an Analysis of the Implications for Survey Design*, London: Department of Employment Research Series, no. 30.

Casto, M. (1994) *Interprofessional Work in the USA – Education and Practice*, in A. Leathard *Going Inter-professional – Working Together for Health and Welfare*, London: Routledge.

CCETSW (1991) *Rules and Requirements for the Diploma in Social Work: Paper 30*, 2nd edn, London: CCETSW.

—— (1993) *Learning for Organisational and Interprofessional Competence in Social Work, Summary Paper 2: General Report*, London and SE Region/King's College, London: CCETSW.

—— (1995) *The Requirements for Post Qualifying Education and Training in the Personal Social Services* (Paper 31), London: CCETSW.

Charles, M. and Stevenson, O. (1990) 'Multidisciplinary is different!' *Child Protection: Working Together Part 1: The Process of Learning and Training*, Nottingham: University of Nottingham.

Clarke, J. (1996) 'After social work', in N. Parton (ed.) *Social Theory, Social Change and Social Work: the State of Welfare*, London: Routledge.

Clarke, P. (1993) 'A typology of inter-disciplinary education in gerontology and geriatrics: are we really doing what we say we are?', *Journal of Inter-professional Care*, 7, 3: 217–27 (Oxfordshire: Carfax).

Claxton, G. (1984) *Live and Learn: an Introduction to the Psychology of Growth and Change in Everyday Life*, Milton Keynes: Open University Press.

—— (1988) *Live and Learn: an Introduction to the Psychology of Growth and Change in Everyday Life*, 2nd edn, Milton Keynes: Open University Press.

Coulshed, V. (1990) *Management in Social Work*, Basingstoke: Macmillan.

Cree, V. and Macauley, C. (1997) *Transfer of Learning: Theory and Practice*. Learning for Competence: CCETSW York Conference, 20–21 February, CCETSW: London.

Critchley, B. and Casey, D. (1984) 'Second thoughts on team building', *Management Education and Development*, 15, 1: 163–75.

Cross, M. (1994) 'Side by side', *Community Care* (20 January): 20–1.

Crouch, M., Riches, P. and Wonnacott, J. (1995) *The Contract Culture: a Survival Guide for Trainers in Children's Services*, London: NSPCC and LBTC Training for Care.

Curry, D., Caplan, P. and Knuppel, J. (1991) *Transfer of Training and Adult Learning*, NE Ohio: Regional Training Centre.

Davenport, J. (1993) 'Is there any way out of the andragogy morass?' in M. Thorpe, R. Edwards and A. Hanson (eds) *Culture and Processes of Adult Learning*, London: Routledge, p. 283.

Davidson, S. (1976) 'Planning and co-ordination of social services in multi-organisational contexts', *Social Service Review*, 50, 1: 117–37.

Davies, S. (1996) 'Evaluating professional nurse training for the impact on practice', in N. Connelly (ed.), *Training Social Services Staff: Evidence from New Research*, London: National Institute for Social Work, pp. 39–42.

Day, M. (1994) 'Racial discrimination – professional implications', *Journal of Interprofessional Care*, 8, 2: 135–55.

Department of Education (1991) 'Competence for a changing world', Guidance Note no. 8.

Department of Health (1991a) *Working Together under the Children Act 1989: A Guide to Arrangements for Inter-agency Co-operation for the Protection of Children from Abuse*, London: HMSO.

—— (1991b) *Working with Child Sexual Abuse. Guidelines for Trainers and Managers in Social Services Departments*, London: HMSO.

—— (1995) *Child Protection: Messages from Research*, London: HMSO.

Department of Health and Social Services Inspectorate (1991) *Training for Community Care: A Joint Approach*, London: HMSO.

Dewey, J. (1938) *Experience and Education*, Kappa Delta Pi.

Dickson, D. and Bamford, D. (1995) 'Improving the interpersonal skills of social work students: the problem of transfer of training and what to do about it', *British Journal of Social Work*, 25, 1 (February).

Doubler, S. (1991) *Change in Elementary School Teachers' Practice in Science in the United States*, PhD thesis, Liverpool University, 42–00370.

ENB/CCETSW (1995) *Shared Learning: a Good Practice Guide*, London: English Nursing Board/CCETSW.

Eraut, M. (1994) *Developing Professional Knowledge and Competence*, London: Falmer Press.

Evers, H., Cameron, E. and Badger, F. (1994) 'Interprofessional work with old and disabled people', in A. Leathard, *Going Inter-professional – Working Together for Health and Welfare*, London: Routledge.

Fisher, T. (1995) 'Child protection: what knowledge do social workers use?', Social Work Research and Development Unit, University of York.

Fletcher, S. (1991) 'Designing competence-based training', ch. 4, *Your Training Design*, London: Kogan Page.

Fox-Harding, L. (1991) 'Underlying themes and contradictions in the Children Act 1989', *Journal of Justice of the Peace*, (September) 15: 591–4.

French, J. and Raven, B. (1959) 'The bases of social power', in D. Cartwright (ed.) *Studies in Social Power*, Ann Arbor: University of Michigan.

Friere, P. (1973) *Education for Critical Consciousness*, London: Sheed and Ward.

Further Education Unit (1988) *Learning by Doing*, London: Elizabeth House, York Road.

Garavan, T. (1991) 'Strategic human resource development', *International Journal of Manpower*, 12, 6: 21–34.

Garrett, B. (1987) *Learning Organisation*, London: Fontana.

—— (1990) *Creating a Learning Organisation: a Guide to Leadership, Learning and Development*, Cambridge: Director Books.

Gist, M., Stevens, C. and Bavetta, A. (1991) 'The effects of self-efficacy and post-training interventions on the acquisition and maintenance of complex interpersonal skills', *Personnel Psychology*, 44: 837–61.

Glennie, S. (1996) 'Managing change', Presentation to 3rd National Interagency Child Protection Training Symposium (December), Leicester NSPCC.

Goble, R. (1994) 'Multi-professional education in Europe: an overview', in A. Leathard, *Going Inter-professional – Working Together for Health and Welfare*, London: Routledge.

Goldstein, I.L. (1993) *Training in Organisations*, 3rd edn, California: Brooks/Cole.

Gray, J. and Gardiner, P. (1989) 'The impact of conceptions of learning on the quality of teaching and learning in social work', *Issues in Social Work Education* 9, 1 and 2: 74–92.

Griffiths, R. (1988) *Community Care; Agenda for Action*, London: HMSO.

Hallett, C. and Birchall, E. (1992a) *Co-ordination of Child Protection: A Literature Review*, London: HMSO.

—— (1992b) *Working Together in Child Protection: Phase 2*, University of Stirling: Report to Department of Health.

Hamblin, A.C. (1974) *The Evaluation and Control of Training*, New York: McGraw-Hill.

Handy, C. (1995) *The Empty Raincoat: Making Sense of the Future*, Sydney: Arrow Business Books.

Haring, N., Lovitt, T., Eaton, M. and Hanson, C. (1978) *The Fourth R.*, Columbus, Ohio: Charles Merrill.

Hatch, J. (1994) 'Women: partners in interprofessional care', *Journal of Interprofessional Care*, 8, 2: 157–62.

Hay, J. (1992) *Transactional Analysis for Trainers*, London: McGraw-Hill.

Hendry, E. and Glennie, S. (eds) (1996) *Promoting Quality. Standards for Inter-agency Child Protection Training*, London: NSPCC/PIAT.

Heron, J. (1989) *The Facilitator's Handbook*, London: Kogan Page.

—— (1993) *Group Facilitation Theories and Models for Practice*, London: Kogan Page.

Hevey, D. (1992) 'The potential of National Vocational Qualifications to make multi-disciplinary training a reality', *Journal of Interprofessional Care*, 6, 3: 215–21 (Oxfordshire: Carfax).

Hinricks, J. (1976) in P. Bramley, *Evaluation of Training: A Practical Guide*, London: Birkbeck College and British Association for Commercial and Industrial Education.

Home Office (1995) *Dealing with Dangerous People: Probation Service and Public Protection: Report of a Thematic Inspection*, London: HM Inspector of Probation.

Honey, P. and Mumford, A. (1982) *The Manual of Learning Styles*, Ardingley House, 10 Linden Ave, Maidenhead, Berks: Honey.

—— (1986) *Using Your Learning Styles*, Ardingley House, 10 Linden Ave, Maidenhead, Berks: Honey.

Hope, P. (1992) *Making the Best Use of Consultants*, 1st edn, Longman.

Hopkins, J. (1996) 'Social work thro' the looking glass', in N. Parton (ed.) *Social Theory Social Change and Social Work: the State of Welfare*, London: Routledge, p. 31.

Horder, J. (1993) 'Conference report: present and future issues in interprofessional education', *Journal of Interprofessional Care*, 7, 1: 17–18.

Horwath, J. (1996) 'Undertaking a training needs analysis within a social care organisation', in N. Connelly (ed.) *Training Social Services Staff: Evidence from New Research*, London: NISW.

—— (1997) 'Issues for inter-agency practice in the late 1990s', *Northern Ireland Journal for Multi-disciplinary Child Care Practice*, Belfast, 3, 4.

—— and Lawson, B. (1996) *Munchausen Syndrome by Proxy: Inter-agency Child Protection and Partnership with Families*, National Children's Bureau.

Howe, D. (1996) 'Surface and depth in social work practice', in N. Parton (ed.) *Social Theory, Social Change and Social Work: the State of Welfare*, London: Routledge, p. 85.

Hughes, L. and Pengelly, P. (1995) 'Who cares if the room is cold? Practicalities, projections and the trainer's authority', in M. Yelloly and M. Henkel (eds) *Learning and Teaching in Social Work*, London: Jessica Kingsley, p. 231.

Husein, E. (1988) 'Evaluation of a staff development process: towards effective education for all', MPhil thesis, Manchester University, 40–0307.

Jacobsen, M. and McKinnon, R. (1989) *Shared Counselling Skills; A Guide to Running a Course for Nurses, Health Visitors, and Midwives*, Edinburgh: Scottish Education Health Group.

Jaques, D. (1992) *Learning in Groups*, 2nd edn, London: Kogan Page.

Jarvis, P. (1983) *Professional Education*, New Patterns of Learning series, London: Croom Helm.

—— (1995) *Adult and Continuing Education Theory and Practice*, 2nd edn, London: Routledge.

Jones, J.F., Stevenson, K.M., Leung, P. and Cheung, K-F.M. (1995) *Call to Competence: Child Protective Services Training and Evaluation*, Englewood, Col: American Humane Association.

Jones, S. and Joss, R. (1995) 'Models of professionalism', ch. 1 in M. Yelloly and M. Henkel, *Learning and Teaching in Social Work: Towards Reflective Practice*, London: Jessica Kingsley Publishers, pp. 15–33.

Joss, R. (1991) 'Professional competence and higher education', ch. 3, quoted in M. Yelloly and M. Henkel (1995) *Learning and Teaching in Social Work: Towards Reflective Practice*, London: Jessica Kingsley Publishers, p. 58.

Kirkpatrick, D.L. (1967) 'Evaluation of training', in Craig and Bittel (eds) *Training and Developmental Handbook*, New York: McGraw-Hill.

Knowles, M.S. (1972) 'Innovations in teaching styles and approaches based upon adult learning', *Education for Social Work*.

—— (1978) *The Adult Learner: a Neglected Species*, Houston, Tex: Gulf Publications.

Kolb, D. (1988) 'The process of experiencial learning', in D. Kolb (ed.) *Experience as the Source of Learning and Development*, London: Prentice-Hall.

Lamberts, H. and Riphagen, F. (1975) 'Working together on a team for primary health care: a guide to dangerous country', *Journal of the Royal College of General Practitioners*, 25: 745–52.

Lancaster, E. (1995) 'Working with sex offenders: where do we go from here', *Probation Journal*, 79–82.

Lawlor, M. and Handley, P. (1996) *The Creative Trainer: Holistic Facilitation Skills for Accelerated Learning*, London: McGraw-Hill.

Leathard, A. (1994) *Going Inter-professional – Working Together for Health and Welfare*, London: Routledge.

LGMB and CCETSW (1997) *Human Resources for Personal Social Services: From Personnel Administration to Human Resources Management*, London: LGMB/CCETSW.

McFarlane, T. and Morrison, T. (1994) 'Learning and change: outcome of interagency networking for child protection', *Northern Ireland Journal of Multi-disciplinary Child Care Practice*, 1, 2: 33–44.

McMahon, F. and Carter, E. (1990) *The Great Training Robbery: a Guide to the Purchasing of Quality Training*, London: Falmer Press.

Manpower Services Commission (1981) *A Glossary of Training Terms*, London: HMSO.

Mansfield, B. (1991) 'Deriving standards of competence', in E. Fennell (ed.) *Development Assessable Standards for National Certification*, London: Employment Department Group.

Margrab, P. (1997) 'Integrated services for children and youth at risk: an international study of multi-disciplinary training', *Journal of Interprofessional Care*, 11, 1: 99–108.

Marsh, I. (1989) *Effectiveness of In-Service Teacher Training: Expectations and Impact*, MEd thesis, Liverpool University, 39–5715.

Marsh, P. and Triseliotis, J. (1996) 'Social workers: their training and first year in work', in N. Connelly (ed.) *Training Social Services Staff: Evidence from New Research*, London: NISW, 4: 54.

Maslow, A.H. (1968) *Towards a Psychology of Being*, New York: D. Van Nostrand.

Menzies, I. (1970) *The Functioning of Groups as a Defence against Anxiety*, London: Tavistock.

Miles, M.B. (1971) *'Learning to Work in Groups': a Program Guide for Educational Leaders*, New York: Teachers College Press.

Miller, A. and Watts, P. (1990) *Planning and Managing Effective Professional Development: a Resource Book for Staff who Work with Children who Have Special Needs*, Harlow: Longman.

Mistry, T. and Brown, A. (1991) 'Black/white co-working in groups', *Groupwork*, 4, 2: 101–18.

Morrison, T. (1993) *Staff Supervision in Social Care*, 1st edn, Harlow: Longman.

—— (1993) *Staff Supervision in Social Care*, Brighton: Pavilion.

—— (1996) 'Partnership and collaboration: rhetoric and realities', *Child Abuse and Neglect*, 20, 2: 127–40 (Pergamon).

—— (1998) 'Collaboration, partnership and change', in M. Adcock and R. White (eds) *Significant Harm*, 2nd rev. edn, London: Significant Publications.

NACRO (1994) *'Strategic role of staff development and training'* Discussion Paper, Bath: NACRO.

Napier, R.W. and Gershenfeld, M.K. (1985) *Groups: Theory and Experience*, Boston: Houghton Mifflin.

Noddings, N. (1984) *Caring: a Feminist Approach to Ethics and Moral Education*, Berkeley: University of California Press.

Parker and Lewis (1980) *Cranfield School of Management*.

Parton, N. (ed.) (1996) *Social Theory, Social Change and Social Work: the State of Welfare*, London: Routledge.

Pavlov, I. (1927) *Conditioned Reflexes*, New York: Oxford University Press.

Pearn, M., Roderick, C. and Mulrooney, C. (1995) *Learning Organisations in Practice*, 1st edn, London: McGraw-Hill.

Peters, T. and Waterman, R. (1982) *In Search of Excellence*, New York: Harper and Row.

Phillipson, J. (1992) *Practising Equality: Women, Men and Social Work*, London: CCETSW.

Piaget, J. (1929) *The Child's Conception of the World*, London: Routledge & Kegan Paul.

Pietroni, M. (1994) 'Inter-professional teamwork: its history and development in hospitals, general practice and community care (UK)', in A. Leathard, *Going Inter-professional – Working Together for Health and Welfare*, London: Routledge.

—— (1995) 'Nature and aims of professional education for social work', in M. Yelloly and M. Henkel *Learning and Teaching in Social Work: Towards Reflective Practice*, London: Jessica Kingsley Publishers, p. 46.

Preston-Shoot, M. (1995) 'Assessing anti-oppressive practice', *Social Work Education*, 14, 2: 11–27.

Rae, L. (1991) *How to Measure Training Effectiveness*, 2nd edn, London: Gower Publishing.

Rawson, D. (1994) 'Models of inter-professional work: likely theories and possibilities', in A. Leathard, *Going Inter-professional – Working Together for Health and Welfare*, London: Routledge.

Reid, K. (1988) 'But I don't want to lead a group! Some common problems of social workers leading groups', *Groupwork*, 2: 124–34.

Richards, M., Payne, C. and Shepperd, W.A. (1990) *Staff Supervision in Child Protection Work*, London: NISW.

Robson, C. (1995) *Real World Research*, 4th edn, Oxford: Blackwell.

Rogers, A. (1996) *Teaching Adults*, 2nd edn, Buckingham: Open University Press.

Rogers, C. (1969) *Freedom to Learn*, Columbus, Ohio: Chas Merrill & Co.

—— (1993) 'The interpersonal relationship in the facilitation of learning', in M. Thorpe, R. Edwards and A. Hanson (eds) *Culture and Processes of Adult Learning*, London: Routledge.

Ryle, G. (1949) *The Concept of Mind*, London: Hutchinson.

Scaife, J. (1995) *Training to Help*, Sheffield: Riding Press.

Schon, D.A. (1987) *Educating the Reflective Practitioner*, 1st edn, San Francisco: Jossey-Bass.

Schultz, B.G. (1989) *Communicating in the Small Group: Theory and Practice*, New York: Harper and Row.

Senge, P.M. (1990a) 'The leader's new work: building learning organisations', *Management Review*, 32, 1 (Fall).

—— (1990b) *The Fifth Discipline: the Art and Practice of the Learning Organisation*, London: Century Business.

—— (1990c) *The Discipline*, New York: Doubleday.

Shardlow, S. and Doel, M. (1996) *Practice Learning and Teaching*, London: BASW Macmillan.

Shaw, I. (1993) 'The politics of interprofessional training: lessons from learning disability', *Journal of Interprofessional Care*, 7, 3: 255–62.

—— (1994) *Evaluating Interprofessional Training*, Aldershot: Avebury.

Sheal, P.R. (1997) *How to Develop and Present Staff Training Courses*, 3rd edn, London: Kogan Page.

Skinner, B. (1951) 'How to teach animals', *Scientific American*, 185 (b).

Smith, G. (1993) *Systemic Approaches to Training in Child Protection*, London: Karnac Books.

Smith, P.B. (1980) *Group Processes and Personal Change*, 1st edn, London: Harper and Row.

Social Services Inspectorate (1994) *Inspection of Management and Resourcing of Training in Social Services Departments: Overview Report 1993–94*, London: Department of Health.

—— (1995) *The Management and Resourcing of Training in Social Services Departments: Overview Reports 1994–95*, London: Department of Health.

—— (1996a) *The Management and Resourcing of Training in Social Services Departments. Overview*, London: Department of Health.

—— (1996b) *Management and Refocusing of Training in Social Services Departments: Overview Report 1994–95*, Nottingham: Department of Health.

—— (1996c) *5th Annual Report of the Chief Inspector 1995–6*, DoH, London: HMSO.

—— (1997) *Training Support Programme: A Report on Targets and Achievements in 1995/6*, London: Department of Health.

Social Services Inspectorate and Department of Health (1995) *The Management and Resourcing of Training in Social Services Departments: Overview Report 1994/5*, London: HMSO.

Somers, M.L. (1971) 'Dimensions and dynamics of engaging the learner', *Education for Social Work* (Fall): 49–57.

Stephenson, J. and Weil, S. (1992) *Quality in Learning*, 1st edn, London: Kogan Page.

Stevenson, O. (ed.) (1989) *Child Abuse: Public Policy and Professional Practice*, London: Harvester Wheatsheaf.

Stevenson, O. and Parsloe, P. (1993) *Community Care and Empowerment*, London: Community Care.

Stickland, G. (1992) 'Positioning training and development departments for organisational change', *Management Education and Development*, 23, 1: 307–16.

Storrie, J. (1992) 'Mastering interprofessionalism: an inquiry into the development of master's programmes with an interprofessional focus', *Journal of Interprofessional Care*, 6, 3: 253–9 (Oxfordshire: Carfax).

Taylor, B. (n.d.) *Experiential Learning: a Framework for Group Skills*, Oasis Communications, Leeds: Beechwood Conference Centre.

Taylor, I. (1996) 'Facilitating reflective learning', in N. Gould and I. Taylor (eds) *Reflective Learning for Social Work*, Aldershot: Arena.

Tempkin-Greener, H. (1983) 'Interprofessional perspectives on teamwork in healthcare: a case study', *Health and Society*, 61, 4: 641–58 (Millbank Memorial Fund Quarterly).

Thompson, N. and Bates, J. (1995) 'In-service training: myth and reality', *Curriculum*, 16, 1: 53–60.

Townsend, R. (1996) 'Learning for change: an exploration of the experience of the implementation of community care', Centre for Labour Market Studies, MSc thesis, Leicester University.

Training Agency (1989) *Training in Britain: a Study of Funding, Activity and Attitudes*, London: HMSO.

Tuckman, B.W. and Jensen, M.A.C. (1977) 'Stages of small-group development', *Journal of Group and Organisational Studies*, 24.

Tuckman, J. and Lorge, I. (1962) 'Individuality as a determinant of group superiority', *Journal of Human Relations*, 15 (1).

UKCC (1986) *Project 2000: A New Preparation for Practice*, London: United Kingdom Central Council.

Vince, R. and Martin, L. (1993) 'Inside action learning: an exploration of the psychology and politics of the action learning model', *Management Education and Development*, 24, 3: 205–15.

Watts, P., Pickles, T. and Miller, A. (1993) *Social Care Professional Development Systems*, 1st edn, Brighton: Pavilion.

Weinstein, J. (1994) *Sewing the Seams for a Seamless Service: A Review of Developments in Interprofessional Education and Training*, London: CCETSW.

Winter, R. (1991) 'Outline of a general theory of professional competences', in M. Maisch and R. Winter (eds) *Asset Programme* (vol. 2), *Development and Assessment of Professional Competences*, Chelmsford: Anglia University and Essex County Council.

Wistow, G. and Hardy, B. (eds) (1996) 'Competition, collaboration and markets', *Journal of Interprofessional Care*, 10, 1: 5–9.

Wood, R. and Power, C. (1987) 'Aspects of the competence performance distinction', *Journal of Curriculum Studies*, 19, 5: 409–24.

Yelloly, M. and Henkel, M. (1995) *Learning and Teaching in Social Work: Towards Reflective Practice*, London: Jessica Kingsley.

Name index

Subject index